QUARANTINE STATIONS
AT PORTS OF ENTRY
Protecting the Public's Health

Committee on Measures to Enhance the Effectiveness of the CDC
Quarantine Station Expansion Plan for U.S. Ports of Entry

Laura B. Sivitz, Kathleen Stratton, and Georges C. Benjamin, Editors

Board on Global Health
Board on Population Health and Public Health Practice

INSTITUTE OF MEDICINE
OF THE NATIONAL ACADEMIES

THE NATIONAL ACADEMIES PRESS
Washington, D.C.
www.nap.edu

THE NATIONAL ACADEMIES PRESS • 500 FIFTH STREET, N.W. • Washington, DC 20001

NOTICE: The project that is the subject of this report was approved by the Governing Board of the National Research Council, whose members are drawn from the councils of the National Academy of Sciences, the National Academy of Engineering, and the Institute of Medicine. The members of the committee responsible for the report were chosen for their special competences and with regard for appropriate balance.

This study was supported by Contract No. 200-2000-00629, Task Order No. 31 between the National Academy of Sciences and the Centers for Disease Control and Prevention. Any opinions, findings, conclusions, or recommendations expressed in this publication are those of the author(s) and do not necessarily reflect the view of the organizations or agencies that provided support for this project.

Library of Congress Cataloging-in-Publication Data

Institute of Medicine (U.S.). Committee on Measures to Enhance the Effectiveness of the CDC Quarantine Station Expansion Plan for U.S. Ports of Entry.
  Quarantine stations at ports of entry : protecting the public's health / Committee on Measures to Enhance the Effectiveness of the CDC Quarantine Station Expansion Plan for U.S. Ports of Entry, Board on Global Health, Board on Population Health and Public Health Practice ; Laura B. Sivitz, Kathleen Stratton, and Georges C. Benjamin, editors.
      p. ; cm.
  "This study was supported by Contract No. 200-2000-00629, Task Order No. 31 between the National Academy of Sciences and the Centers for Disease Control and Prevention"— Galley.
  Includes bibliographical references.
  ISBN 0-309-09951-X (pbk. book)
  1. Quarantine—United States. 2. Bioterrorism—United States—Prevention.
  [DNLM: 1. Quarantine—United States. 2. Bioterrorism—prevention & control—United States. WA 234 I58 2005] I. Sivitz, Laura. II. Stratton, Kathleen R. III. Benjamin, Georges. IV. Title.
  RA665.I57 2005
  363.34'97—dc22
                                    2005033697

Additional copies of this report are available from the National Academies Press, 500 Fifth Street, N.W., Lockbox 285, Washington, DC 20055; (800) 624-6242 or (202) 334-3313 (in the Washington metropolitan area); Internet, http://www.nap.edu.

For more information about the Institute of Medicine, visit the IOM home page at **www.iom.edu.**

Printed in the United States of America.

The serpent has been a symbol of long life, healing, and knowledge among almost all cultures and religions since the beginning of recorded history. The serpent adopted as a logotype by the Institute of Medicine is a relief carving from ancient Greece, now held by the Staatliche Museen in Berlin.

COVER: The cover incorporates images from a colorized transmission electron micrograph taken by C. Goldsmith (CDC) of Avian influenza A H5N1 viruses (seen in gold) grown in MDCK cells (green). Executive Order 13,375 of April 1, 2005, added to the list of quarantinable communicable diseases influenza caused "by novel or reemergent influenza viruses that are causing, or have the potential to cause, a pandemic."

"Knowing is not enough; we must apply. Willing is not enough; we must do."

—Goethe

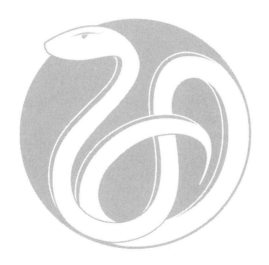

INSTITUTE OF MEDICINE
OF THE NATIONAL ACADEMIES

Advising the Nation. Improving Health.

THE NATIONAL ACADEMIES
Advisers to the Nation on Science, Engineering, and Medicine

The **National Academy of Sciences** is a private, nonprofit, self-perpetuating society of distinguished scholars engaged in scientific and engineering research, dedicated to the furtherance of science and technology and to their use for the general welfare. Upon the authority of the charter granted to it by the Congress in 1863, the Academy has a mandate that requires it to advise the federal government on scientific and technical matters. Dr. Ralph J. Cicerone is president of the National Academy of Sciences.

The **National Academy of Engineering** was established in 1964, under the charter of the National Academy of Sciences, as a parallel organization of outstanding engineers. It is autonomous in its administration and in the selection of its members, sharing with the National Academy of Sciences the responsibility for advising the federal government. The National Academy of Engineering also sponsors engineering programs aimed at meeting national needs, encourages education and research, and recognizes the superior achievements of engineers. Dr. Wm. A. Wulf is president of the National Academy of Engineering.

The **Institute of Medicine** was established in 1970 by the National Academy of Sciences to secure the services of eminent members of appropriate professions in the examination of policy matters pertaining to the health of the public. The Institute acts under the responsibility given to the National Academy of Sciences by its congressional charter to be an adviser to the federal government and, upon its own initiative, to identify issues of medical care, research, and education. Dr. Harvey V. Fineberg is president of the Institute of Medicine.

The **National Research Council** was organized by the National Academy of Sciences in 1916 to associate the broad community of science and technology with the Academy's purposes of furthering knowledge and advising the federal government. Functioning in accordance with general policies determined by the Academy, the Council has become the principal operating agency of both the National Academy of Sciences and the National Academy of Engineering in providing services to the government, the public, and the scientific and engineering communities. The Council is administered jointly by both Academies and the Institute of Medicine. Dr. Ralph J. Cicerone and Dr. Wm. A. Wulf are chair and vice chair, respectively, of the National Research Council.

www.national-academies.org

COMMITTEE ON MEASURES TO ENHANCE THE EFFECTIVENESS OF THE CDC QUARANTINE STATION EXPANSION PLAN FOR U.S. PORTS OF ENTRY

GEORGES C. BENJAMIN, M.D. (*Chair*), Executive Director, American Public Health Association

JOAN M. ARNOLDI, D.V.M.,[1] Retired, Associate Administrator, Animal and Plant Health Inspection Service, U.S. Department of Agriculture

BARBARA A. BLAKENEY, M.S., R.N., President, American Nurses Association

LAWRENCE O. GOSTIN, J.D., L.L.D., Professor of Law, Georgetown University Law Center; Professor of Public Health, Johns Hopkins University; and Director, Center for Law & the Public's Health

MARGARET A. HAMBURG, M.D., Senior Scientist, Nuclear Threat Initiative

FARZAD MOSTASHARI, M.D., M.S.P.H., Assistant Commissioner, Bureau of Epidemiology Services, New York City Department of Health

WILLIAM A. PETRI, JR., M.D., Ph.D., Wade Hampton Frost Professor of Epidemiology, Professor of Medicine, Microbiology, and Pathology, and Chief, Division of Infectious Diseases and International Health, University of Virginia Health System

ARTHUR L. REINGOLD, M.D., Professor of Epidemiology, School of Public Health, University of California at Berkeley

RONALD K. ST. JOHN, M.D., M.P.H., Director General, Centre for Emergency Preparedness and Response, Public Health Agency of Canada

KATHLEEN E. TOOMEY, M.D., M.P.H.,[2] Director, Division of Public Health, Georgia State Health Department

MARY E. WILSON, M.D., Associate Professor of Population and International Health, Harvard School of Public Health and Associate Clinical Professor of Medicine, Harvard Medical School

STUDY STAFF

KATHLEEN STRATTON, Ph.D., Study Director
LAURA B. SIVITZ, M.S.J., Research Associate
DAVID W. GILES, Research Assistant
SHEYI LAWOYIN, M.P.H., Senior Program Assistant
NORMAN GROSSBLATT, ELS (D), Senior Editor
PATRICK KELLEY, M.D., Dr.P.H., Director, Board on Global Health
ROSE MARIE MARTINEZ, Sc.D., Director, Board on Population Health and Public Health Practice

---

[1]Dr. Arnoldi resigned from the committee on December 21, 2004.

[2]Dr. Toomey resigned from the Georgia State Health Department effective January 15, 2005, and from the committee on March 16, 2005.

Reviewers

This report has been reviewed in draft form by persons chosen for their diverse perspectives and technical expertise, in accordance with procedures approved by the National Research Council's Report Review Committee. The purpose of this independent review is to provide candid and critical comments that will assist the institution in making its published report as sound as possible and to ensure that the report meets institutional standards for objectivity, evidence, and responsiveness to the study charge. The review comments and draft manuscript remain confidential to protect the integrity of the deliberative process. We wish to thank the following individuals for their review of this report:

Donald S. Burke, M.D., Bloomberg School of Public Health, Johns Hopkins University

Kathleen F. Gensheimer, M.D., M.P.H., Maine Department of Health and Human Services

David Heymann, M.D., World Health Organization

Ann Marie Kimball, M.D., School of Public Health, University of Washington

Bonnie J. Kostelecky, R.N., M.S., M.P.A., Multnomah County Health Department, Portland, OR

Aileen Plant, Ph.D., M.P.H., Curtin University of Technology, Perth, Australia

K.W. Wheeler, D.V.M., Retired, Animal and Plant Health Inspection Service, U.S. Department of Agriculture

Although the reviewers listed above have provided many constructive comments and suggestions, they were not asked to endorse the conclusions or recommendations nor did they see the final draft of the report before its release. The review of this report was overseen by **Elaine L. Larson, Ph.D., R.N.**, Columbia University. Appointed by the National Research Council, she was responsible for making certain that an independent examination of this report was carried out in accordance with institutional procedures and that all review comments were carefully considered. Responsibility for the final content of this report rests entirely with the authoring committee and the institution.

The committee's letter report released in January 2005 (Appendix A) was also subject to independent review. We wish to thank the following individuals for their review of the letter report:

Ruth L. Berkelman, M.D., M.P.H., Rollins School of Public Health, Emory University

Donald S. Burke, M.D., Bloomberg School of Public Health, Johns Hopkins University

Kathleen F. Gensheimer, M.D., M.P.H., Maine Department of Health and Human Services

Ann Marie Kimball, M.D., School of Public Health, University of Washington

Bonnie J. Kostelecky, R.N., M.S., M.P.A., Multnomah County Health Department, Portland, OR

Monitor appointed by IOM: **Hugh H. Tilson, M.D., Dr.P.H.,** School of Public Health, University of North Carolina.

Contents

Tables, Figures, and Boxes

TABLES

FIGURES

BOXES

Abbreviations

AII	airborne infection isolation
AMS	Automated Manifest System
APHIS	Animal and Plant Health Inspection Service, U.S. Department of Agriculture
APHL	Association of Public Health Laboratories
APIS	Automated Passenger Information System
AQI	Agriculture Quarantine and Inspection, Animal and Plant Health Inspection Service
ASTHO	Association of State and Territorial Health Officials
ATA	Air Transport Association of America Inc.
BIDS	Border Infectious Disease Surveillance Project, Centers for Disease Control and Prevention
CBP	U.S. Customs and Border Protection
CDC	Centers for Disease Control and Prevention
CSTE	Council of State and Territorial Epidemiologists
DGMQ	Division of Global Migration and Quarantine, National Center for Infectious Diseases, Centers for Disease Control and Prevention
DHHS	U.S. Department of Health and Human Services
DHS	U.S. Department of Homeland Security
DOT	U.S. Department of Transportation

DQ   Division of Quarantine, National Center for Infectious
                Diseases, Centers for Disease Control and Prevention

EMS   emergency medical services

FAA   Federal Aviation Administration, U.S. Department of
                Transportation
FBI   Federal Bureau of Investigation
FDA   Food and Drug Administration
FTEs   full-time equivalents

GAO   Government Accountability Office

HIPAA   Health Insurance Portability and Accountability Act
HIV   human immunodeficiency virus

ICD-CM   International Classification of Diseases, Clinical
                Modification
ICU   intensive-care unit
IOM   Institute of Medicine

LPHA   local public health authority

MOA   memorandum of agreement
MSEHPA   Model State Emergency Health Powers Act
MSPHA   Model State Public Health Act

NACCHO   National Association of County and City Health
                Officials
NACO   National Association of Counties
NCID   National Center for Infectious Diseases, Centers for
                Disease Control and Prevention
NHP   nonhuman primates
NIH   National Institutes of Health

OIS   Office of Immigration Statistics, U.S. Department of
                Homeland Security

PHAC   Public Health Agency of Canada
POEs   Ports of Entry

SARS   severe acute respiratory syndrome
State PHA   state public health agency

USCG	U.S. Coast Guard
USDA	U.S. Department of Agriculture
USFWS	U.S. Fish and Wildlife Service, U.S. Department of the Interior
WHO	World Health Organization

QUARANTINE STATIONS
AT PORTS OF ENTRY

Executive Summary

The millions of people and goods that daily traverse the globe disperse microbial threats in their wake, usually without intent to harm. Living things get infected along the way, and the lag time before signs and symptoms appear can be days, weeks, or months. These phenomena and other forces intrinsic in modern technology and ways of life favor the emergence of new diseases and the re-emergence or increased severity of known diseases. Meanwhile, the risk of bioterrorism has become a pressing national security issue. Taken together, these factors have stimulated calls for greater vigilance about microbial threats of public health significance at U.S. gateways. Some of those calls have focused attention on the number and—more important—the role of quarantine stations for human disease at U.S. ports of entry.

The Centers for Disease Control and Prevention (CDC) has quarantine stations at 8 of the 474 U.S. ports of entry (CRS, 2004; DGMQ, 2003). Unlike their namesakes, today's quarantine stations are not stations per se, but rather small groups of individuals located at major U.S. airports. Their core mission remains similar to that of old: mitigate the risks to residents of the United States posed by infectious diseases of public health significance originating abroad. These quarantine station staff, their offices, and their patient isolation rooms are run by CDC's Division of Global Migration and Quarantine (DGMQ).

In fiscal 2003, Congress began to allocate funds for the establishment of new quarantine stations at 17 major U.S. ports of entry that comprise airports, seaports, and land-border crossings. In a significant departure from the recent past, both the preexisting 8 quarantine stations and the new 17 are expected to play an active, anticipatory role in nationwide biosurveillance (DHS, 2004; Gerberding, 2005). Consequently, CDC asked the Institute of Medicine (IOM) to convene an expert committee to assess the present CDC quarantine stations and recommend how they should evolve to meet the challenges posed by microbial threats at the nation's gateways.[1] IOM convened the Committee on Measures to Enhance the Effectiveness of the CDC Quarantine Station Expansion Plan for U.S. Ports of Entry in October 2004; this is the committee's final report to CDC.

STRATEGIC PUBLIC HEALTH LEADERSHIP AT THE NATION'S GATEWAYS

The traditional, primary activities of the CDC quarantine stations no longer protect the U.S. population sufficiently against microbial threats of public health significance that originate abroad, the committee concluded. In 2004, for example, a man suffering from fever, chills, severe sore throat, and diarrhea flew from Sierra Leone to Newark, NJ. By the time he died from Lassa fever less than a week after arrival, he had exposed 188 persons to the disease (CDC, 2004). Another recent failure of the U.S. quarantine system to prevent the importation of serious communicable disease occurred in 2003, when several infected rodents imported from Africa apparently caused a multistate outbreak of human monkeypox (CDC, 2003).

Many of the stations' legacy activities focus on the detection of disease in persons, animals, cargo, and conveyances during the window of time shortly before and during arrival at U.S. gateways. Yet the pace of global trade and travel has narrowed that window dramatically. Consequently, infected individuals and animals do not necessarily develop signs of disease while in transit or by the time of arrival, and available noninvasive diagnostics cannot always identify infected travelers with reasonable sensitivity, specificity, and speed. With 120 million people traveling to and from the United States by air annually (Office of Aviation Policy and Plans, 2005), the quarantine stations face a daunting task in adequately screening arriving passengers and protecting the country from microbial threats of public health significance.

Moreover, the consequences of globalization and the development of the U.S. homeland security infrastructure have increased the complexity of the organizational environment in which the CDC quarantine stations function. This organizational environment, called the Quarantine System in this report, comprises entities that span sectors and jurisdictions. Yet the Quarantine System lacks effective leadership. No entity has principal responsibil-

---

[1]Contract No. 200-2000-00629, Task Order No. 31.

ity, authority, and resources for orchestrating the activities of the Quarantine System to protect the U.S. population from microbial threats of public health significance that originate abroad.

To fill this void, the primary activities of the CDC quarantine stations should shift from the legacy activity of inspection to the provision of strategic national public health leadership for Quarantine System activities. Such leadership, carried out in collaboration with DGMQ and the scientific and organizational capacity of CDC, would improve national preparedness for crises caused by microbial threats of public health significance that originate abroad.

The triad of (1) the CDC quarantine stations, (2) DGMQ headquarters, and (3) the scientific and organizational capacity of CDC form a functional unit in the context of this report. To refer to this unit, the committee coined the term "Quarantine Core." (Additional terminology developed by the committee is presented in the following section). The Quarantine Core should provide strategic public health leadership for the broad, international network of organizations whose actions and decisions affect the CDC quarantine stations at U.S. ports of entry.

BACKGROUND AND FRAMEWORK

Quarantine is the separation and restriction of movement of apparently healthy people or animals that may have been exposed to a microbial threat and therefore may become infectious (DGMQ, 2004). CDC quarantine stations and many of their public health partners have the legal authority to quarantine specific individuals and animals to protect the public's health. In addition, a CDC quarantine station may assure[2] the *isolation* of specific individuals or animals that are reasonably believed to be carrying a communicable disease of public health significance. Through isolation, the infected persons or animals are separated from the population at large, and their movement is restricted to prevent the microbial threat from spreading (DGMQ, 2004). Quarantine and isolation at national borders are non-medical components of the public health toolkit for limiting and containing the spread of microbial threats. Their utility varies, however, depending on the nature of the threat and the extent to which it has spread.

The microbes of concern to the Quarantine Network are bacteria, viruses, protozoa, fungi, and prions that can replicate in humans. A microbial threat of public health significance causes serious or lethal human

---

[2]In this report, "to assure" means to make sure that necessary public health services are provided to all members of society by encouraging the requisite actions, requiring them, or providing the services directly. For an in-depth description of the assurance function in public health, see *The Future of Public Health*, pp. 45-47 (IOM, 1988).

disease and is transmissible from person to person, from animal to person, or potentially both; it also may be transmissible from food or water to people. Because of their potential for wide dispersal, concern is greatest for microbes that spread rapidly from person to person. A microbial threat may be introduced intentionally—as in bioterrorism—or unintentionally.

Additional threats of public health significance of concern to the quarantine stations include the release of chemical or radiological substances and of biological substances other than microbes (e.g., microbial toxins).

The Quarantine Core, System, and Network

As suggested above, the CDC quarantine stations are one component of a large, complex network of organizations whose collective actions provide limited protection to residents of and travelers to the United States from microbial threats of foreign origin. It became apparent to the committee that understanding the role of the CDC quarantine stations in this network would be essential to developing realistic conclusions and recommendations. Consequently, the committee developed a conceptual diagram and vocabulary to visualize and articulate the interrelationships among the stations, the network, and other key actors. The following text describes this diagram, Figure ES.1, as well as the corresponding set of terms coined by the committee for use throughout the report.

Quarantine Core

At the center of the diagram is what the committee has dubbed the "Quarantine Core." As noted above, the Core consists of the CDC quarantine stations, DGMQ headquarters, and the organizational and scientific capacity of CDC. The quarantine stations lie at the center of this diagram because they are the only members of the network whose primary purpose is the mitigation of imported microbial threats at U.S. ports of entry. Any meaningful change in the quarantine stations, however, will involve the resources of DGMQ and the organizational and scientific capacity of CDC. Therefore, the committee's recommendations address the Quarantine Core as a whole.

Quarantine System

In the ring around the Core lies the group of organizations that have (or should have) especially close ties to the Core. Together, this group and the Quarantine Core form what the committee calls the "Quarantine System." The organizations in the System are responsible for performing the critical quarantine functions of planning, surveillance, assessment and response,

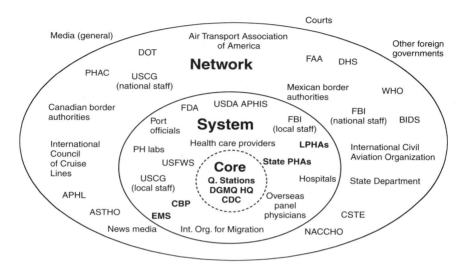

FIGURE ES.1 The relationships among the Quarantine Core, System, and Network for U.S. ports of entry. The circle around the Core is a dotted line to reflect the interdependence of the quarantine stations and their partners in the System. CBP, EMS, LPHAs and State PHAs are bolded to reflect the especially close collaboration of those entities with the stations on virtually a daily basis. Some organizations interact with the quarantine stations at the System level as well as with CDC or DGMQ at the Network level; these organizations appear in both places in the diagram.

and communication to mitigate the risks posed by microbial threats of foreign origin to residents of and travelers to the United States.

In addition to the entities within the Core, the Quarantine System includes local emergency responders and hospitals, local health care providers, local and state health departments, state public health laboratories, port authorities, port staff, airlines, cruise lines, shipping companies, shipping agents, the International Organization for Migration, overseas panel physicians, the U.S. Coast Guard, the Federal Bureau of Investigation, and federal inspectors from U.S. Customs and Border Protection (CBP),[3] U.S. Fish and Wildlife Service, and the Food and Drug Administration. As will be seen in Chapter 4, the consistency and quality of relationships within the System are the subject of several conclusions and recommendations.

Quarantine Network

In the outermost ring lie the organizations and people that interact with DGMQ leadership and the organizational and scientific capacity of CDC, not with individual stations. Together, these entities plus the Quarantine System and Quarantine Core form a multijurisdictional, multisectoral, multinational "Quarantine Network" that protects both travelers entering the United States and the population within U.S. borders from microbial threats of public health significance that originate abroad. In so doing, this Network helps protect the health of the global community.

The members of the Network that lie outside the System include the national-level staff of federal agencies active at the System level, the U.S. Department of State and its embassies, the Department of Homeland Security, national and international transportation industry associations, Mexican and Canadian officials responsible for border activities and disease control, the World Health Organization, and the news media. Although these organizations do not interact with the CDC quarantine stations on a daily basis, they are essential partners whose actions and decisions affect the functioning of the CDC quarantine stations at U.S. ports of entry.

Today's CDC Quarantine Stations at U.S. Ports of Entry

Today, the CDC quarantine station staff at U.S. ports of entry primarily perform the following activities (Committee, 2005;[4] Appendixes D and E):

---

[3]CBP includes veterinary and animal health inspectors from the U.S. Department of Agriculture Animal and Plant Health Inspection Service, as well as the staff of the former Immigration and Naturalization Service and Immigration and Customs Enforcement.

[4]Committee members visited five quarantine stations over the course of the study. This series of site visits, which included meetings with DGMQ field staff as well as federal and

BOX ES.1   Class A and Class B Conditions

In the context of medical examinations of individuals who seek refuge in the United States or want to immigrate to this country:

Class A conditions generally render an alien ineligible for entry into the United States; they include

1. Communicable diseases of public health significance, including chancroid, gonorrhea, granuloma inguinale, human immunodeficiency virus (HIV) infection, leprosy (infectious), lymphogranuloma venereum, syphilis (infectious stage), and tuberculosis (active).
2. A physical or mental disorder and behavior associated with the disorder that may pose, or has posed, a threat to the property, safety, or welfare of the alien or others.
3. A history of such a disorder and behavior that is likely to recur or lead to other harmful behavior.
4. Drug abuse or addiction.
In certain cases, a waiver may be issued to an individual with a Class A condition for entry into the United States. When this occurs, immediate medical follow-up is required.

Class B conditions comprise a "physical or mental abnormality, disease or disability serious in degree or permanent in nature amounting to a substantial departure from normal well-being" (Medical Examination of Aliens. 42 C.F.R. §34.4 [2004]). Individuals with Class B conditions may enter the United States but must receive medical followup soon after arrival.

SOURCES: Medical Examination of Aliens. 42 C.F.R. §34.1–34.8 (2004); Massachusetts Department of Public Health, 2000.

1. Reviewing shipping manifests to identify cargo that may pose a public health threat; ensuring that the shipment is inspected by a quarantine inspector or, more frequently, an inspector from a partner federal agency; ensuring that identified threats are contained, eliminated, or both.
2. Obtaining and reviewing the results of immigrants' overseas medical examinations, identifying immigrants who have Class A or B diseases (Box ES.1), and mailing those results to the state and local health departments with jurisdiction at the immigrants' final destinations.

---

local partners, served as a major means of data collecting for the committee and as an evidence base in writing the report. The citation "Committee, 2005", which appears throughout the report, refers to the committee's notes from these visits. The notes are available in the study's public access file.

BOX ES.2   Quarantinable Communicable Diseases

By executive order of the president of the United States, federal isolation and quarantine are authorized for the following communicable diseases:

1. Cholera.
2. Diphtheria.
3. Infectious tuberculosis.
4. Plague.
5. Smallpox.
6. Yellow fever.
7. Viral hemorrhagic fevers (Lassa, Marburg, Ebola, Crimean-Congo, South American, and others not yet isolated or named).
8. Severe acute respiratory syndrome (SARS).
9. Influenza caused by novel or reemergent influenza viruses that are causing, or have the potential to cause, a pandemic.

SOURCES: Executive Order 13,295 of April 4, 2003: Revised List of Quarantinable Communicable Diseases. *Code of Federal Regulations,* title 3 (2003); Executive Order 13,375 of April 1, 2005: Amendment to Executive Order 13, 295 Relating to Certain Influenza Viruses and Quarantinable Communicable Diseases. *Code of Federal Regulations,* title 3 (2005).

---

3. Meeting arriving refugees and parolees, visually screening them for signs and symptoms of illness, reviewing the results of their overseas medical examinations, giving local health departments notification of their arrival and the results of their overseas examinations, and alerting the health departments to arrivals with Class A or B conditions.

4. Responding to calls from port-based inspectors from other federal agencies about cargo that may pose a public health threat.

5. Visually screening passengers of airplanes arriving from foreign points of origin for signs or symptoms consistent with a quarantinable disease (Box ES.2).

6. Responding to ill passengers (international travelers, immigrants, and refugees) and crew reported by pilots, ship masters, and others.

7. Developing and maintaining relationships with local public health authorities and other System partners at ports within the station's jurisdiction.

8. Overseeing the importation of nonhuman primates to ensure that the process is performed according to a protocol designed to prevent the transmission of zoonotic disease to humans if the nonhuman primates were infected.

9. Inspecting plants and animals that may pose a public health threat and are imported by passengers.

The committee concluded that these activities have public health benefits of various degrees and should continue but should consume only part of quarantine stations' time, for the activities are insufficient in themselves to meet the challenges posed by microbial threats at the nation's gateways.

RECOMMENDATIONS FOR THE QUARANTINE CORE

Strategic Leadership

The United States needs a single entity to exert national strategic public health leadership for the Quarantine Network to successfully protect the U.S. population from microbial threats that originate abroad.

Recommendation 1: The committee recommends that the Quarantine Core strategically lead the United States in its efforts to minimize the risk that microbial threats of public health significance will enter or affect travelers to this country. The Core should have the financial resources and legal authority, consistent with the Constitution and international obligations, to exert this leadership.

As the public health leader for the nation's gateways, the Core should conduct a comprehensive national assessment of the risks posed by microbial threats that have the potential to reach U.S. ports of entry. The Core should then develop a national strategic plan with uniform principles and outcomes designed to mitigate the risks identified in the assessment. If followed, such a plan would help the members of the Quarantine System set priorities for their activities and focus their resources on the people, animals, goods, and conveyances from abroad that pose the greatest risks to the health of the U.S. population.

The committee concluded that the Core alone has the capacity to provide the necessary national public health leadership to the Quarantine Network. Protecting the public's health has traditionally been a function of the states and their localities, however, and the Core should take extra care to collaborate with its state and local partners as it exerts this leadership. Accordingly, as the Core implements its strategic plan, it must assure the local health departments' ability to take on newly delegated responsibilities while continuing to provide essential public health services. In matters not of direct public health concern or in matters of national security, the relevant agency should continue to assume the lead.

Harmonization of Authorities and Functions

Many members of the System appear to lack a clear understanding of the authorities and channels of communication that should be followed to respond to a known or suspect microbial threat of public health significance. Moreover, gaps and overlaps in authority and communication among partners in the System reduce its effectiveness in such areas as identifying cases of zoonotic disease, assuring continuity of care for refugees and immigrants, identifying ill passengers, and conducting contact tracing.

Given sufficient resources and legal authority to exert strategic leadership, the Core could formalize the collaborative relationships that already exist with certain Network partners and establish similar relationships with the remaining Network partners to assure that the responsibilities of the Quarantine Network are executed at all ports of entry on both a routine and emergency basis. The Core also could assure in advance that the responders to microbial threats from abroad would know who is in charge at each location and point in time.

> **Recommendation 2: The committee recommends that, on the basis of its strategic plan, the Quarantine Core work with its partners in the Quarantine Network (and with appropriate agencies in other countries) to delineate or redefine each partner's role, authority, and channel of communication at all locations and specific times in order to minimize the risk that microbial threats of public health significance will enter or affect travelers to the United States.**

Infrastructure

The Quarantine Core relies heavily on port-based inspectors from other federal agencies to identify and report travelers, crew, animals, and cargo that may pose a public health threat at the more than 400 ports that lack quarantine stations and at hours when the quarantine stations are closed. These activities are an official sidebar to the main duties of the port-based officers of the Department of Homeland Security's U.S. Customs and Border Protection (CBP). Although CBP officers receive training for these public health activities during their job orientation and when new diseases emerge, the activities lie outside the domain for which CBP personnel are hired and do not necessarily have high priority for CBP (or other partners of the Core). Further, the quarantine station staff lack the resources to provide CBP with ongoing public health training and reinforcement. The Core will remain reliant on CBP even after the quarantine station expansion is complete, however, because DGMQ will receive insufficient funds to have in-person, round-the-clock coverage at every U.S. port of entry—or even at the most active 10 percent of those ports. Accordingly, the Core should have more opportunities to train its surrogates in the Quarantine System. In addition, it should have up-to-date technology with the capacity for rapid, real-time communication and data-sharing. At present, the infrastructure of the Quarantine System is inadequate to support its current role.

Recommendation 3: The committee recommends enhancements in competences, number of people, training, physical space, and utilization of technology to meet the System's evolving, expanding role.

Location of Stations

DGMQ selected the locations of the 17 new quarantine stations with several goals in mind. Primary among them is to place stations at U.S. ports of entry that receive the greatest volumes of air, sea, and land travelers (DGMQ, 2003). While the committee's expertise and the scope and the timetable of this study precluded a comprehensive review and analysis of DGMQ's plans, the committee offers a set of additional factors DGMQ should consider in its site-selection process, including percentage of international flights covered, amount of coverage during peak arrival times of international flights, coverage of high-risk ports of entry, and the cost-benefit ratio of a robust around-the-clock presence at relatively few, high-risk sites versus a thinner presence at a greater number of sites.

Recommendation 4: The committee recommends that the Core periodically revisit its methodology to ascertain whether the stations are optimally located and staffed and relocate stations or staff as needed. While a volume-based risk assessment seems reasonable, based on available data, the Core should periodically evaluate changes in patterns of global travel and trade, as well as models of infectious disease outbreaks, international spread, and efficacy of interventions.

Surge Capacity

As noted earlier, the quarantine stations' staff currently perform nine primary activities on a routine basis. Although public health emergencies occur sporadically, the committee concluded that the Core should be equally prepared to respond to emergencies as to carry out routine duties.

Recommendation 5: The committee recommends that the Quarantine Core have plans, capacity, resources, and clear and sufficient legal authority to respond rapidly to a surge of activity at any single U.S. port of entry or at multiple U.S. ports simultaneously.

In developing its surge-capacity plans, the Core should collaborate with relevant state and local authorities, many of whom may have already developed emergency response plans for their respective jurisdictions. Furthermore, the committee recommends that the Core build cooperative relationships with agencies that already have extensive experience in emergency response, such as the Federal Emergency Management Agency (FEMA) and U.S. Department of Agriculture (USDA).

Research

The committee found that most practices of the quarantine stations and their surrogates lack a scientific basis. Indeed, much of the practice of detecting infections and controlling outbreaks of disease in the context of the Quarantine Network is based on experience and tradition. It is important that these practices be the subject of systematic research to determine their validity and cost-effectiveness. Further, in the context of new technologies and changing microbial threats, new practices should be developed and tested.

Recommendation 6: The committee recommends that the Core define and devote resources to a research agenda that examines basic public health interventions used or to be developed for use in the System.

The Core should formulate a forward-looking research agenda and should develop plans and protocols for data collection and evaluation during a crisis. This would enable the Core to determine the effectiveness of its practices for containing microbial threats of public health significance.

Measuring Performance

The scientific mindset described above should extend to operational performance.

Recommendation 7: The committee recommends that the Quarantine Core develop scientifically sound tools to measure the effectiveness and quality of all operational aspects of the Quarantine System. The Core should routinely assess the performance of critical quarantine functions by individual CDC quarantine stations, DGMQ headquarters, partner organizations, and the System as a whole. Identified shortfalls should be remedied promptly.

The development and application of measurable standards of effectiveness and quality would yield multiple benefits. It would give members of the System, other policymakers, and the general public clear indicators of the degree to which the U.S. public is protected from microbial threats of public health significance that originate abroad. If the recommended performance metrics become widely accepted, they could stimulate members of the System to strive for operational excellence. Within the Core, performance metrics could set a national standard for the geographically dispersed quarantine stations, especially as new stations are established.

REFERENCES

CDC (Centers for Disease Control and Prevention). 2003. Update: multistate outbreak of monkeypox—Illinois, Indiana, Kansas, Missouri, Ohio, and Wisconsin, 2003. *MMWR Morb Mortal Wkly Rep* 52(27): 642–646.

CDC. 2004. Imported Lassa fever—New Jersey, 2004. *MMWR Morb Mortal Wkly Rep* 53(38): 894–897.

Committee (IOM Committee on Measures to Enhance the Effectiveness of the CDC Quarantine Station Expansion Plan for U.S. Ports of Entry). 2005. Unpublished. *Notes on Site Visits to DGMQ Quarantine Stations.*

CRS (Congressional Research Service, The Library of Congress). 2004. *Border Security: Inspection Practices, Policies, and Issues.* [Online] Available: http://fpc.state.gov/documents/organization/33856.pdf [accessed April 7, 2005].

DGMQ (Division of Global Migration and Quarantine, National Center for Infectious Diseases, Centers for Disease Control and Prevention). 2003. *Reinventing CDC Quarantine Stations: Proposal for CDC Quarantine Station Distribution.* Proposal, September 16, 2003.

DGMQ. 2004. *Fact Sheet: Isolation and Quarantine.* [Online] Available: http://www.cdc.gov/ncidod/dq/sars_facts/isolationquarantine.pdf [accessed May 6, 2005].

DHS (U.S. Department of Homeland Security). 2004. *Bio-Surveillance program initiative remarks by Secretary of Homeland Security Tom Ridge and Secretary of Health and Human Services Secretary Tommy Thompson.* [Online] Available: http://www.dhs.gov/dhspublic/display?theme=43&content=3093 [accessed October 4, 2004].

Gerberding J, Director, Centers for Disease Control and Prevention. 2005. *A Hearing on the Centers for Disease Control and Prevention.* Statement at the Apr. 6, 2005 hearing of the Subcommittee on Labor, Health and Human Services, Education and Related Agencies, Committee on House Appropriations, U.S. House of Representatives.

IOM (Institute of Medicine). 1988. *The Future of Public Health.* Washington, DC: National Academy Press.

Office of Aviation Policy and Plans, Federal Aviation Administration, U.S. Department of Transportation. 2005. *FAA Aerospace Forecasts: Fiscal Years 2005-2006: Table 7 (U.S. and Foreign Flag Carriers: Total Passenger Traffic To/From the United States).* [Online] Available: http://www.api.faa.gov/forecast05/Table7.PDF [accessed April 6, 2005].

1

Introduction

To mitigate the risks posed by microbial threats of public health significance originating abroad, the Centers for Disease Control and Prevention (CDC) places small groups of staff at major U.S. airports. These staff, their offices, and their patient isolation rooms constitute quarantine stations, which are run by CDC's Division of Global Migration and Quarantine (DGMQ).

Positioned at major national gateways, the CDC quarantine stations have experienced first-hand the impact of globalization on public health. The rapid speed and tremendous volume of international and transcontinental travel, commerce, and human migration enable microbial threats to disperse worldwide in 24 hours—less time than the incubation period of most diseases. These and other forces intrinsic to modern technology and ways of life favor the emergence of new diseases and the reemergence or increased severity of known diseases. Meanwhile, the risk of bioterrorism has become a pressing national security issue. Taken together, these factors have stimulated calls for greater vigilance for microbial threats of public health significance at U.S. gateways. Some of those calls have focused attention on the number and role of CDC quarantine stations at U.S. ports of entry.

Congress began to allocate funds in fiscal 2003 for the establishment of new quarantine stations at 17 major U.S. ports of entry that comprise airports, seaports, and land-border crossings. In a significant departure from the recent past, both the preexisting 8 quarantine stations and the new 17 are expected to play an active, anticipatory role in nationwide

BOX 1.1   Statement of Task

Conduct an assessment of the role of the federal quarantine stations given the changes in the global environment, including large increases in international travel, threats posed by bioterrorism and emerging infections, and the movement of animals and cargo. The quarantine stations played a new and important role in the SARS response in 2003. The recognition of their contributions has resulted in increased funding to expand the number and scope of the stations. The assessment is needed to guide the expansion. Issues to be considered include:

1. The current role of quarantine stations as a public health intervention and how the roles should evolve to meet the needs of the 21st century.
2. The role of other agencies and organizations working collaboratively with the CDC's Division of Global Migration and Quarantine at ports of entry (including federal partners such as Customs and Border Protection, Immigration and Customs Enforcement, U.S. Department of Agriculture, and U.S. Fish and Wildlife Service).
3. The role of state and local health departments as partners for public health interventions at the nation's borders (such as activities focused on emergency preparedness and response, disease surveillance, and medical assessment and follow-up of newly arriving immigrants and refugees).
4. Optimal locations for the quarantine stations for efficient and sufficient monitoring and response.
5. Appropriate types of health professionals and necessary skill sets to staff a modern quarantine station.
6. Surge capacity to respond to public health emergencies.

biosurveillance (DHS, 2004; Gerberding, 2005). Consequently, DGMQ asked the Institute of Medicine (IOM) to convene an expert committee to assess the present CDC quarantine stations and recommend how they should evolve to meet the challenges posed by microbial threats at the nation's gateways.[1] DGMQ specifically requested "an assessment of the role of the federal quarantine stations, given the changes in the global environment including large increases in international travel, threats posed by bioterrorism and emerging infections, and the movement of animals and cargo" (Box 1.1).

To conduct this assessment and provide recommendations, IOM convened, in October 2004, the Committee on Measures to Enhance the Effectiveness of the CDC Quarantine Station Expansion Plan for U.S. Ports of Entry. The committee's expertise comprises clinical infectious disease, epi-

---

[1]Contract No. 200-2000-00629, Task Order No. 31.

TABLE 1.1 Locations, Jurisdictions, and Staffing of CDC Quarantine Stations at U.S. Ports of Entry (Established and Nascent), May 2005 and October 2005 Forecast

Location of Quarantine Station	Jurisdiction	No. of Full-Time Equivalents	
		May 2005	Oct. 2005 (forecast)
Anchorage	N/A	1	2
Atlanta* (Hartsfield International Airport)	All ports in Georgia, Alabama, Arkansas, Louisiana, Oklahoma, Mississippi, North Carolina, South Carolina, and Tennessee	3	4
Chicago* (O'Hare International Airport)	All ports in Illinois, Indiana, Iowa, Kansas, Kentucky, Michigan, Minnesota, Missouri, Nebraska, North Dakota, Ohio, South Dakota, and Wisconsin; preclearance port in Toronto[a]	3	6
Dulles, VA[b] (Washington Dulles International Airport)	N/A	1	3
El Paso, TX (Land border crossing)	N/A	2	3
Honolulu* (Honolulu International Airport)	All ports in Hawaii, Guam, and Pacific Trust Territories	3	4
Houston (Houston Intercontinental Airport)	N/A	2	3
Los Angeles* (Tom Bradley International Airport)	All ports in Southern California, Arizona, Colorado, Las Vegas, Nevada, New Mexico, Texas, and the U.S.–Mexico border	4	6

Miami* (*Miami International Airport*)	All ports in Florida, Puerto Rico, and the U.S. Virgin Islands	6	7
Minneapolis	N/A	1	2
Newark	N/A	1	2
New York City* (*John F. Kennedy International Airport*)	All ports in New York, Connecticut, Delaware, District of Columbia, Maine, Maryland, Massachusetts, New Hampshire, New Jersey, Pennsylvania, Rhode Island, Vermont, Virginia, and West Virginia; preclearance ports in Montreal and in Dublin and Shannon, Ireland	7	8
San Diego (*Land border crossing*)	N/A	1	4
San Francisco* (*San Francisco International Airport*)	All ports in Northern California, Nevada (except Las Vegas), Utah, and Wyoming	4	6
San Juan	N/A	1	2
Seattle* (*Seattle-Tacoma International Airport*)	All ports in Washington, Alaska, Idaho, Montana, and Oregon; preclearance ports in Edmonton, Calgary, Vancouver, and Victoria, Canada	4	4
	TOTAL:	44	66

NOTE: N/A = information not yet available; jurisdictions for all stations will be redefined once new stations are fully staffed or nearly so.
*Established station (as of May 2005).
aPreclearance port: A foreign port where individuals who are traveling to the United States undergo—in theory—the same visual screening and other disease surveillance activities conducted at U.S. ports of entry by CDC quarantine station staff.
bDulles, VA, is located approximately 26 miles from Washington, D.C.
SOURCES: DGMQ, 2003; personal communication, M. Remis, DGMQ, May 11, 2005.

demiology, U.S. public health practice, international public health practice, community health education and nursing, and public health law. In addition, three consultants to the committee provided insights into the surveillance, detection, and management of disease in animals and animal products being imported into the United States, CDC quarantine station activities in relation to U.S. seaports, and international laws and regulations relevant to the expansion plans for the CDC quarantine stations.

At the sponsor's request, the committee released the interim letter report *Human Resources at U.S. Ports of Entry to Protect the Public's Health* in January 2005 to provide preliminary suggestions for the priority functions of a modern quarantine station, the competences necessary to carry out those functions, and the types of health professionals who have the requisite competences (Appendix A). This, the committee's final report, assesses the present role of the CDC quarantine stations and articulates a vision of their future role as a public health intervention.

STUDY METHODS

The committee gathered information for this report from journal articles, reports, and news articles; presentations and commentary by constituencies relevant to the study (Appendix B); facts provided by the sponsor at the committee's request; visits by select committee and staff members to five quarantine stations; congressional testimony; and the commissioned papers contained in Appendixes D–F. These information-gathering activities took place between October 2004 and June 2005.

CDC Quarantine Stations: What They Are, What They Do

Quarantine stations have served as a public health intervention at U.S. gateways since the nation's infancy; much has been written about their historic role. Where and how do these stations function today?

Although there are quarantine stations both inside the United States and at its borders, this report deals exclusively with those stations located at ports where people, goods, and conveyances from international points of origin may enter this country. The United States has 474 ports of entry[2] (CRS, 2004); CDC quarantine stations were established at eight of them as of May 2005 (Table 1.1). Figure 1.1 illustrates the present relationship

---

[2]This report uses the term "port of entry" to mean any air, land, or sea port through which people, cargo, and conveyances may legally enter the United States from abroad. It should be noted that "port of entry" has a slightly different meaning when used by the Department of Homeland Security's U.S. Customs and Border Protection (CBP). In CBP's case, a Port of Entry is an administrative center whose jurisdiction may include more than one entry facility

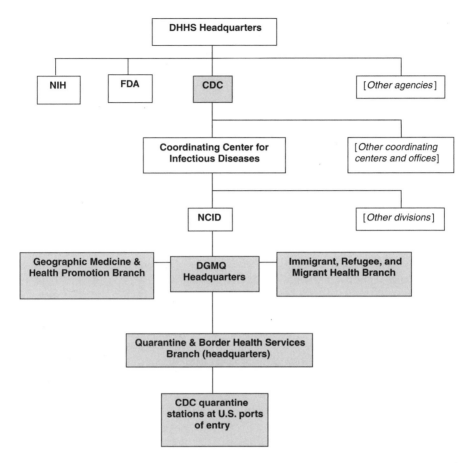

FIGURE 1.1 The relationships among the members of the Quarantine Core (shaded boxes, boldface type) and their partner organizations in the Department of Health and Human Services (white boxes, boldface type). Nonpartner agencies, centers, and divisions within DHHS are also noted in the diagram (white boxes, italicized type).
NOTE: CDC = Centers for Disease Control and Prevention; DHHS = Department of Health and Human Services; DGMQ = Division of Global Migration and Quarantine; FDA = Food and Drug Administration; NCID = National Center for Infectious Diseases; NIH = National Institutes of Health.
SOURCES: CDC, 2005; Cetron, 2004.

---

in a certain geographic area. For instance, the Philadephia Port of Entry services Philadephia International Airport, Philadelphia's seaport, Trenton Mercer Airport, Atlantic City International Airport, and ports in Lehigh Valley, PA (http://www.cbp.gov/xp/cgov/toolbox/contacts/ports/pa/1101.xml). Thus, the United States has fewer CBP Ports of Entry (312) than literal ports of entry (474).

among the CDC quarantine stations, DGMQ and its branches, CDC, and other federal agencies.

Unlike physical areas that travelers pass through, the term "station" in this report refers to a group of one to eight individuals located at an airport, land crossing, or seaport who perform activities designed to help mitigate the risk that microbial and other threats of public health significance may enter the United States or affect travelers to this country. As noted above, all of the established stations (as of May 2005) are located at airports. Although the staff have offices and one or more patient isolation rooms, most interactions between quarantine station staff and travelers or crew take place in public areas of the terminals.

Microbial Threats of Public Health Significance

Microbes in the context of this report are bacteria, viruses, protozoa, fungi, and prions that can replicate in humans. A microbial threat of public health significance causes serious or lethal human disease and is transmissible from person to person, from animal to person, or potentially both; it also may be transmissible from food or water to people. Because of their potential for wide dispersal, concern is greatest for microbes that spread rapidly from person to person. A microbial threat may be introduced intentionally—as in bioterrorism—or unintentionally.

Additional threats of public health significance of concern to the quarantine stations include the release of chemical or radiological substances and of biological substances other than microbes (e.g., microbial toxins).

Overview of Authorities and Activities

Legal Authorities

The quarantine station staff have the delegated authority to detain, medically examine, or conditionally release individuals at U.S. ports of entry who are reasonably believed to be carrying a communicable disease of public health significance. The federal authority vested in DGMQ to order the medical evaluation of such individuals can supersede the public health powers of states and localities under specific circumstances. In addition, DGMQ and CDC can set policies to prevent certain animals that pose a public health threat from entering the country. Chapter 3 contains a more thorough discussion of these legal and regulatory powers, their applications, and their limitations.

Modern Uses of Quarantine and Isolation

The staff of a CDC quarantine station conducts many activities, including ensuring the quarantine of specific individuals and animals. *Quarantine* is the separation and restriction of movement of apparently healthy persons or animals that may have been exposed to a microbial threat and therefore may become infectious (DGMQ, 2004a). On a related note, a CDC quarantine station may also ensure the *isolation* of specific individuals or animals infected by a specific microbial threat. Through isolation, the infected persons or animals are separated from the population at large, and their movement is restricted to prevent the microbial threat from spreading (DGMQ, 2004a). Quarantine and isolation at national borders are important nonmedical components of the public health toolkit for limiting and containing the spread of microbial threats. Their effectiveness varies, however, depending on the nature of the threat and the extent to which it has spread.

Summary of Primary Activities

Today, the CDC quarantine station staff at U.S. ports of entry primarily perform the following activities (Committee, 2005;[3] Appendixes D and E):

1. Reviewing shipping manifests to identify cargo that may pose a public health threat; ensuring that the shipment is inspected by a quarantine inspector or, more frequently, an inspector from a partner federal agency; and ensuring that identified threats are contained.
2. Obtaining and reviewing the results of immigrants' overseas medical examinations, identifying immigrants who have Class A or B diseases (Box 1.2), and mailing those results to the state and local health departments with jurisdiction at the immigrants' final destinations.
3. Meeting arriving refugees and parolees, visually screening them for signs and symptoms of illness, reviewing the results of their overseas medical examinations, giving local health departments notification of their arrival and the results of their overseas examinations, and alerting the health departments to arrivals with Class A or B conditions.
4. Responding to calls from port-based inspectors from other federal agencies about cargo that may pose a public health threat.

---

[3]As already noted in this chapter, committee members visited five quarantine stations over the course of the study. This series of site visits, which included meetings with DGMQ field staff as well as federal and local partners, served as a major means of data collecting for the committee and as an evidence base in writing the report. The citation "Committee, 2005," which appears throughout the report, refers to the committee's notes from these visits. The notes are available in the study's public access file.

BOX 1.2   Class A and Class B Conditions

In the context of medical examinations of individuals who seek refuge in the United States or want to immigrate to this country:

Class A conditions generally render an alien ineligible for entry into the United States; they include

1. Communicable diseases of public health significance, including chancroid, gonorrhea, granuloma inguinale, human immunodeficiency virus (HIV) infection, leprosy (infectious), lymphogranuloma venereum, syphilis (infectious stage), and tuberculosis (active).
2. A physical or mental disorder and behavior associated with the disorder that may pose, or has posed, a threat to the property, safety, or welfare of the alien or others.
3. A history of such a disorder and behavior that is likely to recur or lead to other harmful behavior.
4. Drug abuse or addiction.

In certain cases, a waiver may be issued to an individual with a Class A condition for entry into the United States. When this occurs, immediate medical follow-up is required.

Class B conditions comprise a "physical or mental abnormality, disease or disability serious in degree or permanent in nature amounting to a substantial departure from normal well-being" (Medical Examination of Aliens. 42 C.F.R. §34.4 [2004]). Individuals with Class B conditions may enter the United States, but must receive medical follow-up soon after arrival.

SOURCES: Medical Examination of Aliens. 42 C.F.R. §34.1–34.8 (2004); Massachusetts Department of Public Health, 2000.

5.   Visually screening passengers of airplanes arriving from foreign points of origin for signs or symptoms consistent with a quarantinable disease (Box 1.3).

6.   Responding to ill passengers (international travelers, immigrants, and refugees) and crew reported by pilots, ship masters, and others.

7.   Developing and maintaining relationships with local public health authorities and other System partners at ports within the station's jurisdiction.

8.   Overseeing the importation of nonhuman primates to assure that the process is performed according to a protocol designed to prevent the transmission of zoonotic disease to humans if the nonhuman primates were infected.

BOX 1.3   Quarantinable Communicable Diseases

By executive order of the president of the United States, federal isolation and quarantine are authorized for the following communicable diseases:

1. Cholera.
2. Diphtheria.
3. Infectious tuberculosis.
4. Plague.
5. Smallpox.
6. Yellow fever.
7. Viral hemorrhagic fevers (Lassa, Marburg, Ebola, Crimean-Congo, South American, and others not yet isolated or named).
8. Severe acute respiratory syndrome (SARS).
9. Influenza caused by novel or reemergent influenza viruses that are causing, or have the potential to cause, a pandemic.

SOURCES: Executive Order 13,295 of April 4, 2003: Revised List of Quarantinable Communicable Diseases. *Code of Federal Regulations,* title 3 (2003); Executive Order 13,375 of April 1, 2005: Amendment to Executive Order 13, 295 Relating to Certain Influenza Viruses and Quarantinable Communicable Diseases. *Code of Federal Regulations,* title 3 (2005).

---

9. Inspecting plants and animals that may pose a public health threat and are imported by passengers.

While the staff of all the established stations perform these primary functions, each station's particular priorities are determined by its geographic location, the number of full-time staff and their capabilities, and a range of other factors. Chapter 3 elaborates upon all of these activities in detail.

FRAMING THE ISSUE

As the aviation industry learned from the outbreak of severe acute respiratory syndrome (SARS), the CDC quarantine stations are uniquely positioned to coordinate nationwide responses to global microbial threats of public health significance that have the potential to reach—or cross— U.S. gateways (Meenan, 2005; personal communication, K. Andrus, Air Transport Association, October 21, 2004). Such responses are unusually complex because they often involve multiple organizations that cross sectors, jurisdictions, and nations. As this report will make clear, CDC quarantine stations have the capability in some cases and the potential in others to orchestrate and facilitate these organizationally complex public health responses. Therein lies the stations' chief value to the U.S. population and travelers to this country.

The CDC Quarantine Stations: A National Insurance Policy

In addition to performing the array of daily activities listed above, the CDC quarantine stations serve as part of the United States' national insurance policy against public health catastrophes. As is the case with personal insurance, one hopes never to need it, but if a catastrophe occurs, one is relieved the insurance is there.

Such public health emergencies as the global outbreak of SARS exemplify "low-likelihood, high-consequence events"—a term used in such industries as insurance and emergency management to describe events that are infrequent or have a low probability of occurring but have potentially catastrophic consequences if and when they occur. Uncertainty surrounds low-likelihood, high-consequence events; a cost-benefit assessment is unclear. Efforts to prepare for such events, which may occur years or decades in the future, may be criticized in the present (IOM, 2005).

Strengths and Limitations of Isolation and Quarantine at National Borders

Strengths

Quarantine and isolation at national borders are traditional nonmedical components of the public health toolkit for limiting and containing the spread of microbial threats. The effectiveness of these traditional functional capabilities varies, however, depending on the nature of the threat and the extent to which it has spread. In a recent assessment of the threat of pandemic influenza, the World Health Organization (WHO) concluded that nonmedical interventions, including the health screening of travelers, "can potentially reduce opportunities at the start of a pandemic and slow international spread" (WHO, 2005, p. 52). Such interventions will be the principal protective tools pending the production and distribution of vaccine supplies, the report found.

The presence of trained public health officials at U.S. ports of entry also can have a powerful psychological benefit, particularly for the thousands of port-based workers. The knowledge that a member of the CDC quarantine station staff will board a plane that has reported a case of serious communicable disease and will manage the situation might give port workers the confidence to come to work even during serious outbreaks of disease (Committee, 2005). The confidence-building value of such activities as those performed by the CDC quarantine stations has also been recognized by WHO. Although the health benefit of screening travelers coming from areas affected by serious communicable disease remains unproved, WHO recommends that it be permitted (but not encouraged) before and during an influenza pandemic "for political reasons, to promote public confidence" (WHO, 2005, p. 60).

Limitations

Many of the CDC quarantine stations' present activities focus on the detection of disease in persons, animals, cargo, and conveyances during the window of time shortly before and during arrival at U.S. gateways. Yet the pace of global trade and travel has narrowed that window dramatically. Consequently, infected individuals and animals do not necessarily develop signs of disease while in transit or by the time of arrival, and available noninvasive diagnostics cannot always identify infected travelers with reasonable sensitivity, specificity, and speed. Thus, the quarantine stations can identify only a small percentage of infected people and animals. It is instructive to note that the index case of SARS in Toronto would not have been detected by border quarantine officials had they existed at the time,[4] because that individual was presymptomatic when she returned to Canada from Hong Kong (Personal communication, R. St. John, Public Health Agency of Canada, July 5, 2005).

Microbes incubate undetected in their healthy hosts—whether human, animal, or insect—for widely varied lengths of time before the host exhibits signs of infection. Usually, clinical tests are required to detect infections during the presymptomatic period of disease. Yet there are known diseases for which modern medicine has no clinical diagnostic tools for the presymptomatic state. Moreover, today's diagnostic tools may not recognize novel and dangerous infections in their preclinical state or could lead to misdiagnoses, as happened during the first several months of the SARS outbreak in China (IOM, 2004).

The use of clinical diagnostic tools in general to detect infection in affected travelers takes more time than the present air travel system allows. One quarantine inspector reported he had approximately 30 seconds to determine whether an international traveler displays any signs or symptoms of an infectious disease of public health significance (Committee, 2005; personal communication, R. St. John, Public Health Agency of Canada,

---

[4]The quarantine system that exists today at Canadian ports of entry was created in response to the SARS outbreak.

July 5, 2005). A sea change in social attitudes toward commerce and privacy, as well as an enormous federal investment in public health infrastructure and human resources, would be necessary for presymptomatic tests to become realistic options in the United States.

Refugees and individuals outside the United States applying for an immigrant visa are required to undergo x-ray and diagnostic tests for specific communicable diseases of public health concern before they may receive a U.S. visa and leave their country of origin (DGMQ, 2004b). With the exception of these individuals, however, the Quarantine Network could rarely detect infection in presymptomatic humans and animals entering the United States, even under ideal circumstances.

STRUCTURE OF THIS REPORT

Chapter 2 orients the reader to the recent history of quarantine stations at U.S. ports of entry and to the details of the expansion plan. Chapter 3 contains a description of the committee's findings about the present CDC quarantine stations, including their capacities, methods, operating environment, and linkages. In Chapter 4, the committee presents its conclusions and recommendations on how the quarantine stations should evolve to meet the challenges posed by microbial threats at the nation's gateways.

REFERENCES

CDC (Centers for Disease Control and Prevention, Department of Health and Human Services). 2005. *New CDC Structure.* [Online] Available: http://www.cdc.gov/maso/pdf/CDCOperationalStructure.pdf [accessed June 9, 2005].

Cetron M. 2004. *CDC Division of Global Migration and Quarantine.* Presentation at the October 21, 2004 Meeting of the IOM Committee on Measures to Enhance the Effectiveness of the CDC Quarantine Station Expansion Plan for U.S. Ports of Entry, Washington, DC.

Committee (IOM Committee on Measures to Enhance the Effectiveness of the CDC Quarantine Station Expansion Plan for U.S. Ports of Entry). 2005. Unpublished. *Notes on Site Visits to DGMQ Quarantine Stations.*

CRS (Congressional Research Service, The Library of Congress). 2004. *Border Security: Inspection Practices, Policies, and Issues.* [Online] Available: http://fpc.state.gov/documents/organization/33856.pdf [accessed April 7, 2005].

DGMQ (Division of Global Migration and Quarantine, National Center for Infectious Diseases, Centers for Disease Control and Prevention). 2003. *Quarantine Stations.* [Online] Available: http://www.cdc.gov/ncidod/dq/quarantine_stations.htm [accessed September 20, 2004].

DGMQ. 2004a. *Fact Sheet: Isolation and Quarantine.* [Online] Available: http://www.cdc.gov/ncidod/dq/sars_facts/isolationquarantine.pdf [accessed May 6, 2005].

DGMQ. 2004b. *Medical Examinations.* [Online] Available: http://www.cdc.gov/ncidod/dq/health.htm [accessed January 26, 2005].

DHS (U.S. Department of Homeland Security). 2004. *Bio-Surveillance program initiative remarks by Secretary of Homeland Security Tom Ridge and Secretary of Health and Human Services Secretary Tommy Thompson.* [Online] Available: http://www.dhs.gov/dhspublic/display?theme=43&content=3093 [accessed October 4, 2004].

Gerberding J, Director, Centers for Disease Control and Prevention. 2005. *A Hearing on the Centers for Disease Control and Prevention.* Statement at the Apr. 6, 2005 hearing of the Subcommittee on Labor, Health and Human Services, Education and Related Agencies, Committee on House Appropriations, U.S. House of Representatives.

IOM (Institute of Medicine). 2004. *Learning From SARS: Preparing for the Next Disease Outbreak.* Knobler S, Mahmoud A, Lemon S, Mack A, Sivitz L, Oberholtzer K, Editors. Washington, DC: The National Academies Press.

IOM. 2005. *The Smallpox Vaccination Program: Public Health in an Age of Terrorism.* Washington, DC: The National Academies Press.

Meenan JM, Executive Vice President and Chief Operating Officer, Air Transport Association of America Inc. 2005. *Statement of John M. Meenan.* Statement at the Apr. 6, 2005 hearing of the Subcommittee on Aviation, Committee on Transportation and Infrastructure, U.S. House of Representatives.

WHO (World Health Organization). 2005. *Avian Influenza: Assessing the Pandemic Threat.* Geneva: World Health Organization.

2

Context and Content of the CDC Quarantine Station Expansion Plan

During the late 1960s, more than 500 people staffed the 55 federal quarantine stations then active at U.S. seaports, airports, land-border crossings, consulates, territories, and territorial waters (Cetron, 2004; DGMQ, 2003a). Yet many leaders of the American medical community during those years believed it was "time to close the book on infectious diseases, declare the war against pestilence won, and shift national resources to such chronic problems as cancer and heart disease." This statement, attributed by legend to U.S. Surgeon General William Stewart (Office of the Public Health Service Historian, 2002), reflected the public's confidence in the power of antibiotics and vaccines to eradicate such dreaded communicable diseases as yellow fever, plague, cholera, and especially smallpox, which the quarantine stations had worked to barricade from entering the U.S. population for nearly a century.

The perception that humans had effectively controlled microbial threats led to the dismantling of most of the federal border quarantine system in the 1970s; by the end of that decade, fewer than a dozen active stations remained (Cetron, 2004).

THE EMERGENCE OF NEW INFECTIOUS DISEASES AND THE THREAT OF BIOTERRORISM

At the same time that the border quarantine system was being largely dismantled, new and long-absent infectious diseases were emerging, re-emerging, and spreading in human populations. Nearly 40 newly emerging infectious diseases were identified during the 30 years between 1973 and 2003 (GAO, 2004). The convergence of multiple interrelated factors is responsible for this phenomenon (IOM, 2003). Important factors include

- rapid, high-volume international and transcontinental travel, commerce, and human migration;
- mass relocation of rural populations to cities and the prevalence of overcrowded, unsanitary conditions there;
- exponential growth of population and the number of individuals susceptible to infectious disease;
- widespread changes in climate, ecology, and land use;
- more frequent contact between people and wildlife;
- reduced global investment in public health infrastructure;
- development of antimicrobial resistance.

Numerous scientists, physicians, and public health officers in national and international organizations have voiced concern about these trends and their relationship to such naturally occurring public health threats as West Nile virus, SARS, and pandemic influenza. Also within the past two decades, terrorism in general and bioterrorism in particular have become grave concerns to the U.S. government and its citizens. Consequently, in the late 1990s, DGMQ began to explore ways that the quarantine stations at U.S. ports of entry might help protect U.S. citizens from the unintentional or intentional importation of dangerous infectious agents (Personal communication, D. Kim, DGMQ, October 13, 2004).

EXPANSION PLAN FOR CDC QUARANTINE STATIONS AT U.S. PORTS OF ENTRY

U.S. Government Increases Investment in Quarantine Stations at Ports of Entry

The outbreak of SARS in 2002 and 2003 dramatically demonstrated the need for strong, well-coordinated national and international systems for disease surveillance, detection, and response (DGMQ, 2003b). In the short term, the outbreak led to a modest addition of nine contract employees at the CDC quarantine stations (Personal communications: D. Kim, DGMQ, October 13, 2004; M. Remis, DGMQ, October 21, 2004).

Coupled with the microbial threats described above, SARS reinvigorated interest within the federal government to commit funding to biosecurity initiatives. A portion of the fiscal year 2004 budget appropriation went to DGMQ for the development of three new CDC quarantine stations at U.S. ports of entry: Houston Intercontinental Airport; the Mexico–

U.S. land border crossing in El Paso, Texas; and Dulles International Airport, located 26 miles from Washington, D.C. These three new stations are partially staffed as of this writing (Personal communications: J. Barrow and M. Remis, DGMQ, December 28, 2004; M. Remis, DGMQ, May 11, 2005).

Further expansion of the quarantine stations in number and scope of work was proposed under the biosecurity umbrella of the Administration's fiscal 2005 budget request to Congress (OMB, 2004). This proposal called for expansion to a total of 25 CDC quarantine stations at U.S. ports of entry (Figure 2.1).

Congress allocated $80 million for fiscal 2005 biosecurity activities to the Office of the Secretary of the Department of Health and Human Services (U.S. Congress, 2004), which distributed $10.2 million to DGMQ's Quarantine and Border Health Services Branch, 92% of which was applied to salaries and other personnel expenses (Personal communication, M. Remis, DGMQ, March 21, 2005). The Administration's fiscal 2006 budget request to Congress includes $15.1 million for the quarantine station expansion (Personal communication, M. Remis, DGMQ, March 21, 2005). CDC Director Julie Gerberding forecast that the expansion will be complete by the end of fiscal 2006 if the requested funds are allocated to DGMQ (Gerberding, 2005).

DGMQ's Vision for the Expanded Quarantine System

With its new mandate, DGMQ wants the CDC quarantine stations to do more than respond to and evaluate travelers with suspect or probable illness. It envisions playing an active, anticipatory role in nationwide biosurveillance (DGMQ, 2003b; DGMQ, 2004a). This move may be broadly viewed as a significant step back to the robustness of the U.S. border quarantine station system before 1970, as well as a step forward toward national biosecurity based on today's technology and knowledge of microbial threats to human heath.

"CDC Quarantine Stations are gearing up to make the transition from the current focus on federal inspection services at airports to become a full partner in public health response," reads a 2003 proposal by DGMQ (DGMQ, 2003b, p.1). "The transformed CDC Quarantine Stations will go beyond evaluating ill passengers to encompass a wide range of responses to infectious disease threats, whether intentional—as in the case of bioterrorism—or related to emerging pathogens. . . . [They] will bring new expertise to bridge gaps in public health and clinical practice[1], emergency

---

[1]As of January 18, 2005, seven quarantine medical officers (physicians) are on duty or have accepted offers of employment. Offers of employment have been made to two additional quarantine medical officers. Offers of employment for other staff positions are also pending (Personal communication, M. Remis, DGMQ, January 18, 2005).

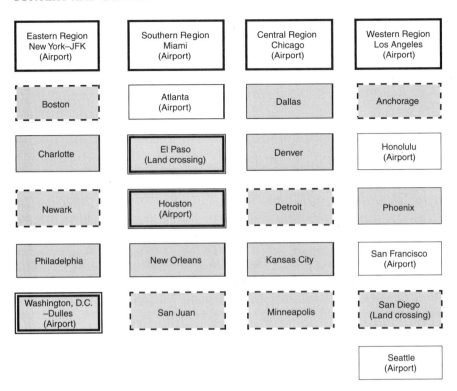

FIGURE 2.1 The proposed geographic distribution of the 25 quarantine stations in the expanded system. The New York, Miami, Chicago, and Los Angeles quarantine stations would have the greatest capacity in both number of people and variety of competences. These staff would support other stations in their geographic region. The white boxes denote the eight cities where quarantine stations have existed prior to 2004. The shaded boxes with a double border identify the 3 cities where the development of new quarantine stations began in 2004; none is fully operational as of this writing. The other shaded boxes represent the 14 cities where DGMQ plans to establish more stations beginning in 2005; those with a dashed border represent the 7 stations slated to open in 2005. The type of port where a quarantine station is or will be located, if known, is indicated in parentheses under the name of each of those cities.
SOURCES: DGMQ, 2004b; personal communication, M. Remis, DGMQ, March 21, 2005.

services, and response management. . . . Improved communications networks will enable passengers to be notified promptly of potential exposures to infectious diseases. These expanded services will be integrated into bioterrorism and emergency preparation and response plans and will be grounded in strengthened collaboration" with state and local health departments, the travel industry, and the health-care community, as well as other federal agencies.

DGMQ also would like the CDC quarantine stations to provide a stronger continuum of health support for refugees, whom the division helps prepare for migration to the United States, and immigrants. Refugees primarily enter the United States through a port with a quarantine station[2], so the stations may be well positioned to monitor the health status of arriving refugees and collaborate with state and local officials on followup health evaluations and treatment. It should be noted that DGMQ does have a program for immigrants and refugees housed in a branch parallel in structure to the branch that houses the quarantine stations staff.

DGMQ's Self-Reported Goals and Accomplishments—Fiscal 2003

In its program review for fiscal 2003, DGMQ articulated its goals for the expanded number and scope of quarantine stations (DGMQ, 2004a). Reflecting on its experience with SARS, DGMQ highlighted the importance of communication and linkages with partner organizations in both routine and emergency contexts. The program review also noted the importance of risk communication with travelers through travel health recommendations and specific travel alerts. The review presented a long list of the quarantine stations' accomplishments in fiscal 2003; those that pertain directly to the committee's findings and conclusions include the following:

- Met 31 flights arriving from Africa to inspect Liberian and Somali Bantu refugees; met 23 flights with adoptees arriving from China to assess their general state of health and rash illnesses and to facilitate notification of state health departments for medical follow-up.
- Reviewed or responded to more than 2,000 cases of reported illnesses among travelers arriving in the United States and implemented control measures.
- Oversaw arrivals of 6,663 immigrants and 36,163 refugees; oversaw shipments of 2,245 nonhuman primates, 1,402 dogs, and 54,268 etiologic agents.
- Performed or oversaw the performance of 2,077 inspections of maritime vessels for rodent infestation.

---

[2]A large number of refugees enter the United States at Newark Liberty International Airport, which lacks a quarantine station at present. The International Office for Migration does the initial processing of these refugees and gives their documentation to quarantine station staff at John F. Kennedy International Airport in New York City, who notify appropriate health departments. Newark is one of the 14 cities designated for a quarantine station (Personal communication, M. Remis, DGMQ, January 18, 2005).

Selection of Ports for the New CDC Quarantine Stations

Figure 2.1 illustrates the proposed geographic distribution of CDC quarantine stations at U.S. ports of entry. DGMQ's plan groups the 25 stations into four regions. Each region will have one station—those in New York, Miami, Chicago, and Los Angeles—with relatively robust capacity. Other stations in the region may draw upon this capacity as needed.

DGMQ used the following criteria to select the cities that have received or will receive a new quarantine station (DGMQ, 2003b):

1. Volume of international human travelers:
   - Airports with >500,000 arriving international air travelers per year.
   - Seaports in major cities with >150,000 arriving international maritime travelers per year.
   - Land crossings in major cities with >10 million arriving international travelers.
2. Total volume of human travelers, airports:
   - Airports with >25 million arriving international and domestic air travelers per year.
3. Volume of imported wildlife:
   - Major cities that serve as designated or nondesignated ports of entry by the U.S. Fish and Wildlife Service to receive international shipments of wildlife.
4. National security considerations:
   - The selected cities are among the 83 so-called Tier 1 U.S. cities, which are believed to be strategic destinations from a national security standpoint (Personal communication, M. Cetron, DGMQ, September 22, 2004).

According to fiscal 2002 data gathered by DGMQ, the 25 cities in the expanded system receive around 75 percent of international air travelers arriving in the United States, or approximately 52 million people, and 48 percent of arriving international sea travelers, or 5.9 million people (DGMQ, 2003b). In addition, more than 78 million people enter the United States through the land-border crossings in El Paso, Texas, and San Diego (DGMQ, 2003b). The 25 cities in the expanded system also receive around 32 percent of the maritime cargo annually imported to the United States; this was equivalent to approximately 275 million short tons of cargo in 2003, as illustrated in Appendix D, Table D.6 (1 short ton = 2,000 pounds).

For a complete description of DGMQ's methodology and data, see Appendix C.

Proposed Workforce for Expanded Stations

DGMQ has proposed a workforce plan to support the activities of 25 CDC quarantine stations at U.S. ports of entry (DGMQ, 2004c). This plan has changed over time; the version presented here dates to July 2004. It appears that, to some extent, DGMQ has begun to act on the plan. Notably, medical officer-epidemiologists have been hired for many of the existing stations, and the title "quarantine public health advisor" has recently replaced "quarantine inspector." We decided to use the title "inspector" in this report because, for the most part, it still reflects a principal activity of those workers.

The proposed workforce comprises eight full-time equivalents (FTEs) located at the Quarantine & Border Health Services Branch headquarters and 158 FTEs in the field. Headquarters would have a chief, a deputy chief, an administrative officer, a training coordinator, a technical writer-editor, a lead medical officer-epidemiologist, an epidemiologist, and a mathematical statistician.

The four regional stations (Chicago, Los Angeles, Miami, and New York-JFK) would each have eight FTEs: a regional supervisor, a medical officer-epidemiologist, four public health advisors at the GS-11 or GS-12 level, and two public health advisors at the GS-9 level. The remaining 21 stations would have six FTEs each: a lead public health advisor (the station's supervisor), a medical officer-epidemiologist, three public health advisors at the GS-11 or GS-12 level, and one public health advisor at the GS-9 level. The field medical officer-epidemiologists would report to the lead medical officer-epidemiologist, and the regional supervisors would report to the chief of the Quarantine & Border Health Services Branch.

Field staff would support operations from 8:00 A.M. to 4:30 P.M. on Mondays through Fridays. One or more FTEs would always be on call after hours to provide around-the-clock coverage. It is unclear how many after-hours officers there would be and where they would be located. DGMQ projected that extending the hours of operation to nearly all day, every day, would require a 25 percent increase, or 39 more FTEs.

REFERENCES

Cetron M. 2004. *CDC Division of Global Migration and Quarantine.* Presentation at the October 21, 2004, Meeting of the IOM Committee on Measures to Enhance the Effectiveness of the CDC Quarantine Station Expansion Plan for U.S. Ports of Entry, Washington, DC.

DGMQ (Division of Global Migration and Quarantine, National Center for Infectious Diseases, Centers for Disease Control and Prevention). 2003a. *CDC–History of Quarantine–DQ.* [Online] Available: http://www.cdc.gov/ncidod/dq/history.htm [accessed September 20, 2004].

DGMQ. 2003b. *Reinventing CDC Quarantine Stations: Proposal for CDC Quarantine Station Distribution.* Proposal, September 16, 2003.

DGMQ. 2004a. *Program Review Fiscal Year 2003.* Program review, May 7, 2004.

DGMQ. 2004b. *Proposed Organization Chart.* Organizational chart, July 8, 2004.

DGMQ. 2004c. *Proposed Organization Chart Breakout.* Organizational chart, July 8, 2004.

GAO (United States Government Accountability Office). 2004. *Emerging Infectious Diseases: Review of State and Federal Disease Surveillance Efforts.* GAO–04–877. Washington, DC: GAO.

Gerberding J, Director, Centers for Disease Control and Prevention. 2005. *A Hearing on the Centers for Disease Control and Prevention.* Statement at the Apr. 6, 2005 hearing of the Subcommittee on Labor, Health and Human Services, Education and Related Agencies, Committee on House Appropriations, U.S. House of Representatives.

IOM (Institute of Medicine). 2003. *Microbial Threats to Health: Emergency, Detection, and Response.* Smolinski MS, Hamburg MA, Lederberg J, Editors. Washington, DC: The National Academies Press.

Office of the Public Health Service Historian. 2002. *FAQ's.* [Online] Available: http://lhncbc.nlm.nih.gov/apdb/phsHistory/faqs_text.html [accessed January 10, 2005].

OMB (Office of Management and Budget, The Executive Office of the President of the United States). 2004. *Budget of the U.S. Government, Fiscal Year 2005.* [Online] Available: http://www.whitehouse.gov/omb/budget/fy2005/budget.html [accessed December 9, 2004].

U.S. Congress, House of Representatives, Committee of Conference. 2004. *Making Appropriations for Foreign Operations, Export Financing, and Related Programs for the Fiscal Year Ending September 30, 2005, and for Other Purposes: Conference Report to Accompany H.R. 4818.* 108th Cong., 2nd Sess. Report 108-792. November 20, 2004.

3

Today's CDC Quarantine Stations at U.S. Ports of Entry

This chapter presents the committee's findings about the activities and composition of the present CDC quarantine stations at U.S. ports of entry and the nature of their relationships with other organizations. Most of the available information is qualitative in nature, deriving from direct observation and interviews. The chapter begins with a description of the broad statutory and regulatory foundation of the CDC quarantine stations' activities. A conceptual framework for understanding the stations' organizational environment follows. Then the committee discusses its findings about the processes and outcomes of four fundamental activities:

1. Identification of ill passengers and crew.
2. Responding to reports of ill passengers.
3. Assuring immigrant and refugee health.
4. Inspection of animals, animal products, etiologic agents, hosts, and vectors.

The conclusions and recommendations in Chapter 4 are based upon these findings.

STATUTORY AND REGULATORY FOUNDATION OF CDC QUARANTINE STATION ACTIVITIES

The secretary of the Department of Health and Human Services (DHHS) has statutory responsibility for preventing the introduction, transmission, and spread of communicable diseases from foreign countries into the United States and its possessions (42 U.S.C. §264). To implement this statute, the secretary develops and enforces regulations through the Centers for Disease Control and Prevention (CDC) (8 U.S.C., 42 U.S.C. §70 and §71). CDC has authorized its Division of Global Migration and Quarantine (DGMQ) to carry out many of these regulations through a variety of activities, including the operation of quarantine stations at select ports of entry and the administration of regulations that govern the movement of people, animals, cargo, and conveyances into the United States. For example, DGMQ can detain, medically examine, or conditionally release individuals at U.S. ports of entry who are reasonably believed to be carrying a communicable disease of public health significance (42 CFR §70 –71). Also, DGMQ and CDC can set policies to prevent certain animals that pose a public health threat from entering the country (42 CFR §71.32).

QUARANTINE CORE, SYSTEM, AND NETWORK

The committee found the CDC quarantine stations to be one component of a large, complex network of organizations whose collective actions provide limited protection to residents of and travelers to the United States from microbial threats of foreign origin. It became apparent that understanding the role of the CDC quarantine stations in this network would be essential to developing realistic conclusions and recommendations. Consequently, the committee developed a conceptual diagram and vocabulary to visualize and articulate the interrelationships among the stations, the network, and other key actors. The committee used this diagram and vocabulary both during its deliberations and in its report.

The committee found that some members of the network interact primarily or exclusively with the headquarters staff of DGMQ, rather than with individual stations. For instance, the Director of DGMQ has direct contact with the World Health Organization and the Air Transport Association of America.

Other members of the network interact with CDC's quarantine operations at multiple levels. For example, the issuance of a joint FDA–CDC ban on the importation and interstate trade of African rodents in the wake of the monkeypox outbreak was accomplished through communication among DGMQ leadership, relevant officials at CDC headquarters, and their counterparts at FDA's main offices in the Washington, DC, area. By contrast, FDA's field inspectors at U.S. ports of entry interact primarily with the CDC quarantine station in their region.

In addition, the committee found, a subgroup of organizations in the network interacts with the quarantine stations more closely and frequently than the rest of the network. Within this subgroup, some organizations and individuals have weekly or even daily contact with the quarantine station staff. The FDA field inspectors are a part of this subgroup.

Figure 3.1 presents the visual schematic created by the committee to illustrate these findings. The following text describes this diagram in detail, as well as the corresponding set of terms coined by the committee for use throughout the report.

The Quarantine Core

At the center of the diagram is what the committee has dubbed the "Quarantine Core," which consists of the CDC quarantine stations, DGMQ headquarters, and the organizational and scientific capacity of CDC (Figure 1.1 illustrates the relationship among these entities). The quarantine stations lie at the center of this diagram because they are the only members of the network whose primary purpose is the mitigation of imported microbial threats at U.S. ports of entry.

The Quarantine System

In the ring around the Core lies the subgroup of organizations that have (or should have) especially close ties to the Core. Together, this subgroup and the Quarantine Core form what the committee calls the "Quarantine System." The organizations within the System are responsible for performing the critical quarantine functions of planning, surveillance, assessment and response, and communication to mitigate the risks posed by microbial threats of foreign origin to residents of and travelers to the United States.

In addition to the entities within the Core, the Quarantine System includes local emergency responders and hospitals, local health care providers, local and state health departments, state public health laboratories, port authorities, port staff, airlines, cruise lines, shipping companies, shipping agents, the International Organization for Migration, overseas panel physicians, the U.S. Coast Guard, the Federal Bureau of Investigation, and federal inspectors from U.S. Customs and Border Protection (CBP),[1] the U.S. Fish and Wildlife Service, and the Food and Drug Administration. As will be seen in Chapter 4, the consistency and quality of relationships within the System are the subject of several conclusions and recommendations.

The Quarantine Network

In the outermost ring lie the organizations and people that interact with DGMQ leadership and the organizational and scientific capacity of CDC,

---

[1]CBP includes veterinary and animal health inspectors from the U.S. Department of Agriculture Animal and Plant Health Inspection Service, as well as the staff of the former Immigration and Naturalization Service and Immigration and Customs Enforcement.

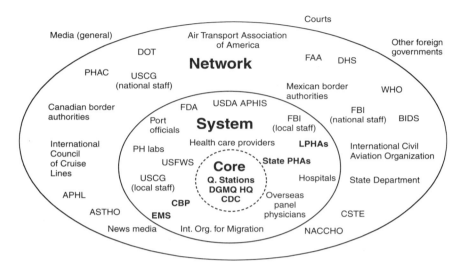

Abbreviation	Full Name
APHL	Association of Public Health Laboratories
ASTHO	Association of State and Territorial Health Officials
BIDS	Border Infectious Disease Surveillance Project, Centers for Disease Control and Prevention
CBP	U.S. Customs and Border Protection, U.S. Department of Homeland Security
CDC	Centers for Disease Control and Prevention
CSTE	Council of State and Territorial Epidemiologists
DGMQ HQ	Division of Global Migration and Quarantine headquarters
DHS	U.S. Department of Homeland Security
DOT	U.S. Department of Transportation
EMS	emergency medical services
FAA	Federal Aviation Administration, U.S. Department of Transportation
FBI	Federal Bureau of Investigation
FDA	U.S. Food and Drug Administration
LPHA	local pubic health authority
NACCHO	National Association of County and City Health Officials
PH labs	state public health labs
PHAC	Public Health Agency of Canada
State PHA	state public health agency (U.S.)
USCG	U.S. Coast Guard
USDA APHIS	U.S. Department of Agriculture Animal and Plant Health Inspection Service
USFWS	U.S. Fish and Wildlife Service, U.S. Department of the Interior
WHO	World Health Organization

FIGURE 3.1 The relationships among the Quarantine Core, System, and Network for U.S. ports of entry. The circle around the Core is a dotted line to reflect the interdependence of the quarantine stations and their partners in the System. CBP, EMS, LPHAs, and State PHAs are bolded to reflect the especially close collaboration of those entities with the stations on virtually a daily basis. Some organizations interact with the quarantine stations at the System level as well as with CDC or DGMQ at the Network level; these organizations appear in both places in the diagram.

not with individual stations. Together, these entities plus the Quarantine System and Core form a multijurisdictional, multisectoral, multinational "Quarantine Network" that protects both travelers entering the United States and the population within U.S. borders from microbial threats of public health significance[2] that originate abroad. In so doing, this Network helps protect the health of the global community.

The members of the Network that lie outside the System include the national-level staff of federal agencies active at the System level, the U.S. Department of State and its embassies, the Department of Homeland Security, national and international transportation industry associations, Mexican and Canadian officials responsible for border activities and disease control, the World Health Organization, and the news media. Although these organizations do not interact with the CDC quarantine stations on a daily basis, they are essential partners whose actions and decisions affect the functioning of the CDC quarantine stations at U.S. ports of entry.

IDENTIFICATION OF AND RESPONSE TO
ILL PASSENGERS AND CREW

While the United States has 474 ports of entry[3] (CRS, 2004), CDC quarantine stations were established at only 8 of them as of May 2005 (Table 1.1, Table 3.1).The absence of Quarantine Core personnel at most U.S. ports of entry impedes the establishment of critical relationships, plans, and protocols with members of the System to lay the groundwork for identifying and responding to cases of illness there (Committee, 2005). As a

---

[2]Definition: A microbial threat of public health significance causes serious or lethal human disease and is transmissible from person to person, from animal to person, or potentially both; it also may be transmissible from food or water to people. Because of their potential for wide dispersal, concern is greatest for microbes that spread readily from person to person. A microbial threat may be introduced intentionally—as in bioterrorism—or unintentionally. Additional threats of public health significance of concern to the quarantine stations include the release of chemical or radiological substances and of biological substances other than microbes (e.g., microbial toxins).

[3]This report uses the term "port of entry" to mean any air, land, or sea port through which people, cargo and conveyances may legally enter the United States from abroad. It should be noted that "port of entry" has a slightly different meaning when used by the Department of Homeland Security's U.S. Customs and Border Protection (CBP). In CBP's case, a Port of Entry is an administrative center whose jurisdiction may include more than one entry facility in a certain geographic area. For instance, the Philadelphia Port of Entry services Philadelphia International Airport, Philadelphia's seaport, Trenton Mercer Airport, Atlantic City International Airport, and ports in Lehigh Valley, PA (http://www.cbp.gov/xp/cgov/toolbox/contacts/ports/pa/1101.xml). Thus, the United States has fewer CBP Ports of Entry (331) than literal ports of entry (474).

TABLE 3.1   Number of Ports of Entry to the United States Compared with Number of Official Ports of Entry (POEs) Defined by U.S. Customs and Border Protection, 2005

	Air	Sea	Land	TOTAL
No. of ports of entry	216	143	115	474
No. of official POEs	—	—	—	331[a]

NOTE: Official U.S. Ports of Entry (POEs) are determined by U.S. Customs and Border Protection (CBP). According to CBP, "a 'Port of Entry' is an officially designated location (seaports, airports, and or land border locations) where CBP officers or employees are assigned to accept entries of merchandise, clear passengers, collect duties, and enforce the various provisions of CBP and related laws." Some POEs are not staffed. Staffed POEs may be responsible for overseeing inspections at multiple entry facilities (airports, seaports, and land crossings) within a single geographic area. Thus, the total number of entry facilities is greater than the total number of ports of entry.

[a]Fourteen of these are CBP preclearance stations in Canada and the Caribbean.

SOURCES: CBP, 2005d; CBP, 2005e; CRS, 2004.

result, identification and responses to signs of microbial threats in persons, animals, cargo and conveyances generally are unsystematic.

For example, in one recent experience, an inbound international ship reported to the U.S. Coast Guard that a crew member had a fever and rash, potentially signs of a quarantinable disease (Personal communication, P. Edelson, DGMQ, March 24, 2005). The potential microbial threat is typically isolated in such cases by having the ship anchor offshore and transporting a clinician there to examine the patient and decide whether the sailor's illness is likely a communicable disease of public health concern. Because of lack of preparation for such an event, however, the local health department could not identify a clinician in the county to examine the sailor. The quarantine station with jurisdiction over the case believes that clinicians with relevant expertise were present in the county at the time, but the local health department lacked the resources and planning to identify an appropriate clinician on the spot. Consequently, the ship docked at port before the patient underwent clinical evaluation. Had the sailor been infected with a microbial threat of public health significance, the community might have suffered an outbreak that cost lives. The larger the port and community, the greater the likely impact of an ineffective Quarantine System.

Visual Screening of Passengers and Crew for Signs of Illness

With tremendous growth in the volume of international air traffic, significant cuts in the Quarantine Core's resources, and limited federal investment to fill the gap, the CDC quarantine stations inspect just a small fraction of arriving international air travelers and crew for clinical signs of a communicable disease of public health significance. To make the most of its limited resources at airports where there is a quarantine station, the CDC staff sets priorities for which international flights it will meet to screen disembarking passengers and crew. The highest-priority flights are those arriving from points of origin where an infectious disease outbreak is known or believed to have occurred and flights whose pilot has reported a suspect or probable case of disease or injury on board. High-priority flights at the present time include those arriving from Africa and from the Southeast Asian countries where avian influenza is endemic (Committee, 2005).

In addition to inspecting travelers who self-identify or are identified prior to arrival by crew members, quarantine inspectors screen arriving travelers for physical signs suggestive of quarantinable communicable disease: rash, unusually flushed or pale complexion, jaundice, shivering, profuse sweating, diarrhea, and inability to walk without assistance (DQ, 2000). So as not to impede the movement of travelers through airports and customs stations, the brief visual inspections are conducted from a distance of several feet (Committee, 2005). The inspectors stand at various locations in the terminal, depending on the airport. In many locations, the travelers are walking past the staff member while the inspection takes place. Such locations include

- The gate where arriving passengers enter the terminal.
- Hallways where passengers from multiple arriving flights walk toward customs (or through which international travelers pass en route to connecting flights).
- The side of passport control booths located inside U.S. territory.

Partners in the Identification of Ill Passengers

Aircraft Commanders and Ship Masters

The quarantine stations rely not only on CBP but also on airline crews and ship masters to identify ill passengers. The commanders of aircraft destined for the United States have a regulatory responsibility for notifying the quarantine station nearest their first U.S. destination of "the occurrence, on board, of any death or ill person among passengers or crew" (42 CFR §71.21b). Similarly, the masters of ships sailing to the United States have a regulatory responsibility for immediately notifying the quarantine station nearest the port of arrival of "the occurrence, on board, of any death or any ill person among passengers or crew (including those who have disembarked or been removed) during the 15-day period preceding the date of expected arrival" (42 CFR §71.21a). Ideally, when a quarantine station receives prearrival notification of illness or death, a quarantine inspector, a local emergency responder, a clinician, or a combination of the three boards the conveyance to evaluate the ill passenger before anyone disembarks, thus containing the potential microbial threat (Committee, 2005).

Anecdotal evidence suggests that pilots and ship masters fail to comply with these prearrival reporting regulations out of ignorance, neglect, or other factors (Committee, 2005; personal communication, P. Edelson, DGMQ, March 24, 2005). The penalty for sidestepping this regulation—$5,000 or less per vessel—is inconsequential (42 U.S.C. §271b). Officers of CBP and the U.S. Coast Guard (USCG) have statutory responsibility "to aid in the enforcement of quarantine rules and regulations" (42 U.S.C. §268b); it is unclear how they do so in relation to the aforementioned regulations.

A 2001 report by CDC found that many pilots were unfamiliar with the requirement to report arriving ill passengers aboard a flight (CDC, 2001). More recently, flight attendants aboard a plane en route from London to the United States failed to identify a man with signs and symptoms of chills, fever, diarrhea, and severe sore throat. The man was hospitalized within hours of his arrival and diagnosed with Lassa fever, a quarantinable communicable disease, after having exposed 19 passengers in flight (CDC, 2004c; personal communication, M. Cetron, DGMQ, October 21, 2004). Three of the five quarantine stations visited by the committee, as well as DGMQ HQ officials, agreed that many pilots do not follow the regulatory notification procedures and instead radio intermediaries, such as MedLink, a service available to most commercial airlines that directly links pilots to emergency care physicians[4] (Committee, 2005; MedAire, 2005). When radioed, MedLink's physicians give the pilots medical instructions, contact emergency response teams to meet the plane when it lands, and contact hospitals to receive the patient or patients. The company that owns MedLink, MedAire Inc. of Tempe, Arizona, offers a similar service called MAS to cargo vessels.

The executive vice president of the Air Transport Association of America Inc. (ATA) recently testified that CDC and his staff "have made sure that our members fully understand the reporting requirements for passengers with suspected communicable diseases" (Meenan, 2005, p.3). To further encourage airline pilots to comply with prearrival notification procedures, CDC quarantine station personnel make an effort to meet any plane reporting an ill passenger, even if (as is frequently the case) the reported signs and symptoms clearly indicate that the passenger does not have a quarantinable communicable disease (Committee, 2005).

---

[4]The JFK-based quarantine station receives approximately two prearrival notification calls per week from aircraft pilots (Committee, 2005).

ATA's members are reportedly trying to train their crews better to recognize and report passengers who display signs of communicable disease of public health concern (Personal communication, K. Andrus, ATA, October 21, 2004). The 2001 CDC report mentioned above recommended that commercial in-flight manuals be updated to include procedures for managing an ill passenger and detailed information on how to contact the closest quarantine station (CDC, 2001); whether such action has been taken is unclear.

The quarantine stations receive such infrequent prearrival notifications from ship masters that some CDC staff believe only the veteran ship masters are aware of the regulation (Appendix D). As noted above, USCG is responsible for assisting in the enforcement of prearrival notification rules among ships, and federal regulation requires vessels to immediately notify the nearest USCG group office of hazardous conditions. Such conditions include injury or illness to persons aboard the vessel (33 CFR 160.1–160.215). For a thorough description of the relationship between the CDC quarantine stations and U.S. seaports, see Appendix D.

The failure to notify a quarantine station of on-board illness could, in certain cases, represent a missed opportunity for the Quarantine Core to contain a potential outbreak of a serious communicable disease, compromising public health and national security.

U.S. Customs and Border Protection (CBP)

More than 460 U.S. ports of entry and preclearance ports lack personnel from the Quarantine Core to screen arriving travelers for signs of communicable disease of public health significance. For every full-time-equivalent quarantine station staff member, there are approximately 300 CBP field officers.[5] Consequently, the Core relies on CBP inspectors to watch for ill passengers at most ports and to carry out other regulatory responsibilities on their behalf. In addition, because the CDC quarantine stations are not open 24 hours a day, 7 days a week, on-site CBP personnel sometimes act as surrogates for quarantine inspectors during their off-hours. The Core has created a field manual for these surrogates (DQ, 2000).

Port-based CBP officials are officially responsible for performing this surrogate function for CDC among their "duties as assigned" (Personal communication, P. Gaddini, CBP, June 3, 2005). The officers receive

---

[5]Calculation based on DGMQ forecast of 66 field staff in October 2005 (see Chapter 1) and assumption that the number of CBP inspection staff at ports of entry in fiscal 2004—19,230—remained approximately the same in fiscal 2005 (see Appendix E, Table E.4) (CRS, 2004).

BOX 3.1   The Role of U.S. Ports of Entry as Defined by the Department of Homeland Security

Ports of entry are responsible for daily port specific operations. There are 317 official ports of entry in the United States and 14 preclearance stations in Canada and the Caribbean, a total of 331 official manned and unmanned ports. Port personnel are the face at the border for most cargo and visitors entering the United States. Here CBP enforces the import and export laws and regulations of the U.S. federal government and conducts immigration policy and programs. Ports also perform agriculture inspections to protect the USA from potential carriers of animal and plant pests or diseases that could cause serious damage to America's crops, livestock, pets, and the environment.

SOURCE: CBP, 2005d.

on-the-job training for this function when they are newly hired; they receive additional training from CDC quarantine station staff when new diseases of public health significance are detected. Job performance in the area of "public health measures" is discussed with these officers during their mid-year and year-end performance reviews.

The primary duties of port-based CBP officials are summarized in Box 3.1. The protection of humans from infectious disease of public health concern—whether introduced intentionally or unintentionally—is absent from this statement, as well as from the public mission statements of CBP and its Immigration Inspection Program (Boxes 3.2 and 3.3). This function also was absent from the CBP Commissioner's 2005 testimony outlining his department's duties and functions to the U.S. House of Representatives Committee on Appropriations (Bonner, 2005). By contrast, the protection of U.S. agriculture—and, by extension, the U.S. economy—from "potential carriers of animal and plant pests or diseases" appears explicitly in the mission statement of CBP Ports of Entry (CBP, 2005d).

Data were unavailable for the committee to quantitatively measure the extent and quality of disease surveillance conducted at U.S. ports of entry. On the basis of the committee's observations, CBP does conduct disease inspection to varying degrees at some ports (Committee, 2005). CBP inspectors collocated at airports with a CDC quarantine station tend to be trained by station staff to conduct public health screening. The DGMQ 2003 Program Review lists 157 public health training sessions for 2,034 federal inspection service inspectors and other agencies (DGMQ, 2004). These CBP inspectors appear to take the responsibility seriously as much for their own safety as for the health of the public. By contrast, anecdotal

---

**BOX 3.2   Mission Statement of
U.S. Customs and Border Protection**

We are the guardians of our Nation's Border.

We are America's frontline.

We safeguard the American homeland at and beyond our borders.

We protect the American public against terrorists and the instruments of terror.

We steadfastly enforce the laws of the United States while fostering our Nation's economic security through lawful international trade and travel.

We serve the American public with vigilance, integrity, and professionalism.

SOURCE: CBP, 2005b.

---

evidence indicates that quarantine station staff can provide only minimal training to CBP inspectors at subports—the majority of U.S. air, sea, and land ports of entry—because of limited travel budgets, frequent turnover among CBP personnel, and unclear lines of authority due to reorganization within the U.S. Department of Homeland Security (DHS) (Committee, 2005). The Core has for more than a decade lacked sufficient funds for quarantine station staff to visit subports[6] with reasonable frequency (Personal communication, M. Becker, DGMQ, March 24, 2005).

The extent to which CBP staff inspect passengers, animals, and cargo for disease appears to be influenced in part by the goodwill that quarantine station staff have fostered through relationships with their CBP counterparts; these relationships are strongest at ports that contain quarantine stations or that quarantine station staff have recently visited to conduct on-site training sessions. Concern among CBP inspectors of contracting a serious communicable disease that originates abroad also seems to motivate them to perform disease inspections on the Quarantine Core's behalf (Committee, 2005; personal communication, A. Lombardi and P. Gaddini, CBP, January 20, 2005).

On the basis of the information presented above, the committee concluded that the CBP function as a surrogate to the CDC quarantine stations

---

[6]Subport: DGMQ refers to ports of entry without a CDC quarantine station located on site as subports. The eight established CDC quarantine stations are responsible for the subports located within their jurisdictions (Table 1.1).

BOX 3.3   Immigration Inspection Program: Mission and Role

Mission

The mission of the inspections program is to control and guard the boundaries and borders of the United States against the illegal entry of aliens. In a way that:

- Functions as the initial component of a comprehensive, immigration enforcement system;
- Prevents the entry of terrorists, drug traffickers, criminals, and other persons who may subvert the national interest;
- Deters illegal immigration through the detection of fraudulent documents and entry schemes;
- Initiates prosecutions against individuals who attempt or aid and abet illegal entry;
- Cooperates with international, Federal, state and local law enforcement agencies to achieve mutual objectives;
- Contributes to the development and implementation of foreign policy related to the entry of persons;
- Facilitates the entry of persons engaged in commerce, tourism, and/or other lawful pursuits;
- Respects the rights and dignity of individuals;
- Examines individuals and their related documents in a professional manner;
- Assists the transportation industry to meet its requirements;
- Responds to private sector interests, in conformance with immigration law;
- Continues to employ innovative methods to improve the efficiency and cost effectiveness of the inspections process.

Role

Individuals seeking entry into the United States are inspected at Ports-of-Entry (POEs) by CBP officers who determine their admissibility. The inspection process includes all work performed in connection with the entry of aliens and United States citizens into the United States, including preinspection performed by the Immigration Inspectors outside the United States. "An officer is responsible for determining the nationality and identity of each applicant for admission and for preventing the entry of ineligible aliens, including criminals, terrorists, and drug traffickers, among others. U.S. citizens are automatically admitted upon verification of citizenship; aliens are questioned and their documents are examined to determine admissibility based on the requirements of the U.S. immigration law."

SOURCE: CBP, 2005c.

is an inherited role historically performed as well as possible given the limitations of training, time, and resources. But the back-up that CBP provides to the CDC quarantine stations clearly falls outside the domain for which CBP officials are hired and for which they are best trained. The port-based staff of CBP and other federal agencies have multiple responsibilities that, from their perspective, take precedence over the duties of the Core. The committee addresses this shortcoming in its recommendations in Chapter 4.

Overview of Response

The Quarantine System lacks a nationally standard protocol for responding to suspect and probable cases of quarantinable communicable disease that have been reported to or identified by a quarantine station. Although states and localities bear primary responsibility for the management and monitoring of these cases, local public health laws governing the response to and treatment of infectious disease in general vary widely across the United States (IOM, 2003, pp. 101-111). The following paragraphs provide an overview of the System's response to ill passengers, then focus on the robust role played by local public health and health care entities.

If an ill passenger (reported during travel) arrives at a U.S. port of entry that has a quarantine station, CDC staff evaluate the individual for signs, symptoms, and travel history consistent with a quarantinable communicable disease (Box 1.3). If the passenger arrives at a port of entry lacking a CDC quarantine station and a station is notified of the passenger, the station with jurisdiction[7] over the port (see Table 1.1) consults the physician on call at DGMQ headquarters or alerts the local health department to evaluate the individual for signs and symptoms of a quarantinable disease. If the index of suspicion is high, the individual is sent to a health care facility for diagnosis (Personal communications: J. Barrow and M. Remis, DGMQ, December 28, 2004; S. Maloney, DGMQ, January 18, 2005).

Recently identified diseases of public health concern among air travelers include measles, meningitis, viral hemorrhagic fevers, and tuberculosis (CDC, 2004c; Lasher et al., 2004; LoBue and Moser, 2004). Many of the illnesses identified by pilots or quarantine inspectors, however, are found to be either noncommunicable diseases or communicable diseases of insignificant public health concern. Table 3.2 presents the number of cases of illness reported to or found by the quarantine stations in 2003 and the types of medical control measures taken in response.

Although the Quarantine Core does not have jurisdiction over departing flights, the quarantine stations provide advice upon request to CBP, port authorities, or airlines regarding suspected cases of illness among passengers on departing flights (Committee, 2005). CBP, which has jurisdic-

---

[7]Each quarantine station is responsible for many ports of entry without a quarantine station located within a specific geographic area. For example, Hartsfield International Airport in Atlanta has jurisdiction over all ports in Georgia, Alabama, Arkansas, Louisiana, Oklahoma, Mississippi, North Carolina, South Carolina, and Tennessee (Table 1.1).

TABLE 3.2 All Cases of Illness Reported to or Found by DGMQ in 2003 and Medical Control Measures Taken

	Number of Cases	
	At U.S. Ports with a CDC Quarantine Station	At U.S. Ports without a CDC Quarantine Station (Subports)
All cases reported to or found by DGMQ	1,919	176
Reported prior to arrival	219	102
Meeting foreign quarantine criteria	67	85
Medical control measures taken		
Persons placed in isolation	4	3
Surveillance orders issued	607	422
Medical holds issued	121	1

NOTE: It is impossible to indicate the total number of ill passengers entering the United States, as screening measures do not—and cannot—identify every case.
SOURCE: DGMQ, 2004.

tion over international departures, can contact the Quarantine Core for medical advice if an ill passenger is identified on an outbound flight. Local public health authorities also will occasionally contact a quarantine station to alert the staff that a departing passenger may be infectious. In such cases, the quarantine station notifies the airline, which almost always follows the Quarantine Core's advice regarding the health risk posed by the passenger (Committee, 2005).

Partners in Response: Local Public Health and Health Care Entities

Certain state and local entities appear to be involved most of the time in the response to suspect or probable cases of quarantinable communicable disease that come to the attention of the Quarantine Core. Below is a description of these entities and their roles, in rough chronological order (CDC, 2004a; Checko and Libbey, 2005; Committee, 2005; personal communication, P. Edelson, DGMQ, March 24, 2005):

- The local public health authority (LPHA) is notified.
- At airports, local emergency medical services (EMS) personnel provide urgent medical care, if necessary, and conduct a preliminary clinical evaluation.
- At seaports, a local physician is dispatched to the ship at anchor to provide urgent medical care, if necessary, and to conduct a preliminary clinical evaluation.

- The LPHA and the CDC quarantine station staff (in consultation with a physician at DGMQ headquarters) share their conclusions and decide what steps should be taken next.
- Most of the time, the Quarantine Core and the LPHA agree upon next steps. Infrequently, the Quarantine Core believes a patient should be hospitalized for evaluation, but the LPHA either disagrees or lacks the resources and authority to mandate such evaluation. Under these circumstances, the Core has the federal authority to order hospital-based evaluation and monitoring of the patient. To prepare for such eventualities, the Core has entered into memoranda of agreement (MOAs) with more than 130 hospitals near ports of entry around the country (DGMQ, 2004; personal communications: P. Edelson, DGMQ, March 24, 2005, and M. Remis, DGMQ, August 29, 2005). Participating hospitals must accept suspect or probable cases of quarantinable communicable diseases or "other conditions of urgent public health significance" for diagnosis and management (CDC, 2004a). An abbreviated MOA appears in Appendix G.
- If the case calls for hospitalization, a local ambulance transports the patient to the hospital, where local physicians examine the patient and collect tissue samples for laboratory tests by a hospital or state public health laboratory.[8]
- The LPHA, the CDC quarantine station, or both sometimes receive follow-up calls from the laboratory and hospital with the patient's diagnosis. At other times, the CDC quarantine station must call the hospital to learn the diagnosis; however, some operators at hospitals do not recognize the station's authority to obtain health information and refuse to provide it due to Health Insurance Portability and Accountability Act (HIPAA) regulations.

Suspect and probable cases of quarantinable communicable disease remain under federal jurisdiction for a very short period of time. In general, the transfer of the patient to EMS personnel represents the transfer of legal authority from the Quarantine Core—the federal government—to the locality or state. From that point forward, the locality or state bears ultimate responsibility for medical care administered by EMS, the choice of hospital to which the patient is delivered, the medical care provided by the hospital, laboratory tests conducted by public health laboratories, and medical follow-up conducted by local or state public health authorities.

The CDC quarantine station staff do not provide medical treatment, even since the decision in 2004 to begin hiring physicians (generally one per

---

[8]In cases when the patient is thought to carry one of the most lethal kinds of infectious agents, such as Ebola virus, the samples would be sent to a biosafety level 4 laboratory, which might be located out of state.

station) for the first time in decades (Committee, 2005). Before then, no one on the quarantine station staff had medical training, although some of the inspectors had been trained as nurses or in provision of EMS in an earlier career. The staff could always consult by phone with a physician at DGMQ HQ. The relevance of clinically trained staff for the stations is discussed in Chapter 4 and Appendix A.

Both reported and anecdotal evidence suggests that small numbers of commercial travelers routinely enter the United States during the symptomatic stage of quarantinable communicable diseases without coming to the attention of air commanders, ship masters, or CDC quarantine station staff at U.S. ports of entry. Such cases have been identified through retrospective studies (CDC, 2001; CDC, 2004c).

Obtaining Passengers' Contact Information During an Outbreak Investigation

At present, the process of obtaining passengers' contact information for contact tracing is a labor-intensive, time-consuming process. When this information is obtained from the airlines, it arrives by mail or fax in a lengthy paper form called a passenger manifest. The handover of this information to the Quarantine Core appears to be delayed by logistical obstacles and legal concerns. Customs declarations, which contain travelers' local contact addresses, also are challenging to obtain (Committee, 2005; DGMQ, 2004; Meenan, 2005; personal communications: K. Andrus, ATA, October 21, 2004, and P. Edelson, DGMQ, March 18, 2005).

The difficulty in obtaining passengers' contact information to alert them to a microbial threat of public health significance has several detrimental consequences: first, the quarantine stations cannot identify or locate a significant percentage of potentially exposed passengers; second, by the time many passengers are contacted, it may be too late to implement effective preventive measures; and third, affected passengers may spread the disease among their close contacts, as happened during the outbreak of SARS (Personal communication, P. Edelson, DGMQ, March 18, 2005).

The airline industry, as represented by the ATA, and the Federal Aviation Administration (FAA) have been collaborating with DGMQ and CDC on both intermediate and long-term solutions to expedite the transfer of passenger contact information to the quarantine stations (Meenan, 2005; Jordan, 2005).

Intermediate Solution: Passenger Locator Card

The intermediate solution has been to develop a card on which passengers' contact information is collected in a machine-readable format

(DGMQ, 2004; Meenan, 2005). When needed, these so-called passenger locator cards would be quickly scanned and the data transmitted electronically to a quarantine station or to DGMQ headquarters. One advantage of these cards over passenger manifests is that the traveler records his or her actual seat, which sometimes differs from the assigned seat listed in the manifest (Personal communication, K. Andrus, ATA, October 21, 2004). The intended use of passenger locator cards appears to be confined to two particular circumstances (Meenan, 2005):

• During an outbreak of communicable disease of public health significance that affects international travelers, CDC would identify affected countries and, in conjunction with airlines, would identify specific flights on which cards should be distributed.
• When a pilot has reported an ill passenger or crew member while the flight is in the air, cards could be distributed.

Passenger locator cards had not been field-tested as of April 2005 (Personal communication, M. Remis, DGMQ, April 7, 2005). The International Air Transport Association and the International Civil Aviation Organization are reportedly reviewing and modifying the cards for international use (DGMQ, 2004). The member airlines of ATA are prepared to use passenger locator cards when and if directed by CDC to do so (Meenan, 2005).

Long-Term Solution 1: eManifest

In the long run, both the airline industry and CDC would prefer that passenger contact information already collected by airlines be transmitted electronically to public health officials for contact tracing to contain a microbial threat. This information is stored in so-called electronic passenger manifests (eManifest). DGMQ and Delta Airlines have been working for the past few years on a model system for the transmittal of eManifests from Delta to the Quarantine Core (DGMQ, 2004). In general, legal, technical and political challenges must be overcome to make eManifests from any airline accessible to the Quarantine Core (Meenan, 2005).

One challenge is the issue of privacy in the electronic age. As the Core and its airline partners pursue the idea of utilizing eManifests for contact tracing, they face important concerns over who may obtain the manifest's content, for what purposes, and for how long. The privacy policies of airlines based in the United States require that they maintain the confidentiality of passengers' personal information unless compelled to disclose it by law. The American airline industry would reportedly welcome a regulatory change that compels airlines to give the quarantine stations access to electronic passenger manifests during an outbreak investigation (Personal communication, K. Andrus, ATA, October 21, 2004). The privacy issue is more challenging in the European Union, however, and a solution to the issue there remains unclear (DGMQ, 2004).

Other challenges to the use of eManifests for contact tracing include incompatible computer systems in use by airlines and the Quarantine Core and the question of reciprocity with other countries (Meenan, 2005).

Collaboration among the Quarantine Core, CBP, the Transportation Security Administration, and other federal entities that seek passenger information—and face similar obstacles to obtaining it—may expedite the development of solutions to these challenges (Meenan, 2005).

Passenger manifests alone—whether delivered electronically or on paper—do not always provide sufficient or accurate information for contact tracing, the committee found. A study conducted by the CDC quarantine station in Hawaii and the Hawaii Department of Health concluded that the information from passenger manifests should be supplemented by other information sources to conduct rapid contact tracing of airline passengers after they have disembarked (Lasher et al., 2004). In another case, the director of DGMQ reported that a cell-phone number, not usually contained in passenger manifests, was one of the most useful tools for tracing 20 contacts of a man who was ill with Lassa fever while traveling from London to Newark, NJ (Personal communication, M. Cetron, DGMQ, October 21 2004). Also, as noted above, passenger manifests list travelers' assigned seats, which may differ from where they actually sat during the flight.

Long-Term Solution 2: National Architecture for Collecting Passenger Information

In parallel with its work on eManifests, the Core reportedly has begun to develop a national information architecture that may be an alternative source of passengers' contact information in the future (DGMQ, 2004). This information would be extracted from the Advanced Passenger Information System,[9] the Global Distribution System, the computerized passenger profile system, and other sources. The Core is collaborating on this project with the John A. Volpe National Transportation Systems Center, a research and development organization within the U.S. Department of Transportation, and MITRE Corporation, a not-for-profit, federally char-

---

[9]CBP electronically collects pertinent information on international passengers and houses it in a national database called the Advanced Passenger Information System (APIS) (CBP, 2005a).

HEALTH ALERT NOTICE
FOR INTERNATIONAL TRAVELERS ARRIVING IN OR RETURNING TO THE UNITED STATES

TO THE TRAVELER: You could have been exposed to a communicable disease prior to your arrival in the United States. You should monitor your health for at least 6 weeks. If you become ill with fever accompanied by rash, stiff neck, yellowing of the skin or eyes, or unusual bleeding; or severe diarrhea with or without fever, you should consult your physician. To help your physician make a diagnosis, tell him or her about your recent travel outside the United States and whether you were in contact with someone who had any of these conditions. Please save this card and give it to your physician if you become ill.

TO THE PHYSICIAN: The patient presenting this card recently traveled outside the United States and could have been exposed to a communicable disease that is not commonly seen in the United States. If you suspect a communicable disease such as measles, smallpox, bacterial meningitis, yellow fever, viral hemorrhagic fever, or cholera, please notify your city, county, or state health officer (http://www.cdc.gov/other.htm#states), and the Division of Global Migration and Quarantine, Centers for Disease Control and Prevention (404-498-1600 or 404-639-2888 after business hours; http://www.cdc.gov/ncidod/dq/contactus.htm).

U.S. DEPARTMENT OF HEALTH AND HUMAN SERVICES
Centers for Disease Control and Prevention
National Center for Infectious Diseases
Division of Global Migration and Quarantine

CDC 75.8 REV 2-02

FIGURE 3.2   CDC Health Alert Notice. The staff of CDC quarantine stations distribute Health Alert Notices to passengers arriving at a U.S. port of entry from an area experiencing an outbreak of communicable disease of public health significance. These paper notices are one of the Quarantine Core's principal tools for educating international travelers who have potentially been exposed to a microbial threat.
SOURCE: DGMQ, 2002.

tered organization whose expertise includes systems engineering, information technology, and operational concepts.

Response Protocols During Public Health Emergencies

During the outbreak of severe acute respiratory syndrome (SARS), the Quarantine Core and a multitude of volunteers spent hundreds of hours educating international travelers about the new disease and appropriate forms of health care and distributing health alert cards (Figure 3.2), which provided educational and contact information (DGMQ, 2004; Meenan, 2005). For years, the Core has monitored electronic sentinel surveillance systems for reports of infectious disease outbreaks around the world. Since U.S. residents generally lack immunity to diseases that are not endemic in this country, outbreaks of communicable diseases that are common in other parts of the world can pose a serious risk to the health of Americans (CDC, 2004c; Ndao et al., 2005; Shu, 2005). In addition, outbreaks of infectious disease of public health concern to individuals of any nationality come to the Core's attention; one example is meningitis (CDC, 2001). To the extent possible, given the quarantine stations' limited human resources and geographic reach, the staff meet such flights upon arrival and inform travelers of how to identify and report signs and symptoms of the disease. The CDC quarantine station staff are expected to participate in emergency responses that affect their entire airport, and a station's role differs from one airport to the next according to the nature of the emergency plan. John F. Kennedy International Airport in New York City (JFK), for instance, establishes an operations center in the event of a large-scale emergency. The staff of all federal inspection agencies located at JFK must coordinate their response activities through the operations center, which manages media relations so as to communicate consistent messages to the public with one voice (Committee, 2005).

IMMIGRANTS AND REFUGEES: ROLE OF THE QUARANTINE CORE

The scope of this study precluded a thorough examination of the many complex issues surrounding the health of migrants to the United States in relation to the Quarantine Core. Thus, the following discussion is limited, and the topic is ripe for further study.

Some quarantine stations spend more time on immigrant and refugee health than any other issue (Committee, 2005). Table 3.3 presents the total number of immigrants, refugees, and asylees admitted into the United States in 2003. These populations, particularly refugees, generally carry a greater burden of disease than the average traveler because they tend to come from developing nations where access to preventive and curative care is limited and where a relatively high number of communicable diseases of public health concern are endemic. As a rule, refugees enter the United States through a port with a CDC quarantine station (8 U.S.C. §1522).

To protect the health of U.S. communities, immigrants and refugees

TABLE 3.3 Numbers of Immigrants, Refugees, and Asylees Accepted into the United States, 2003

Category of Arrivals	Number Admitted in 2003
Immigrants	705,827
Refugees	28,306
Persons granted asylum	15,470

SOURCE: OIS, 2004.

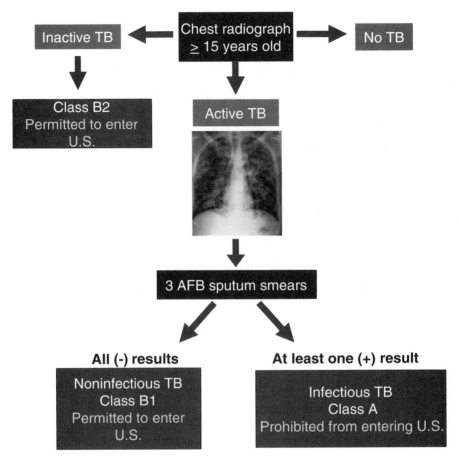

FIGURE 3.3 Algorithm for screening prospective immigrants, refugees, and asylees to the United States for tuberculosis (TB). First, individuals who are 15 years old or older must have a chest x ray. An overseas physician selected by the U.S. Department of State examines the x ray to determine whether the person has tuberculosis (TB), and if so, whether the *Mycobacterium tuberculosis* complex is active or inactive. Individuals who are diagnosed with inactive TB receive Class B2 status and may enter the United States but are required to undergo medical follow-up after arrival. Individuals who are diagnosed with active TB then undergo a laboratory test to determine whether the infectious agent is communicable. If sputum smears are negative for acid-fast bacilli (AFB) on 3 consecutive days, the individual has a noninfectious form of TB and may enter the United States with Class B1 status. These individuals may begin a course of treatment before leaving their home country and must receive medical follow-up in the United States. If one or more sputum samples test positive, the individual has infectious TB—a Class A communicable disease—and may not enter the United States without a special waiver (DQ, 1991; LoBue and Moser, 2004; Royce, 2005).
SOURCE: Maloney, 2001.

TABLE 3.4 Communicable Diseases of Public Health Concern Diagnosed in Immigrants and Refugees to the United States by Panel Physicians, 1999–2003

Health Condition	Immigrants	Refugees	Total
Infectious (AFB+) active TB: class A	29	7	36
Noninfectious (AFB-) active TB: class B1	19,206	2,140	21,346
Inactive TB: class B2	17,026	8,025	25,051
HIV	102	735	837
Syphilis	209	62	271
Hansen's disease (leprosy)	13	4	17
TOTAL	36,585	10,973	47,558

SOURCE: Adapted from personal communication, S. Maloney, DGMQ, August 29, 2005.

applying for a visa to the United States are required to undergo medical screening in their country of origin. The purpose of screening is to identify foreign-born individuals who have a communicable disease of public health concern classified as a Class A or B disease (Box 1.2). The screening process includes a physical exam and an x ray of the lungs to identify signs of tuberculosis (Figure 3.3). U.S. embassy staff select the clinicians, known as panel physicians, who perform these medical evaluations (DQ, 1991; LoBue and Moser, 2004) (42 CFR §34.1–34.8).

Panel physicians identified more than 46,000 suspect cases of noninfectious active tuberculosis (TB) and inactive TB among the 2 million immigrants and 280,000 refugees who came to the United States between 1999 and 2003 (Table 3.4).

The effectiveness of overseas medical screening depends on accurate diagnoses by the clinicians overseas as well as further medical evaluation and follow-up by LPHAs of foreign-born individuals after their arrival in the United States. The CDC quarantine stations at U.S. ports of entry facilitate the follow-up of immigrants and refugees by notifying the LPHAs and forwarding medical paperwork of all refugees and of immigrants who have admissible, medically notifiable conditions. The stations are responsible for identifying such immigrants who enter the United States through a port that contains a quarantine station, while CBP personnel are responsible for identifying those individuals who enter through all other ports and forwarding their paperwork to one of the stations (Cetron, 2004b; Committee, 2005; Royce, 2005; personal communication, S. Maloney, DGMQ, January 18, 2005).

A small-scale, unpublished study conducted by DGMQ in 1999, as well as anecdotal evidence, suggests that both the CDC quarantine stations at ports of entry and CBP miss a significant percentage of immigrants who have medically notifiable conditions and are admissible into the United

States (Royce, 2005; personal communication, P. Edelson, DGMQ, March 24, 2005). Because CBP personnel are under pressure to move through immigrants' paperwork quickly, the quarantine station staff must reportedly "scramble" to obtain the Class B forms from subports (Personal communication, P. Edelson, DGMQ, March 24, 2005).

Flights carrying refugees and parolees generally enter the United States at an airport with a quarantine station (8 U.S.C. §1522). In theory, CDC quarantine station staff meet every arriving refugee flight, visually screen the passengers for signs and symptoms of illness, and notify local health departments of their arrival. Because of the number of demands on a small workforce, however, the quarantine inspectors at JFK meet only the refugee flights known to carry passengers with medical histories of concern. All other refugee flights are met by the International Organization for Migration, which acts on DGMQ's behalf (Committee, 2005; personal communication, M. Becker, DGMQ, April 19, 2005).

In addition to visual screening, the quarantine station staff review the results of refugees' and parolees' overseas medical examinations to identify individuals with Class A or Class B conditions. If such cases are identified, local public health authorities receive notification so they may monitor the patients' health and health care for the safety of the individual and his or her community (Personal communication, S. Maloney, DGMQ, January 18, 2005). The hard copies of refugees' and parolees' medical exams are mailed in batches to the appropriate public health authority (Committee, 2005).

To reduce the volume of refugees arriving at JFK, they have been permitted for several years to enter the country through Newark's international airport. There, personnel from the International Organization for Migration review the medical paperwork and send it in batches to the quarantine station at JFK (Personal communication, M. Remis, DGMQ, January 18, 2005).

Immigrants may enter the United States through any port, and they are not visually screened upon arrival; only their medical paperwork is reviewed by federal authorities. The CDC quarantine stations are ultimately responsible for identifying immigrants with Class A or B diseases. Anecdotal evidence suggests that a significant number of immigrants who have Class A or B diseases are missed because of human error in the scanning of paperwork (Committee, 2005; personal communication, P. Edelson, DGMQ, March 24, 2005). This appears to be particularly true at subports.

If the immigrant enters through a subport, CBP personnel in the Immigration Inspection Program collect and scan the overseas medical exam reports for conditions of public health concern; the paperwork of individuals found to have Class A or B diseases is sent to the CDC quarantine station with jurisdiction over the subport (Table 1.1). The station then sends the paperwork to the local health department where the immigrant will reside. If the immigrant arrives at a port with a CDC quarantine station, a quarantine inspector reviews the paperwork. Should the immigrant's overseas medical exam identify a disease of public health significance, the quarantine station mails information to the relevant state and local health departments about the immigrant's final destination, the suspect disease, and the results of his or her overseas medical exams. The station also notifies the immigrant, advising him or her to report to the local health department (Committee, 2005; personal communications: J. Barrow and M. Remis, DGMQ, December 28, 2004, and S. Maloney, DGMQ, January 18, 2005).

One of DGMQ's three branches (Figure 1.1) is dedicated to immigrant and refugee health. Many of this branch's accomplishments in 2003 illustrate overlap and potential synergy with the branch containing the quarantine stations. These accomplishments include (DGMQ, 2004):

- Screening and treatment for malaria, varicella, and measles of Liberians in Cote d'Ivoire who were awaiting transport to the United States.
- Provision of full antimalarial and anti-intestinal parasitosis treatment for 1,030 (out of 1,468) refugees from sub-Saharan Africa prior to departure for the United States during fiscal year 2002.
- Strengthening the training of overseas panel physicians and improving standardization of U.S. visa applicant medical screening by providing guidelines for interpreting chest radiographs suggestive of active TB.
- Finalizing of new and more complete technical instructions for medical examination of aliens in the United States (performed by licensed physicians known as civil surgeons) for tuberculosis.

This information demonstrates how another branch of DGMQ also has responsibilities that help protect the U.S. population and travelers to this country from microbial threats of public health significance that originate abroad.

INSPECTION OF ANIMALS AND ANIMAL PRODUCTS, ETIOLOGIC AGENTS, HOSTS, AND VECTORS[10]

Jurisdiction of the Quarantine Core

A small number of imported animal species are regulated by the Quarantine Core: domestic dogs, domestic cats, nonhuman primates (NHPs), turtles, tortoises, and terrapins (Foreign Quarantine—Importations, 42 CFR

---

[10]Much of the information in this section comes from interviews that the authors of a commissioned paper conducted with DGMQ and staff at partner agencies. The paper, *Microbial Threats of Public Health Significance Originating in Animals or Animal Products at U.S. Ports of Entry* appears in Appendix E and includes a list of interviewees.

§71.51–71.53, §71.56). The Core can add other animals or animal groups to its authority on the basis of a specific threat or through the federal rule-making process (42 CFR §71.32). Two contemporary examples of restrictions on the import of specific animals perceived to pose a public health threat are the bans on the importation of civet cats, an important potential source of the SARS coronavirus (Zhong, 2004), and African rodents, the probable source of human monkeypox virus that emerged in the United States in 2003 (Di Giulio and Eckburg, 2004).

The CDC quarantine stations are technically responsible for inspecting all imports of animals under their authority to ensure that the animals do not display signs of communicable disease. In practice, however, this responsibility usually is carried out by CBP veterinary and animal health inspectors on behalf of the Quarantine Core (Appendix E). The principal exception is the inspection of shipments of NHPs, which must be imported according to a strict protocol intended to protect the people involved from contracting a zoonotic disease, as discussed below (Cetron, 2004a; Committee, 2005). Legal and illegal imports of animal products, etiologic agents, hosts, and vectors that may pose a public health threat also lie within CDC jurisdiction (42 CFR §71.54).

Jurisdictions of CBP and the U.S. Fish and Wildlife Service

Agricultural Imports

In March 2003, following the establishment of the Department of Homeland Security (DHS), the Agriculture Quarantine and Inspection unit (AQI) of the U.S. Department of Agriculture's Animal and Plant Health Inspection Service (APHIS), was shifted to CBP (APHIS, 2003). AQI's veterinary and animal health inspectors continue to screen agricultural imports to protect the United States from potential carriers of animal and plant pests or diseases that could cause serious damage to America's crops, livestock, pets, and the environment (CBP, 2005d). Such pests and diseases may be naturally occurring or intentionally introduced.

CBP inspectors generally notify a CDC quarantine station when they have identified importations of animals, animal products, etiologic agents, and other items under DGMQ's jurisdiction. These inspectors sometimes notify a CDC quarantine station when they believe they have identified other animals or animal products of possible public health significance, although the high volume of imports frequently impedes CBP in doing so (Appendix E).

The transfer of AQI from USDA to DHS has created additional layers of communication that have impeded the rapid delivery of critical information to port inspectors (Appendix E). The Government Accountability Office (GAO) found that CBP's agricultural inspectors do not always receive timely information about high-risk cargo that should be held for inspection (GAO, 2005). For instance, CBP inspectors at a seaport in a major agricultural state did not receive an alert in 2004 about an outbreak of a highly pathogenic, zoonotic strain of avian influenza until a week after the warning was issued (GAO, 2005). In addition, farm groups and some members of Congress have questioned whether CBP officers will receive sufficient training to properly inspect agricultural imports (FASS, 2003). Despite an overall increase in the number of agricultural imports to the United States during the past 2 years, GAO reported a decrease in the number of these imports that have been inspected since CBP assumed primary responsibility for the inspection of farm animals and agricultural products at U.S. ports of entry (GAO, 2005).

Inspection of Wildlife

The Department of the Interior's U.S. Fish and Wildlife Service (USFWS) is yet another agency involved in the regulation and inspection of animal imports. USFWS enforces U.S. and international laws regarding the trade and transport of wildlife (Division of Law Enforcement, 2002). The service has statutory authorities over the importation of nonfarm animals, including birds, fish, reptiles, and amphibians, and such animal byproducts as pelts, skins, coats, and game trophies. These authorities derive from the Endangered Species Act (16 U.S.C. §1531–1543), the Lacey Act (18 U.S.C. §703–712), and the Migratory Bird Treaty Act (16 U.S.C. §668–668C).

Passengers and conveyances arriving in the United States from a foreign point of origin are required by law to declare all wildlife importations to USFWS. Port-based USFWS officers inspect international cargo, baggage, and passengers for endangered and protected species of wildlife (Division of Law Enforcement, 2002). If an officer of USFWS is unavailable, CBP employees inspect and process the imported wildlife instead (PPQ, 2005). When a specific animal or animal product for importation to the United States poses a potential threat to public health, USFWS coordinates the inspection and response to the item with DGMQ, as discussed below (Appendix E).

Jurisdictional Overlap and Zoonotic Disease

When cases of jurisdictional overlap arise, the agencies involved must decide how to apportion operational responsibilities or knit complementary responsibilities together (Personal communication, P. Edelson, DGMQ, March 18, 2005). For example, DGMQ and USFWS both have an interest in responding to importations of goatskin because it may carry spores of *Bacillus anthracis*, the causative agent of anthrax.

No federal agency has a mandate and mission that cover all imported animals and zoonoses (Personal communication, P. Arguin, DGMQ, April 8, 2005). In general, a strict protocol defining which agency has jurisdiction over a perceived zoonotic threat does not exist; the decision is made by the local officers in charge from the three agencies on the basis of the nature of the particular situation (Appendix E). The exceptions to this practice occur when such high-profile microbial threats as avian influenza or monkeypox arise. In these cases, the Quarantine Core and the relevant agency collaborate at the federal level to formulate a national response and resolve questions of jurisdictional overlap (Personal communication, R. Koppaka, DGMQ, March 18, 2005). For instance, USDA APHIS and CDC issued complementary orders banning the import of birds from Southeast Asia to guard against avian influenza (CDC, 2004b). In the wake of the monkeypox outbreak, collaboration between CDC and FDA led the agencies to issue a joint order banning the interstate shipment of African rodents (FDA, 2003). In the same order, CDC banned the importation of these rodents into the United States (CDC and FDA, 2003).

A liaison from Veterinary Services frequently visits the CDC quarantine stations and speaks with them about zoonotic diseases. This person then will pass the information on to the other federal groups in making his rounds (Appendix E). It appears that this individual is one of the main means of communication about zoonotic disease among the inspectors from the three agencies.

Jurisdictional Overlap and the Seizure of Bush Meat

Bush meat is a term broadly applied to game meat from wild animals that are hunted for consumption, typically in the bush of Africa but also elsewhere in the world. The illegal importation and trade in bush meat has burgeoned in recent years, along with an increased demand for farmed game meats (Klein, 2005). Bush meat has the potential to carry microbial threats of public health concern, as described below; consequently, CDC quarantine inspectors have found or have been alerted with growing frequency to the presence of bush meat in passengers' baggage (Committee, 2005). CDC is only one of four federal agencies that have regulatory authority over domestic and imported game meats, however. The following paragraphs explain how CDC, USFWS, USDA APHIS, and CBP manage their overlapping responsibilities for bush meat (Klein, 2005; Appendix E).

Bush meat comes from a wide variety of animals, including NHPs, hoofed animals, reptiles, birds, and rodents, many of which are protected by international wildlife and trade laws. The consumption of bush meat may pose a public health risk because the animals' health and origin are often unknown and because any pathogens that lie in bush meat from NHPs have the potential to cross the species barrier into humans with relative ease. Communicable diseases of public health concern that may originate in bush meat include Ebola, HIV/simian immunodeficiency virus (SIV), monkeypox, herpes B, Rift Valley fever, tuberculosis, salmonellosis, and brucellosis. Animal diseases of concern in bush meat may include transmissible spongiform encephalopathies, such as mad cow disease and scrapie (Klein, 2005).

The commercial harvest and importation of bush meat into the United States is often illegal and a violation of international laws. The total amount of bush meat entering the United States is unknown, but USFWS, USDA, and CBP estimate that only a small fraction is intercepted. The United Kingdom's Department of Food and Rural Affairs estimates that about 12,000 tons of smuggled bush meat enters that country annually (Klein, 2005; Appendix E).

USDA APHIS, USFWS, FDA, and CDC all have jurisdiction over bush meat based on the following laws and regulations (Klein, 2005):[11]

- USDA APHIS has jurisdiction under the Animal Health Protection Act to inspect, detain, quarantine, seize, and destroy animals, meat, and meat products in interstate commerce or those being imported into the United States that pose a risk of introducing a pest or foreign animal disease, such as foot-and-mouth disease or avian influenza.

- USFWS has authority under the Endangered Species Act, the Lacey Act, the Convention on International Trade in Endangered Species of Wild Fauna and Flora (CITES), and the Wild Bird Conservation Act to prohibit the importation of any wild animals or animal products that may threaten native wildlife or violate state, federal, or local wildlife laws.

- CDC has jurisdiction under the Public Health Service Act to prohibit the importation of animals and animal products and to regulate foreign quarantine to prevent introduction of communicable diseases that threaten public health. CDC bans include importation of all NHPs, African rodents (42 CFR §71.56), civets, and Asian birds. These bans are specifically designed to protect the U.S. population from Ebola, SIV, monkeypox, SARS, and avian influenza.

- FDA has jurisdiction under the Federal Food, Drug, and Cosmetic Act, which says that all foods not covered by standard meat and poultry inspections must meet the same safety standards applied to all domestic

---

[11]See Table E.1 in Appendix E for further details.

foods. In addition, under the Public Health Safety Act, the FDA can prohibit the interstate commerce of animal products to prevent the transmission of communicable disease harmful to humans.

When multiple federal agencies have jurisdictions over a single product (such as bush meat), determining responsibility is based primarily on the particular situation at hand. The local heads of each agency will contact one another and determine whose jurisdiction involves the most stringent regulation. For example, if endangered monkey meat is discovered at a port of entry, the risk posed by pathogens that could be in the meat leads CDC to have primary responsibility even though endangered species are the responsibility of USFWS.

Since CDC has very few local inspectors and no disposal facilities, it will often rely on inspectors from other groups (usually APHIS) to notify it of any confiscated bush meat. Then, CDC can either seize the product or instruct APHIS to seize and dispose of the product on its behalf, since APHIS would have access to the proper disposal facilities (Appendix E).

The CDC Animal Inspection Process

Paper shipping manifests—lists of cargo coming into a port—are the principal tool employed by the CDC quarantine stations at ports of entry to identify the animals, animal products, etiologic agents, and so on that warrant inspection. The staff study these lists each day and often ask CBP field staff to conduct the physical inspections of specific shipments on the Core's behalf. CDC is infrequently called by other agencies to conduct a physical inspection of these imports (Appendix E).

In addition to shipping manifests, the CDC quarantine staff review the vaccination certificates of imported dogs and cats, answer telephone queries, and follow up on calls from officials of other federal inspection agencies—particularly CBP's veterinary inspectors and USFWS inspectors—who have identified items that appear to fall within the Quarantine Core's jurisdiction. CBP inspectors do not actively seek animal products and related items of public health concern, but as a courtesy, they generally notify CDC quarantine station staff if they come across such an item in the course of their work. At times, local law enforcement officials, individuals from airlines and cargo carriers, local veterinarians, and local health groups also inform the Quarantine Core when they perceive a possible public health threat in imported animals or animal products (Appendix E).

When quarantine station staff inspect an animal in person, they conduct a visual inspection for outward signs of illness. If such signs are visible, the animal is confined until a veterinarian from CBP or the private sector conducts a clinical examination at the importer's cost (Appendix E).

The Core's Reliance on Federal Partners

Since the Quarantine Core lacks sufficient staff to conduct all the necessary physical inspections of cargo and items carried by passengers, it often delegates this responsibility to other parties, most often CBP. Some imports are cleared by telephone and others by fax (Personal communication, J. Barrow and M. Remis, DGMQ, November 9, 2004). The CDC quarantine stations allow CBP inspectors to sign through their materials and goods when the stations are closed (in general, CDC quarantine stations are open only during regular business hours). The station staff occasionally train CBP inspectors to recognize outward signs of disease of public health concern in animals, but the stations' small workforce and travel budget limit the frequency of such training. CDC quarantine stations that have jurisdiction over an especially large volume of cargo shipments frequently request assistance from state and local partners to enforce quarantine regulations over imported animals and animal products perceived to be a potential public health threat. The Quarantine Core also requests assistance at times from private individuals, such as local veterinarians, or from local law enforcement officers. The need for assistance is particularly acute at subports. In such cases, a product will be held until a CDC quarantine inspector either arrives or communicates directions on how to proceed (Appendix E).

Some at-risk cargo enters the United States without being inspected or cleared (Personal communication, J. Barrow and M. Remis, DGMQ, November 9, 2004). In addition to the factors noted above, this is a result of the tremendous volume of imports, the stations' broad geographical jurisdictions, the inefficiency of the paper-based process, and the inability to identify intentionally or unintentionally mislabeled cargo. For instance, if the samples of the 1957 pandemic strain of influenza virus accidentally shipped worldwide by a private U.S. company in early 2005 had been imported to the United States, those shipments would not have captured the attention of the Quarantine Core because they were not labeled as pandemic strains (Stein and Vedantam, 2005).

Electronic Cargo Manifest Systems

The Trade Act of 2002, slowly being implemented at the ports of entry, is converting to paperless shipping manifests. DGMQ is pursuing the possibility of accessing the International Trade Data System with the goal of reviewing incoming cargo at all ports and identifying those items that might need further scrutiny (Personal communication, J. Barrow and M. Remis, DGMQ, November 9, 2004). At present CBP has access to the Automated Manifest System (AMS), another electronic manifest tool whose utility depends in part on the accuracy of the importer's labeling. According to staff at every quarantine station the committee visited, having access to AMS would significantly enhance their ability to identify cargo that poses a public health threat (Committee, 2005). The major barrier to access is financial. Security clearance is required for anyone who accesses this system and DGMQ has not allocated resources for this yet, although the committee understands it is under active consideration. In addition, stations might require updated communications links.

Inspection of Nonhuman Primates

CDC quarantine station staff always observe the importation of NHPs to determine whether regulations designed to protect people are followed. These animals are so genetically similar to humans that an infectious agent in an NHP could cross the species barrier to humans relatively easily. NHP importers are reportedly diligent about notifying USFWS of a pending shipment, and procedures are in place for both USFWS and CBP to notify CDC of such shipments. When the animals arrive, inspectors from the Quarantine Core

- Ensure that people remain 10 feet or more from the NHPs.
- Check that the aircraft door separating the crew from the NHPs is securely closed to prevent air exchange, which could potentially transport respiratory droplets containing microbial threats.
- Check that no animal excretions remain in the aircraft once the animals are offloaded.

Clearing a shipment of NHPs takes 3 to 4 hours. One shipment consists on average of 120 NHPs. Los Angeles International Airport receives approximately 10,000 NHPs per year, more than any other CDC quarantine station (Cetron, 2004a; Committee, 2005; personal communication, M. Marty, DGMQ, May 16, 2005; Appendix E).

CONCLUSION

This chapter has illustrated the complexity of the Network within which the CDC quarantine stations operate. Clearly, the actions of the Core alone do not assure the effective protection of travelers to and people within the United States from microbial threats of public health significance that originate abroad. In the next chapter, the committee presents a vision that encompasses the entire Quarantine Network. The subsequent recommendations are designed to help the Core achieve its part of that vision and influence its partners in the Network to do the same.

REFERENCES

APHIS (Animal and Plant Health Inspection Service, United States Department of Agriculture). 2003. *APHIS Fact Sheet. The Animal and Plant Health Inspection Service and Department of Homeland Security: Working Together to Protect Agriculture.* [Online] Available: http://www.aphis.usda.gov/lpa/pubs/fsheet_faq_notice/fs_aphis_homeland.pdf [accessed April 4, 2005].

Bonner RC, Commissioner, U.S. Customs and Border Protection. 2005. *Fiscal 2006 Appropriations: Homeland Security: Statement of Robert C. Bonner, Commissioner, U.S. Customs and Border Protection.* Statement at the March 15, 2005 hearing of the Subcommittee on Homeland Security, Committee on House Appropriations, U.S. House of Representatives.

CBP (U.S. Customs and Border Protection, Department of Homeland Security). 2005a. *Advance Passenger Information System (APIS) Fact Sheet.* [Online] Available: http://www.customs.gov/xp/cgov/travel/inspections_carriers_facilities/apis/apis_factsheet.xml [accessed Jun 14, 2005].

CBP. 2005b. *CBP Mission Statement and Core Values.* [Online] Available: http://www.cbp.gov/xp/cgov/toolbox/about/mission/guardians.xml [accessed April 19, 2005].

CBP. 2005c. *Immigration Inspection Program.* [Online] Available: http://www.cbp.gov/xp/cgov/border_security/port_activities/overview.xml [accessed April 19, 2005].

CBP. 2005d. *Ports of Entry.* [Online] Available: http://www.cbp.gov/xp/cgov/toolbox/ports/ [accessed April 19, 2005].

CBP. 2005e. *Ports of Entry and User Fee Airports.* [Online] Available: http://www.cbp.gov/xp/cgov/import/communications_to_industry/ports.xml [accessed July 11, 2005].

CDC (Centers for Disease Control and Prevention). 2001. Exposure to Patients with Meningococcal Disease on Aircrafts—United States, 1999-2001. *MMWR Weekly* 50(23): 485-489.

CDC. 2004a. *Memorandum of Agreement to Prevent the Introduction, Transmission, and Spread of Communicable Diseases in the United States (Version 4).* Memorandum of Agreement, 2004.

CDC. 2004b. *Order of the Centers for Disease Control and Prevention, Department of Health and Human Services.* [Online] Available: http://www.cdc.gov/flu/avian/pdf/embargo.pdf [accessed June 14, 2005].

CDC. 2004c. Imported Lassa fever—New Jersey, 2004. *MMWR Morb Mortal Wkly Rep* 53(38): 894–897.

CDC, FDA. 2003. Control of communicable diseases; restrictions on African rodents, prairie dogs, and certain other animals. *Federal Register* 68(213): 62353–62369.

Cetron M. 2004a. *Animal Importations.* Presentation at the October 21, 2004, Meeting of the IOM Committee on Measures to Enhance the Effectiveness of the CDC Quarantine Station Expansion Plan for U.S. Ports of Entry, Washington, DC.

Cetron M. 2004b. *Immigrant Refugee and Migrant Health Branch, DGMQ.* Presentation at the October 21, 2004, Meeting of the IOM Committee on Measures to Enhance the Effectiveness of the CDC Quarantine Station Expansion Plan for U.S. Ports of Entry, Washington, DC.

Checko P, Libbey P. 2005. *Measures to Enhance the Effectiveness of CDC Quarantine Station Expansion Plan for U.S. Ports of Entry.* Presentation at the January 20, 2005, Meeting of the IOM Committee on Measures to Enhance the Effectiveness of the CDC Quarantine Station Expansion Plan for U.S. Ports of Entry, Baltimore, MD.

Committee (IOM Committee on Measures to Enhance the Effectiveness of the CDC Quarantine Station Expansion Plan for U.S. Ports of Entry). 2005. Unpublished. *Notes on Site Visits to DGMQ Quarantine Stations.*

CRS (Congressional Research Service, The Library of Congress). 2004. *Border Security: Inspection Practices, Policies, and Issues.* [Online] Available: http://fpc.state.gov/documents/organization/33856.pdf [accessed April 7, 2005].

DGMQ (Division of Global Migration and Quarantine, National Center for Infectious Diseases, Centers for Disease Control and Prevention). 2002. *Health Alert Notice.* Informational card for public distribution.

DGMQ. 2004. *Program Review Fiscal Year 2003.* Program review, May 7, 2004.

Di Giulio DB, Eckburg PB. 2004. Human monkeypox: an emerging zoonosis. *The Lancet Infectious Diseases* 4(1): 15–25.

Division of Law Enforcement, U.S. Fish & Wildlife Service. 2002. *Annual Report FY 2001.* [Online] Available: http://library.fws.gov/Pubs9/LEannual01.pdf [accessed August 16, 2005].

DQ (Division of Quarantine, National Center for Infectious Diseases, Centers for Disease Control and Prevention). 1991. *Technical Instructions for Medical Examination of Aliens.* [Online] Available: http://www.cdc.gov/ncidod/dq/pdf/ti-alien.pdf [accessed May 5, 2005].

DQ. 2000. *Public Health Screening at U.S. Ports of Entry: A Guide for Federal Inspectors.* [Online] Available: http://www.cdc.gov/ncidod/dq/pdf/hguide.pdf [accessed January 25, 2005].

FASS (Federation of Animal Science Societies). 2003. *No Retraining for Agriculture Inspectors in Border Agency Plan.* [Online] Available: http://www.fass.org/fasstrack/news_item.asp?news_id=1646 [accessed August 16, 2005].

FDA (U.S. Food and Drug Administration, Department of Health and Human Services). 2003. *Joint Order of the Centers for Disease Control and Prevention and the Food and Drug Administration, Department of Health and Human Services.* [Online] Available: http://www.fda.gov/oc/opacom/hottopics/monkeypox/monkeypox.html [accessed June 15, 2005].

GAO (United States Government Accountability Office). 2005. *Homeland Security: Much Is Being Done to Protect Agriculture From a Terrorist Attack, but Important Challenges Remain.* GAO–05–214. Washington, DC: GAO.

IOM (Institute of Medicine). 2003. *The Future of the Public's Health in the 21st Century.* Washington, DC: The National Academies Press.

Jordan JL, Federal Air Surgeon, Federal Aviation Administration. 2005. *Efforts to Prevent Pandemics by Air Travel.* Statement at the Apr. 6, 2005 hearing of the Subcommittee on Aviation, Committee on Transportation and Infrastructure, U.S. House of Representatives.

Klein PN. 2005. Regulatory report: game meat: a complex food safety and animal health issue. *Food Safety Magazine* 10(96).

Lasher LE, Ayers TL, Amornkul PN, Nakatab MN, Effler PV. 2004. Contacting passengers after exposure to measles on an international flight: implications for responding to new disease threats and bioterrorism. *Public Health Reports* 119(5): 458–463.

LoBue PA, Moser KS. 2004. Screening of immigrants and refugees for pulmonary tuberculosis in San Diego County, California. *Chest* 126(6): 1777–1782.

Maloney, SA. 2001. *Overseas Screening and Stateside Evaluation of Immigrants and Refugees with Tuberculosis.* Presentation at the July 2001 Annual Meeting of the Tuberculosis and Respiratory Diseases Institute, American Lung Association of North Carolina, Black Mountain, NC.

MedAire. 2005. *MedAire: A Health and Security Company.* [Online] Available: www.medaire.com [accessed April 13, 2005].

Meenan JM, Executive Vice President and Chief Operating Officer, Air Transport Association of America Inc. 2005. *Statement of John M. Meenan.* Statement at the Apr. 6, 2005 hearing of the Subcommittee on Aviation, Committee on Transportation and Infrastructure, U.S. House of Representatives.

Ndao M, Bandyayera E, Kokoskin E, Diemart D. 2005. Malaria "epidemic" in Quebec: diagnosis and response to imported malaria. *Canadian Medical Association Journal* 172(1): 46–50.

OIS (Office of Immigration Statistics, U.S. Department of Homeland Security). 2004. *2003 Yearbook of Immigration Statistics.* [Online] Available: http://uscis.gov/graphics/shared/statistics/yearbook/2003/2003Yearbook.pdf [accessed April 6, 2005].

PPQ (Plant Protection and Quarantine, Animal and Plant Health Insepction Service, United States Department of Agriculture). 2005. *Animal Product Manual.* [Online] Available: http://www.aphis.usda.gov/ppq/manuals/pdf_files/APM.pdf [accessed August 16, 2005].

Royce S. 2005. *Quarantine Stations and the Control of M. tuberculosis.* Presentation at the January 20, 2005, Meeting of the IOM Committee on Measures to Enhance the Effectiveness of the CDC Quarantine Station Expansion Plan for U.S. Ports of Entry, Baltimore, MD.

Shu P. 2005. Fever screening at airports and imported dengue. *Emerging Infectious Diseases* 11(3): 460–462.

Stein R, Vedantam S. 2005, Apr. 13. Deadly flu strain shipped worldwide: officials race to destroy samples. *The Washington Post.* A1.

Zhong N. 2004. Management and prevention of SARS in China. *Philosophical Transactions of the Royal Society of London. Series B: Biological Sciences* 359(1447): 1115–1116.

4

Bridge from Present to Future: Vision and Recommendations

The traditional, primary activities of the quarantine stations run by the Centers for Disease Control and Prevention (CDC) no longer protect the U.S. population sufficiently against microbial threats of public health significance[1] that originate abroad, the committee concluded. Many of the stations' legacy activities focus on the detection of disease in persons, animals, cargo, and conveyances during the window of time shortly before and during arrival at U.S. gateways. Yet the pace of global trade and travel has narrowed that window dramatically. Consequently, infected people and animals do not necessarily develop signs of disease while in transit or by the time of arrival, and available noninvasive diagnostics cannot always identify infected travelers with reasonable sensitivity, specificity, and speed.

Moreover, the consequences of globalization and the development of the U.S. homeland security infrastructure have increased the complexity of the organizational environment in which the CDC quarantine stations function. This organizational environment, the Quarantine System, lacks effec-

---

[1]Definition: A microbial threat of public health significance causes serious or lethal human disease and is transmissible from person to person, from animal to person, or potentially both; it also may be transmissible from food or water to people. Because of their potential for wide dispersal, concern is greatest for microbes that spread readily from person to person. A microbial threat may be introduced intentionally—as in bioterrorism—or unintentionally. Other threats of public health significance include the release of chemical or radiological substances and of biological substances other than microbes (e.g., bacterial toxins).

70

tive leadership. No single entity has the responsibility, the authority, and the resources for orchestrating the activities of the System to protect the U.S. population from microbial threats of public health significance that originate abroad.

To fill this void, the primary activities of the CDC quarantine stations should shift from the legacy and historical activity of inspection to the provision of strategic national public health leadership for Quarantine System activities. Such leadership, carried out in collaboration with the Division of Global Migration and Quarantine (DGMQ) and the scientific and organizational capacity of CDC, would improve national preparedness for crises caused by microbial threats of public health significance that originate abroad. The Quarantine Core should provide similar strategic leadership to the Quarantine Network. The committee concluded that the stations' traditional primary activities should continue but should consume only a fraction of their time.

The Core's leadership role stems naturally from the unique responsibility of federal government to assure[2] action for health (IOM, 2003, p. 34) as well as from CDC's position as a lead federal agency for protecting the health of Americans. The Core alone has the appropriate expertise, resources, and experience to provide strategic national public health leadership to the Quarantine Network. At the same time, the committee recognizes that from both a historical and a constitutional perspective, protecting the public's health has primarily been a function of the states and their localities[3] (IOM, 2003). Accordingly, the Core must take extra care to collaborate with—as well as respect the jurisdictional authorities of—its state and local partners as it assumes this leadership role. In addition, the Core should be careful to respect preexisting systems and infrastructures that states and localities may have already developed and put into place. The committee emphasizes the need for cooperation, flexibility, and partnership among the Core and its partners in the recommendations that follow.

This chapter begins with a vision of a Quarantine Network that reflects the committee's sense of how best to protect against microbial threats of public health significance at U.S. ports of entry. Subsequently, the committee presents seven recommendations designed to help the quarantine sta-

---

[2]In this report, "to assure" means to make sure that necessary public health services are provided to all members of society by encouraging the requisite actions, requiring them, or providing the services directly. For an in-depth description of the assurance function in public health, see *The Future of Public Health*, pp. 45-47 (IOM, 1988).

[3]It should be noted, however, that while the Constitution grants states and localities primary responsibility for protecting the public's health, the federal government has specific legal authorities over quarantine in the United States (Gostin, 2000).

tions and Quarantine Core effectively lead the System and the Network. Given the desire to transform the CDC quarantine stations into a more robust component of the U.S. public health infrastructure, these recommendations address core functions of public health: assessment, policy development, and assurance (IOM, 2003).

COMMITEE'S VISION OF THE 21ST CENTURY QUARANTINE NETWORK FOR U.S. PORTS OF ENTRY

A multijurisdictional, multisectoral, multinational Quarantine Network protects both travelers entering the United States and the population within U.S. borders from microbial and other threats of public health significance that originate abroad. In so doing, this Network helps protect the health of the global community. Central to the Quarantine Network from a domestic perspective is a System that comprises the people and organizations on the front lines of public health activities at U.S ports of entry. The Core consists of the quarantine stations, DGMQ headquarters, and the national scientific and organizational capacity of CDC. Figure 3.1 illustrates the relationships among the Quarantine Core, System, and Network.

The Quarantine Network will **minimize the risk** that microbial threats of public health significance may enter the United States.

The Quarantine System will **detect and respond** to such threats in travelers who are en route to the United States and who arrive at a U.S. port of entry. The System will **manage** index cases and **monitor** suspect cases, probable cases, and close contacts.[4] The Quarantine System also will **participate in public health emergency planning and response activities** for biological, chemical, and radiological threats and other disasters.

The Core will **anticipate** microbial and other threats of public health significance and will **collaborate** with the other members of the Network to prevent their arrival. The Quarantine Core will routinely **measure and evaluate** its performance and will **adapt and change** in response to its findings, as well as to the rapidly changing global environment. The Core will not only **carry out statutory responsibilities but also provide strategic public health leadership** to the Quarantine Network on matters at the intersection of international travel, global trade, and public health. As noted above, this leadership role stems naturally from the unique responsibility of the federal government to assure action for health (IOM, 2003, p. 34) and from CDC's position as a lead federal agency for protecting the health of Americans.

---

[4]For purposes of this report, "close contacts" refers to fellow travelers, border guards, port employees, and family members.

RECOMMENDATIONS

Strategic Leadership

Recommendation 1: The committee recommends that the Quarantine Core strategically lead the United States in its efforts to minimize the risk that microbial threats of public health significance will enter or affect travelers to this country. The Core should have the financial resources and legal authority, consistent with the Constitution and international obligations, to exert this leadership.

Development of a National Strategic Plan by the Quarantine Core

On the basis of its collective experience in public health practice, law, and governance, the committee concluded that a national strategic plan developed by the Core would provide the people of the United States with the best possible framework for protection against importation of microbial threats of public health significance. With its focus on human communicable disease, the Quarantine Core's national strategic plan would complement those plans formulated by the Department of Homeland Security to protect the American public.

The Quarantine Core should begin developing its strategic plan by conducting a comprehensive assessment of the risks posed at multiple types of ports of entry to this country by microbial and other threats of public health significance. As noted in Appendix D, airports and seaports vary in their physical and institutional structures. The same is true of U.S. land-border crossings (Personal communication, R. St. John, Public Health Agency of Canada, July 5, 2005). The types of imported goods and conveyances and the points of origin of travelers and crew also vary widely from one port to the next. The comprehensive risk assessment should examine the implications of these variations. No such assessment of the Quarantine System has been conducted for at least 10 years (Bozzi, 1995).

Once the risk assessment is complete, the Core should collaborate with its partners in the Quarantine System to develop a strategic plan for mitigating the risks identified in the assessment. The plan should have a set of nationally uniform principles and outcomes as well as malleable elements that localities can shape to their unique circumstances. An important part of this plan will be the development of public health protocols for managing and monitoring persons, goods, and conveyances.

Since colonial times, tension over the control of U.S. quarantine functions has existed between states and localities on one side and the federal government on the other (DGMQ, 2003a; Gostin, 2000; Mullan, 1989). The committee is cognizant of this tension and of the reality that states and localities carry out most of the public health functions required by federal quarantine laws. By recommending a strategic plan that is uniform only in its principles and outcomes, the committee intends to give states and localities enough latitude to decide on the details of execution.[5]

The uniformity of the plan will facilitate the flow of essential communication and data among all stations and their System partners nationwide. As an earlier Institute of Medicine report concluded, "a public health system that can assure the nation's health requires an alignment of policy and practice of governmental public health agencies at the national, state, and local levels" (IOM, 2003, p.96). In addition, a plan that promotes a uniform level of outcomes has the potential to prevent terrorists and some commercial interests from finding ports of entry whose public health protection mechanisms are substandard.

The malleable elements of the strategic plan should help the members of the system, including each of the nearly 3,000 U.S. local public health authorities (NACCHO, 2003), tailor the implementation of the plan to their unique circumstances (Figure 4.1).

Legal Authority and Resources Necessary to Implement the Strategic Plan

Domestic law

The Core will need sufficient legal authority to implement the strategic plan. As the Institute of Medicine noted in an earlier report, U.S. federal and state public health laws are frequently antiquated, fragmented, and inconsistent (IOM, 2003). These broad observations certainly characterize quarantine authority, which may suffer from such deficiencies as the narrow application to specified diseases, lack of clear criteria for implementation, and absence of adequate procedural due process as required under the Constitution (Gostin, 2000).

To help states remedy some of these deficiencies not only in their quarantine authority, but also in their overall legal preparedness for public health, two model laws have been written: the Model State Emergency Health Powers Act (MSEHPA) and the "Turning Point" Model State Public Health Act (MSPHA) (Gostin et al., 2002). MSEHPA was drafted by

---

[5]The committee is also cognizant of a similar tension at the federal level. As noted earlier, the Core alone possesses the appropriate expertise, resources, and experience to provide strategic national public health leadership to the Quarantine Network. The Core should, however, collaborate closely with its federal partners while strategically leading the country's efforts to minimize the risk of microbial threats of public health significance entering the United States. In matters not of direct public health concern or in matters of national security, the relevant agency should continue to assume the lead.

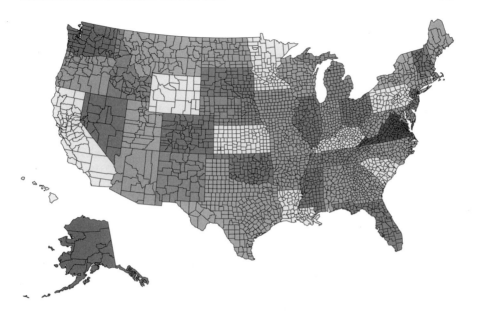

FIGURE 4.1 The geographic boundaries of the United States' 3,066 counties. Because the majority of the nation's nearly 3,000 local public health agencies (LPHAs) serve single counties, this map approximates a visual representation of LPHAs—each of which has unique characteristics that would influence how it executes elements of a national strategic plan.
SOURCES: IOM, 2003; NACO, 2005.

the Center for Law and the Public's Health at the request of the CDC after September 11, 2001. MSPHA was drafted as part of the Robert Wood Johnson "Turning Point" initiative and has detailed provisions for isolation, quarantine, and other health powers. These provisions provide a strong model for states to consider when modernizing their public health legislation.

Thirty-three states and the District of Columbia have passed bills or resolutions that include provisions from or closely related to MSEHPA; 21 of those bills or resolutions include the modernization of isolation and quarantine powers in a public health emergency (http://www. publichealthlaw.net/MSEHPA/MSEHPA%20Surveillance.pdf). The committee encourages all states to examine and modernize their public health laws, particularly for isolation and quarantine.

For the Core to exercise national strategic public health leadership, there is a need for coordination of federal, state, and local authority for the exercise of public health powers. At present, legal and regulatory authority, as well as practice and implementation, are fragmented at the various levels of government.

Laws at the federal and state level should ensure that the Quarantine Core has clear authority to carry out all its essential functions, including inspection, disinfection, nuisance abatement, medical examination, vaccination, treatment, isolation, and quarantine. In particular, the law should ensure at least the following:

- The Core has adequate power and duties to isolate and quarantine with respect to all diseases of public health importance at specific places and times, including enforcement of isolation or quarantine orders in a timely fashion.
- There are clear lines of authority within the Quarantine Core and among the various levels of government—among the various federal agencies and among federal, tribal, state, and local governments.
- The Core has the authority to obtain all relevant information from domestic and transnational sources to carry out its responsibilities for protecting the public (e.g., electronic passenger manifests).
- The Core operates under standards of procedural and substantive fairness as established under the Constitution and applied by the Supreme Court, including the provision of procedural due process.
- The Core has the legal authority to track and control the state-to-state spread of disease resulting from international travelers, animals, and cargo arriving at U.S. ports of entry and moving across state lines.

International law

The Quarantine Core must also comply with the United States' international obligations. This is particularly important because of the expanded role for DGMQ. The revised International Health Regulations, adopted by the World Health Assembly in May 2005, should receive special attention. For a complete discussion of the international laws and obligations relevant to this report, see Appendix F.

Financial resources

Along with sufficient legal authority, the Core should have sufficient funds for both DGMQ HQ and the quarantine station staff to carry out their responsibilities under the strategic plan. The Core also should make every effort to assure that all of its partners are fully aware of and trained to carry out any public health functions delegated to them under the strategic plan. These functions will be discussed in more detail in connection with Recommendation 3, but the allocation of sufficient funds in an effective manner is integral to assuring the capacity and competence of state, tribal, and local public health authorities, laboratories, and health care providers to carry out their duties under the strategic plan.

Although appropriate levels of funding and methods of allocating funds fall outside the committee's expertise and scope of work, some general observations about financial allocations are appropriate here. First, all financial arrangements between the Core and states and localities should take into account the structural and functional diversity of the country's numerous local health departments. In addition, the Core should consider allocating federal funds from the Core to states and localities through a multiyear financing mechanism that gives them adequate "discretion and flexibility to plan and implement multiyear efforts" (IOM, 2000, pp.16–17). The U.S. Government Accountability Office (GAO) recently made similar observations regarding bioterrorism funds (GAO, 2005). GAO noted that state and local administrative processes slowed the obligation and expenditure of bioterrorism funds and urged federal authorities to consider the time-consuming planning process that precedes the obligation and spending of funds at the state and local levels.

Another general observation is that formalized funding arrangements could be useful in strengthening collaboration between the Core and its state and local partners. The provision of funds could be tied to specific performance indicators, such as the regularity of scheduled interaction and partnering activities. Under such arrangements, the quarantine stations should be held just as accountable as the states and localities.

Finally, as the Core implements the strategic plan, it must assure the local health departments' ability to take on delegated responsibilities while continuing to provide essential public health services. Unfunded mandates will only impose greater financial burdens on localities.

Harmonization of Authorities and Functions

Recommendation 2: The committee recommends that, on the basis of its strategic plan, the Quarantine Core work with its partners in the Quarantine Network (and with appropriate agencies in other countries) to delineate or redefine each partner's role, authority, and channel of communication at all locations and specific times in order to minimize the risk that microbial threats of public health significance will enter or affect travelers to the United States.

The Quarantine Network is a very complex environment, as Figure 3.1 suggests. The multiplicity of missions, players, skill sets, systems, laws, rules, and regulations at play in the Network appears to reduce its effectiveness. The wide array of potential sources of microbial threats further complicates the Network. This environment would become more effective if roles were clarified and harmonized, eliminating some of the present breaks in the lines of authority and communication described in Chapter 3.

As a first step toward harmonizing the authorities and functions within the Network, the Core should articulate gaps in authority and function. Some of the gaps identified by the committee or the Quarantine Core are described below. Through the risk assessment described in the strategic plan, the Core could identify additional gaps.

Electronic Passenger Manifests

One gap DGMQ has clearly identified is the difficulty of collecting passenger information in a timely manner in connection with a communicable disease investigation, as discussed in Chapter 3. Local public health authorities and the quarantine stations usually can trace only a fraction of exposed passengers, even with a great effort, increasing the risk of dispersal of microbial threats of public health significance and endangering the health of travelers after they arrive in this country. Although U.S. Customs and Border Protection (CBP) and DGMQ staff working at several ports of entry thought that during an extreme public health emergency such information would likely be made available to DGMQ, this is not assured (Committee, 2005). The Quarantine Core has been working with numerous partners in the System and the Network to overcome the barriers to accessing passengers' contact information. An interim solution—the targeted use of passenger locator cards—appears to be close at hand.

Identification of Ill Passengers

Another gap in the Network pertains to a mismatch between the responsibility for screening ill travelers and the role of the individuals informally assigned to this task (such as CBP staff). These individuals act as the Core's surrogates at most U.S. ports of entry, yet CBP does not count microbial threats of public health significance among its principal threats of concern at U.S. borders, as described in Chapter 3. Moreover, the quarantine stations have lacked adequate budgets to routinely visit all subports to train CBP staff and evaluate their effectiveness (Personal communication, M. Becker, DGMQ, March 24, 2005). Consequently, the surveillance conducted for ill travelers (and certain animals) arriving from international points of origin is largely passive in nature at most U.S. ports of entry (Committee, 2005).

Furthermore, as discussed in Chapter 3, pilots and captains of U.S.-bound airplanes and ships do not always notify a CDC quarantine station of ill persons on board, even though the law requires them to do so (42 CFR § 71.21a,b; Committee, 2005; Appendix D).

Continuity of Care for Refugees and Immigrants

Refugee health is another gap in the Network. The U.S. Department of State is responsible for refugees before their resettlement but has limited capacity to cope with their health issues. The Quarantine System is not designed to provide refugees with comprehensive preventive health care abroad. Consequently, many refugees with infectious diseases, some of public health concern, arrive at U.S. ports of entry (Catanzaro and Moser, 1982; CDC, 1998; CDC, 2002; Miller et al., 2000). Local public health authorities—a component of the System—bear the burden of any adverse impact the refugees may have upon the health of their new communities. Because some illnesses of refugees are not typically seen in the United States, their signs and symptoms often fall below the index of suspicion of American clinicians, leading to delays in treatment that may be life-threatening and contributing to the dispersal of microbial threats. Ultimately, the cost of treating such illnesses in the United States could be much greater than effective preventive care administered to refugees before their resettlement in this country.

As pictured in Figure 1.1 and noted in Chapter 3, DGMQ has a distinct branch that is dedicated to immigrant and refugee health. The research portfolio of the Immigrant, Refugee, and Migrant Health Branch aims to improve the health status of or health information regarding some immigrants and refugees prior to their arrival in the United States (DGMQ, 2004a). This work will likely reduce the number of people infected with microbial threats of public health significance who reach U.S. gateways. This work also will likely improve the quality and accuracy of the health information evaluated and processed by quarantine inspectors or their CBP surrogates. In summary, measures that strengthen the Immigrant, Refugee, and Migrant Health Branch are likely to promote and support the goals of the quarantine stations.

Zoonotic Diseases

The adequacy of animal health screening for zoonotic[6] diseases is another weakness in the Quarantine System. No federal agency has a mandate and mission that covers all imported animals and zoonoses (Personal communication, P. Arguin, DGMQ, April 8, 2005). Although the Quarantine Core has the authority to respond to a specific perceived threat of zoonotic disease on a conveyance (42 C.F.R. §71.32), the Core's standing to screen all imported animals for zoonoses is questionable (Personal communication, P. Arguin, DGMQ, April 8, 2005). Yet an estimated 75 percent of

---

[6]A zoonotic disease is one that can be transmitted from animals to humans.

emerging microbial threats to human health and 61 percent of all human pathogens are zoonotic (Taylor et al., 2001). Newly emergent zoonoses include monkeypox, severe acute respiratory syndrome (SARS), West Nile virus, and mad cow disease (variant Creutzfeldt-Jakob disease in humans). Many predictions about the nature of future novel pathogens anticipate the emergence of zoonoses (IOM, 2004).

Harmonization of Functions and Protocols Among Countries

The revised International Health Regulations will help to ensure harmonization on a global level, especially during crises. For the Network to function most effectively, however, all countries' approaches and activities should be routinely harmonized and coordinated. Routine cooperation will foster learning and sharing opportunities, ultimately ensuring that countries institute the most effective practices and procedures. For example, the Core's capacity to perform effective global disease surveillance would be enhance by increased collaboration and information-sharing among countries. In addition, public confidence in the Network will increase as the international community observes similar and coordinated responses taking place across the globe.

Conclusions

The Core should initiate efforts to bridge these and other gaps in the Quarantine Network. To a great extent, the success of these efforts will be contingent upon cooperation from relevant partners. The Core should continue to explore ways to jointly develop with the Department of State a more comprehensive public health approach to managing immigrants and refugees to improve their health, reduce costs, and prevent the spread of infectious disease. Through its relationships with CBP, the U.S. Department of Agriculture (USDA), and the U.S. Fish and Wildlife Service (USFWS), the Core should work toward a comprehensive national strategy for preventing the importation of zoonotic disease. In addition, the highest ranking officials of the Core should continue to highlight the absence of sufficient staff who are qualified, trained, and tasked to inspect arriving travelers and crews for signs of communicable disease of public health significance. Meanwhile, the Core should continue to pursue strategies at all levels to alleviate this shortfall. The Core also should work with appropriate authorities to ensure prearrival notification that sick persons are aboard conveyances and to obtain access to electronic passenger manifests. Effective contact tracing during disease outbreaks will be possible only with the information included in these manifests; access, however must be subject to the high standards of health information privacy and security. These are but a few examples of the numerous clarifying and harmonizing activities that would improve the Network's effectiveness and efficiency.

Infrastructure

Recommendation 3: The committee recommends enhancements in competences, number of people, training, physical space, and utilization of technology to meet the System's evolving, expanding role.

The infrastructure of the Quarantine System is inadequate to support its current role, let alone the role envisioned for it under the expansion plan. Only a limited amount of resources are available to the quarantine stations and their partners in the System for their work in mitigating the risks posed by microbial threats of public health significance at U.S. ports of entry. These limits (and mismatches) in people, tools, training, physical space, and use of technology keep the System far from achieving what is realistically possible in relation to both its present regulatory responsibilities and any sort of expanded public health role. Enhancements in the Quarantine System's infrastructure will be especially important in today's dynamic regulatory environments, both domestic and international.

People and Training

One of the most glaring problems with the infrastructure of the System pertains to its human resources. The Core's field staff numbers approximately 40 (Personal communication, M. Remis, DGMQ, May 11, 2005). By contrast, 120 million people traveled to and from the United States by air in 2003—a ratio of 1 CDC inspector per 3 million travelers (Office of Aviation Policy and Plans, 2005). With its severely limited human resources, the Quarantine Core also is unable to oversee the vast majority of imported cargo either on paper or in person and must accept on faith that most cargo is imported with appropriate permits or is innocuous (Committee, 2005; personal communication, J., Barrow and M. Remis, DGMQ, November 9, 2004; Appendixes D and E).

If the Core expands to 25 stations, DGMQ's plan calls for a field staff of 158 (DGMQ, 2004b), reducing this ratio to about 1 CDC inspector per 750,000 travelers. Adding the 19,000-some CBP field inspectors approaches a more reasonable balance of 1 federal official per 6,300 travelers (CRS, 2004); however, only those inspectors located at CDC-staffed airports appear to receive adequate training to actually identify ill passengers.

As noted earlier, while port-based CBP officials have a duty to act as surrogates for the CDC quarantine stations, they also have multiple responsibilities of their own that (from their perspective) take precedence over the duties of the Core (see Boxes 3.1 and 3.2). Furthermore, the committee is concerned that a significant percentage of these CBP officers lack appropriate and sufficient competences, training, and resources to perform this surrogate function. These issues represent serious weaknesses in the Quarantine System. While conducting its risk assessment and developing a national strategic plan, the Quarantine Core should define these deficiencies and assure they are corrected.

The present obstacles to improving training are both internal and external to the Core. Internal obstacles include the small workforce at existing field stations, an insufficient travel budget for visiting subports to conduct training sessions (as noted in Recommendation 2), lack of videoconferencing capabilities among stations and substations, and insufficient security clearance to enter many substations, particularly seaports (Appendix D). External obstacles include the high level of turnover among CBP officials, irregular hours of airline crews, and multiple demands and priorities that compete for the attention of private sector and federal partners (Committee, 2005).

Competences

DGMQ should assure that every station has access to individuals who possess all the competences required to carry out the responsibilities of the new and expanded Quarantine System. As discussed in Chapter 1, the committee issued an interim letter report on competences for the Core's staff. That report was done prior to the committee's complete analysis of the Network and the development of its vision. However, the competences outlined in the interim letter report, reprinted in Appendix A, remain compelling to the committee.

The CDC quarantine station staff and their colleagues at headquarters require competences to execute historical and statutory functions, to plan, to conduct surveillance for public health threats, to perform clinical and public health assessment and response, to perform health and risk communication, and to develop collaborative relationships with all members of the Network. Several points made in the interim report bear repeating here:

• Each station should have access to individuals with the competences outlined by the committee. These individuals could be located either on-site or off-site. Potential off-site human resources could be based at the regional stations, DGMQ headquarters, the private sector, partner agencies, or elsewhere. In general, using partners as a resource for some of the competences could help the stations build collaborative relationships that enhance the stations' overall effectiveness. A regional station might need staff on-site who collectively possess all the competences necessary to execute all of the priority functions.

• Many combinations of health professionals and others could, as a team, have all the competences necessary to conduct the priority functions necessary for the surveillance, detection, and response to microbial threats of public health significance at U.S. ports of entry.

• Today's quarantine inspectors and officers have extensive knowledge about—and experience in—the historical functions of the quarantine stations. As new staff with expanded backgrounds in public health are hired, DGMQ should ensure that the important experiences of its outstanding and long-serving staff are not lost. Because many techniques, practices, and knowledge of the quarantine station staff have not been codified in a serious way, the stations' continued functioning depends on the people who have fulfilled their roles so well for decades. These experienced individuals should be involved in the development of training modules for new staff who will carry out historical functions at new stations as the expansion progresses.

• The quarantine stations should have access to translators in the languages of the travelers and crews who typically arrive at their ports. In addition, the quarantine station staff should be able to demonstrate knowledge of and sensitivity to the cultural norms in interpersonal communication and health care of travelers and crews who typically arrive at their port.

• Finally, DGMQ should make as a priority the hiring of clerical support for the quarantine stations. This will allow the quarantine inspectors to perform functions well matched to their competence and to meet the competences laid out by the committee. As the stations, the Core, and the Network evolve, the inspectors will need to take on greater and more complex responsibilities and will need strong clerical support.

While developing this report, the committee learned that none of the Core's field staff have formal veterinary backgrounds (Appendix E), although they have regulatory responsibility for screening an array of pets, exotic imports of animal origin, and live animals that might harbor a zoonotic disease, as described in Chapter 3. The station staff usually reviews paperwork about these animals and sometimes does brief visual exams, but physical examinations of the animals would be more informative, according to the analysis commissioned by the committee (Appendix E). The Core should examine and rectify this mismatch between competences and statutory responsibilities in the realm of animal inspection.

Physical Space

The location and layout of the quarantine stations are ideal in some airports and suboptimal in others (Committee, 2005). DGMQ has no financial leverage to influence where the airport authority places stations, because airports are required by regulation to provide quarantine station space free (42 CFR §71.47). Airport real estate comes at a premium to their landlords, so nonprofit operations, such as DGMQ, are sometimes viewed as an undue burden (Borrone, 2005). The Core should be cognizant of these financial and regulatory issues as it continues to build relationships with its System partners at airports. As more of these partners appreciate the complete role the Core plays, perhaps negotiations over space will become easier and more fruitful.

Use of Technology

DGMQ should attempt to acquire electronic communication and data systems that are more robust, modern, and redundant than those currently in place. Such technological enhancements would facilitate the rapid, effective exchange of electronic information that is integrated with CDC's headquarters-based systems. DGMQ also should acquire electronic information-gathering and advanced transmission systems to help compensate for its cirumscribed geographic reach. In addition, it should continue to seek access to databases and systems that contain information to protect the public's health, such as the Automated Manifest System (AMS), Notification of Arrivals, and the Automated Passenger Information System (APIS). Although the stations may need new administrative support as a result of these enhancements, they already need substantial clerical help in their current configuration.

The ability to receive and transmit digital images could yield important public health rewards. Obtaining access to the chest x rays of immigrants and refugees, for instance, can be a slow and difficult process for the Core. The transmittal of these x rays as digital images should, at the very least, expedite the process, and the committee urges the Core to assess the feasibility and benefits of utilizing digital imagery in screening immigrants and refugees for active tuberculosis. Relaying digital images could also be useful in assessing skin lesions and other clinical findings. Furthermore, electronically scanned medical records of immigrant and refugees could be transmitted to the quarantine stations and local public health departments before the individuals arrive in the United States, creating an opportunity to review the records in advance. The electronic transmittal of immigrant and refugee medical records would also reduce the processing delays and errors noted in Chapter 3.

With the ability to transmit and receive digital images throughout the System, more travelers and crews with signs, such as rashes, that might indicate an infection of public health concern could be screened remotely by the quarantine stations, DGMQ HQ, and available physicians. The same technology could increase the number of animals inspected for zoonoses.

The transmission of digital images from off-site locations also would expand the capacity of the geographically confined quarantine station staff to inspect contraband, tissues, etiologic agents, and so on.

The Quarantine Core and its state, tribal, and local partners should develop and maintain shared data and data systems to improve the monitoring of numerous outcomes and processes. In the case of routine screening and management of immigrants and refugees, for instance, shared databases would help the Core oversee

- Medical follow-up determined to be medically indicated for individuals with active or inactive tuberculosis.
- The administration of necessary vaccinations.
- The treatment of parasitic infections.

To cite another example, shared data and data systems would help the Core and local public health authorities exchange surveillance data and information on exposed persons during contact tracing and outbreak management. As noted in Recommendation 2, the sharing of data systems among countries would amplify the Core's global surveillance capacity.

Location of Stations

Recommendation 4: The Committee recommends that the Core periodically revisit its methodology to ascertain whether the stations are optimally located and staffed and relocate stations or staff as needed. While a volume-based risk assessment seems reasonable, based on available data, the Core should periodically evaluate changes in patterns of global travel and trade, as well as models of infectious disease outbreaks, international spread, and efficacy of interventions.

DGMQ selected the locations of the 17 new quarantine stations with several goals in mind. Primary among them is to place stations at U.S. ports of entry that receive the greatest volumes of air, sea, and land travelers (DGMQ, 2003b). Both the committee's expertise and the scope and timetable of this study precluded a comprehensive review and analysis of DGMQ's data and methods for selecting the cities and ports for the new quarantine stations. The committee recommends, however, that DGMQ consider these additional factors in its site-selection process:

- Percentage of international flights covered.
- Amount of coverage during peak arrival times of international flights.

- The cost-benefit ratio of a robust, round-the-clock presence at relatively few, high-risk sites versus a thinner presence at a greater number of sites.
- Coverage of high-risk ports of entry identified in the risk assessment described in Recommendation 1.

In addition, the Core should develop virtual or mobile teams to supplement permanent stations, should the need arise, because of resource constraints or changing threat assessments. Finally, the Core should continue to strengthen existing stations as it builds new ones.

Surge Capacity

Recommendation 5: The committee recommends that the Quarantine Core have plans, capacity, resources, and clear and sufficient legal authority to respond rapidly to a surge of activity at any single U.S. port of entry or at multiple U.S. ports simultaneously.

The Core should assure that a surge-capacity plan for public health emergencies at U.S. ports of entry is part of the emergency plan of the municipalities that contain such ports. One way to accomplish this could be to make it a prerequisite to the receipt of CDC funds for emergency preparedness and bioterrorism planning at the state level and for those cities that receive direct CDC funds. In addition, DGMQ should consider having its staff participate—as resources allow—in response and planning efforts for local public health emergencies. This would not only help foster closer relationships and stronger partnerships with state and local partners but also ensure that DGMQ staff maintain and develop important emergency response skills.

Tools that would be useful in planning for surges include:

- Streamlined protocols for transferring staff from one quarantine station to another.[7]
- Emergency hiring plans.
- Contracts and agreements with local hospitals,[8] emergency respond-

---

[7]The ability to transfer staff is a slow and bureaucratic process in general. Furthermore, relocation will be disruptive to the staff members' personal lives. The protocols should address these challenges.

[8]The committee realizes that some hospitals, fearing stigmatization as "the quarantine facility," may be hesitant to enter into agreements with DGMQ. The committee encourages DGMQ to take this concern into account as it continues to establish partnerships with local hospitals. As noted in Chapter 3, however, DGMQ has already entered into memoranda of agreement with more than 130 hospitals near ports of entry throughout the United States.

ers (fire and ambulance), social service providers, local public health authorities and laboratories, and airport and seaport authorities (to facilitate rapid security clearance).

- Locations to isolate all passengers of a flight for a reasonable period.
- Push-packs (cots, blankets, toiletries, and towels) for quarantine support.
- Virtual teams, mobile teams, or both that can nimbly shift their attention and resources to any one of numerous ports of entry as risks or real events dictate.[9] Such teams could be based at DGMQ headquarters, regional quarantine stations, or other stations. CDC could assemble a team from its emergency command center via videoconference, or a quarantine station could temporarily relocate staff to a port of entry that lacks a permanent station.
- Communication plans and designated, trained personnel to interface with the media and health care providers and to communicate to the public.

Furthermore, the Core should build cooperative relationships with other federal agencies that have extensive experience in emergency response, such as the Federal Emergency Management Agency (FEMA) and USDA. Given their experience in assembling personnel and materials during emergencies, such agencies could serve as valuable resources for the Core as it works to strengthen its surge capacity.

Research

Recommendation 6: The committee recommends that the Core define and devote resources to a research agenda that examines basic public health interventions used or to be developed for use in the System.

Much of the practice of detecting infections and controlling outbreaks of disease in the context of the Quarantine Network has a basis in experience and tradition. It is important that these practices be the subject of systematic research to determine their validity and cost effectiveness. Further, in the context of new technologies and changing microbial threats, new practices should be developed and tested.

---

[9]One such risk could be intelligence data suggesting the potential for an attack at a certain port.

Determining the Effectiveness of the Stations' Practices

The visual screening of arriving international travelers at airports has evolved from laws dating back to 1891 that mandated the medical inspection of all arriving immigrants one person at a time. Then, as now, the public health service was severely understaffed—even at Ellis Island (Mullan, 1989). To cope with multiple duties and huge influxes of hopeful journeyers, the medical officers of the time resorted to cursory visual screening of immigrants for signs of unwanted disease. According to one seasoned public health officer conducting inspections at Ellis Island in 1917, "experience enables [me] in that one glance to take in six details, namely, the scalp, face, neck, hands, gait, and general condition, both mental and physical" (Mullan, 1989, p.45). The system was very inefficient. Fifteen to 20 percent of new arrivals were detained for further medical examination, but less than 1 percent ultimately were found to have an infection that was grounds for refusing entry into the United States (Mullan, 1989).

In today's fast-paced world, thousands of travelers rush through the international terminals of major U.S. airports every day. The culture is loath to stop or slow its pace for anything that isn't absolutely necessary. Logically, in this environment, it would seem to be the exception and not the rule for a quarantine inspector with or (more often) without clinical training to successfully spot signs of a serious communicable disease in one or more individuals hurrying by. Only an infected individual whose illness has progressed to a symptomatic stage that severely impairs his or her ability to function precisely during the hours in flight, when disembarking, or shortly after would clearly stand out from the crowd. On the basis of this reasoning and data gathered on site visits, the committee concluded that visual inspections identify a small percentage of travelers who have communicable diseases of public health significance. Therefore, the stations should devote only a small fraction of their time to the visual inspection of disembarking passengers.

Just as consumers and payers of medical care increasingly base their choices on data about the efficacy of drugs and treatment regimens, so the quarantine stations should scrutinize their methods in a scientific, quantitative way. Designing studies to carefully measure the sensitivity and specificity of current techniques will generate data that either validate or debunk the methods in use. Questions to be asked and answered should include:

- How effective is the current process for screening the health of immigrants and refugees? Could it be improved, and if so, how?
- What is the veracity of self-reported health information?
- What are the most effective methods of tracing exposed travelers or possibly infectious animals?

For example, if passenger locator cards are to be used for contact tracing, the Core should evaluate their effectiveness and continue to research alternative methods.

Developing a Forward-Looking Research Agenda

The Core also should formulate a forward-looking research agenda to develop a scientific foundation for decisions that may need to be made in the future. For instance, many countries would have saved money and time during the SARS outbreak had they previously conducted small studies of the efficacy, cost effectiveness, and efficiency of thermal scanners in identifying individuals with a specific, fever-inducing disease. Such studies would have revealed that the predictive value of a positive thermal scan was zero (St. John et al., 2005; personal communication, R. St. John, Public Health Agency of Canada, July 5, 2005). Questions to be asked and answered should include:

- Given an array of perceived microbial threats, each of a different nature, which method or methods of exit screening[10] would most effectively identify infected individuals? A questionnaire? If so, what questions should be asked? A medical exam? What would be of any use at all?
- What are the environmental factors that contribute to or prevent the transmission of infectious agents on airplanes, cruise ships, cargo ships, and other conveyances?
- How sensitive, specific, and costeffective are existing rapid diagnostic tests, and how and where should those tests be applied? What basic research is needed to develop new rapid diagnostic tests?
- What are the best methods to reduce postarrival diseases, such as tuberculosis, in immigrants and refugees?

In developing this research agenda, the Core should collaborate with its national and international partners to ensure mechanisms for closer cooperation and a better exchange of knowledge and information in the research process.

Developing Data-Collection and Data-Evaluation Plans

In addition, the Core should develop, in advance, data-collection and data-evaluation plans to apply when an incident occurs. The very process of

---

[10]The screening of persons departing from a location where there is a diagnosed outbreak (WHO, 2005).

responding to an incident generates data, but it is extremely difficult to design a data-collection scheme and obtain the necessary clearances (for human-subject studies) in the midst of a crisis. Having such plans and tools at the ready would make it possible to collect and analyze data generated during the crisis. This will be especially important if the incident involves a microbial threat about which many important characteristics are unknown.

Measuring Performance

Recommendation 7: The committee recommends that the Quarantine Core develop scientifically sound tools to measure the effectiveness and quality of all operational aspects of the Quarantine System. The Core should routinely assess the performance of critical quarantine functions by individual CDC quarantine stations, DGMQ headquarters, partner organizations, and the System as a whole. Identified shortfalls should be remedied promptly.

As described in Chapter 3, the absence of evidence-based performance standards and measurement in the present Quarantine System made it virtually impossible for the committee to objectively evaluate most of the System's performance. This weakness in the System would be remedied by the development of scientifically sound metrics for assessing effectiveness and quality.

The Core should catalog all the components of System processes and operations that influence the detection of microbial threats of public health significance at ports of entry. Next, the Core should identify a rational set of measures of the effectiveness and quality of the identified processes and operations. A standard set of tools should be developed for performing measurement. Finally, the Core should use these tools to routinely evaluate its own performance, the performance of individual partner organizations, and the performance of the entire System in concert. The difficulty of conducting objective self-assessments suggests that the Core should consider identifying an unbiased advisory group to perform this activity.

The use of a nationally uniform, evidence-based toolkit to assess the System's performance will help maintain a consistent level of quality and effectiveness in efforts to mitigate the risk that microbial and other threats of public health significance will enter or affect travelers to the United States. Moreover, consistently high quality and effectiveness across all ports of entry will have the positive externality of boosting public confidence in the federal government's ability to protect public health. Below are eight examples of the types of questions that the evaluations should answer.

1. What is the completeness of ascertainment of passengers with conditions of public health concern?

2. What proportion of refugees receives appropriate immunizations or other indicated disease screening, prevention, and treatment prior to arrival in the United States?

3. What proportion of immigrants with a notifiable communicable disease identified overseas completes treatment?

4. What is the quality and effectiveness of the relationships within the Quarantine System?

5. Are the new stations on track to establish relationships with key System partners within a predefined period?

6. Does the training given to CBP, emergency medical services (EMS), and port staff enhance their ability to identify and respond to potential infectious disease threats?

7. How often and completely do members of the System follow response and notification protocols?

8. Do these protocols reduce morbidity and mortality when applied during drills and tabletop exercises?

Questions 4 and 5 call for further explanation. Informal relationships are the glue that holds the System together—a finding documented by the committee (Committee, 2005) and the commissioned paper titled *U.S. Seaports and the CDC Quarantine System* (Appendix D). For this reason, DGMQ headquarters should hold new stations accountable for establishing critical relationships with System partners within a defined period; otherwise, the stations are not fully functional. Metrics for evaluating critical relationships may be difficult to formulate; the disciplines of sociology and organizational dynamics may be helpful in this regard. But the task of measuring the quality and effectiveness of relationships is as important as it may be challenging, because their ongoing evaluation and improvement will help assure that the System is fully functional and operating effectively.

Recommendation 3 discusses the infrastructure of the Quarantine System. Given the weaknesses identified by the committee in this area and the significant impact of staffing, technology, and space on operational performance, the Core should also routinely assess the adequacy of the System's infrastructure and its resources. Through regular evaluation, the Core could better identify, for example, appropriate staffing levels and hours of operation for the quarantine stations.

CONCLUSION

The U.S. Quarantine Network needs strategic public health leadership. The CDC quarantine stations at U.S. ports of entry should provide this leadership to the Quarantine System, and the Quarantine Core should provide it to the Network as a whole. In so doing, the Core could assure the flow of essential communication and data among all CDC quarantine stations and their System partners, promoting rapid, effective, nationally coordinated public health responses to microbial threats that originate abroad.

Given sufficient resources and legal authority to exert strategic national public health leadership, the Core could formalize the collaborative relationships it already has and could establish new linkages to assure that the responsibilities of the Network are executed at all ports of entry on both a routine and emergency basis. In particular, the Quarantine System must be capable of preventing, anticipating, preparing for, and responding to foreign-origin microbial threats that reach U.S. ports of entry when and where CDC quarantine station staff are absent. To achieve this capability, the Core needs sufficient financial and human resources to train its surrogates and acquire information technology that permits rapid, real-time communication and data-sharing among the stations and their System partners.

Finally, the Quarantine Core should build for today and for 50 years hence. Microbial threats of public health significance have been increasing in number and severity for decades; this trend will likely continue for the foreseeable future. The nation must prepare—now—to meet future microbial threats at its gates.

REFERENCES

Borrone L. 2005. *U.S. Seaports and the CDC Quarantine Station System.* Comments received in response to the IOM Report "Human Resources at U.S. Ports of Entry to Protect the Public's Health". Unpublished.

Bozzi C. 1995. *Final Report: Review and Evaluation of CDC's Quarantine and Immigration Programs.* Program evaluation, June 21, 1995.

Catanzaro A, Moser RJ. 1982. Health status of refugees from Vietnam, Laos, and Cambodia. *Journal of the American Medical Association* 247(9): 1303–1308.

CDC (Centers for Disease Control and Prevention). 1998. Enhanced medical assessment strategy for Barawan Somali refugees—Kenya, 1997. *MMWR. Morbidity and Mortality Weekly Report* 46(52–53): 1250–1254.

CDC. 2002. Increase in African immigrants and refugees with tuberculosis—Seattle-King County, Washington, 1998-2001. *MMWR. Morbidity and Mortality Weekly Report* 51(39): 882–883.

Committee (IOM Committee on Measures to Enhance the Effectiveness of the CDC Quarantine Station Expansion Plan for U.S. Ports of Entry). 2005. Unpublished. *Notes on Site Visits to DGMQ Quarantine Stations.*

CRS (Congressional Research Service, The Library of Congress). 2004. *Border Security: Inspection Practices, Policies, and Issues.* [Online] Available: http://fpc.state.gov/documents/organization/33856.pdf [accessed April 7, 2005].

DGMQ (Division of Global Migration and Quarantine, National Center for Infectious Diseases, Centers for Disease Control and Prevention). 2003a. *CDC–History of Quarantine–DQ.* [Online] Available: http://www.cdc.gov/ncidod/dq/history.htm [accessed September 20, 2004].

DGMQ. 2003b. *Reinventing CDC Quarantine Stations: Proposal for CDC Quarantine Station Distribution.* Proposal, September 16, 2004.
DGMQ. 2004a. *Program Review Fiscal Year 2003.* Program review, May 7, 2004.
DGMQ. 2004b. *Proposed Organization Chart Breakout.* Organizational chart, July 8, 2004.
GAO (United States Government Accountability Office). 2005. *Bioterrorism: Information on Jurisdictions' Expenditure and Reported Obligation of Program Funds.* GAO–05–239. Washington, DC: GAO.
Gostin LO. 2000. *Public Health Law: Power, Duty, Restraint.* Berkeley: University of California Press.
Gostin LO, Sapsin JW, Teret SP, Burris S, Mair JS, Hodge JG Jr, Vernick JS. 2002. The Model State Emergency Health Powers Act: planning for and response to bioterrorism and naturally occurring infectious diseases. *JAMA* 288(5): 622–628.
IOM (Institute of Medicine). 1988. *The Future of Public Health.* Washington, DC: National Academy Press.
IOM. 2000. *Calling the Shots: Immunization Finance Policies and Practice.* Washington, DC: National Academy Press.
IOM. 2003. *The Future of the Public's Health in the 21st Century.* Washington, DC: The National Academies Press.
IOM. 2004. *Learning from SARS: Preparing for the Next Disease Outbreak.* Knobler S, Mahmoud A, Lemon S, Mack A, Sivitz L, Oberholtzer K, Editors. Washington, DC: The National Academies Press.
Miller JM, Boyd HA, Ostrowski SR, Cookson ST, Parise ME, Gonzaga PS, Addiss DG, Wilson M, Nguyen-Dinh P, Wahlquist SP, Weld LH, Wainwright RB, Gushulak BD, Cetron MS. 2000. Malaria, intestinal parasites, and schistosomiasis among Barawan Somali refugees resettling to the United States: a strategy to reduce morbidity and decrease the risk of imported infections. *American Journal of Tropical Medicine and Hygiene* 62(1): 115–121.
Mullan F. 1989. *Plagues and Politics: The Story of the United States Public Health Service.* New York: Basic Books, Inc.
NACCHO (National Association of County and City Health Officials). 2003. *NACCHO Annual Report 2003.* [Online] Available: http://archive.naccho.org/Documents/annual_report_2003.pdf [accessed 2005 April 27, 2005].
NACO (National Association of Counties). 2005. *About Counties Overview.* [Online] Available: http://www.naco.org/Template.cfm?Section=About_Counties [accessed June 14, 2005].
Office of Aviation Policy and Plans, Federal Aviation Administration, U.S. Department of Transportation. 2005. *FAA Aerospace Forecasts: Fiscal Years 2005-2006: Table 7 (U.S. and Foreign Flag Carriers: Total Passenger Traffic To/From the United States).* [Online] Available: http://www.api.faa.gov/forecast05/Table7.PDF [accessed April 6, 2005].
St. John RK, King A, de Jong D, Bodie-Collins M, Squires SG, Tam TWS. 2005. Border screening for SARS. *Emerging Infectious Diseases* 11(1): 6–10.
Taylor LH, Latham SM, Woolhouse ME. 2001. Risk factors for human disease emergence. *Philosophical Transactions of the Royal Society of London. Series B: Biological Sciences* 356(1411): 983–989.
WHO (World Health Organization). 2005. *Avian Influenza: Assessing the Pandemic Threat.* Geneva: World Health Organization.

APPENDIXES

A

Human Resources at U.S. Ports of Entry to Protect the Public's Health: Interim Letter Report

January 13, 2005

Dr. Martin Cetron
Director
Division of Global Migration and Quarantine
National Center for Infectious Disease
Centers for Disease Control and Prevention
1600 Clifton Road, Mailstop E-03
Atlanta, GA 30333

Dear Dr. Cetron:

This interim letter report contains the competences[1] and types of health professionals suggested for the CDC quarantine station system by the Institute of Medicine's Committee on Measures to Enhance the Effectiveness of the CDC Quarantine Station Expansion Plan for U.S. Ports of Entry. These suggestions fulfill the first deliverable requested by the CDC Division of Global Migration and Quarantine (DGMQ) in Contract No. 200-2000-00629, Task Order No. 31.

---

[1]To be consistent with current workforce terminology, the committee uses the terms "competences" or "abilities" for skills belonging to individuals and "capacities" or "capabilities" for collections of skills posessed by the human resources of an organization.

BOX A.1   Statement of Task

The factors to be considered in an assessment of current and future border quarantine functions would include:

    1. The current role of quarantine stations as a public health intervention and how the roles should evolve to meet the needs of the 21st century.
    2. The role of other agencies and organizations working collaboratively with the CDC's Division of Global Migration and Quarantine at ports of entry (including federal partners such as Customs and Border Protection, Immigration and Customs Enforcement, U.S. Department of Agriculture, and U.S. Fish and Wildlife Service).
    3. The role of state and local health departments as partners for public health interventions at the nation's borders (such as activities focused on emergency preparedness and response, disease surveillance, and medical assessment and follow-up of newly arriving immigrants and refugees).
    4. Optimal locations for the quarantine stations for efficient and sufficient monitoring and response.
    5. Appropriate types of health professionals and necessary skill sets to staff a modern quarantine station.
    6. Surge capacity to respond to public health emergencies.

Form naturally follows function; however, our committee has been challenged to recommend a human-resource structure for the expanding quarantine station system before developing a robust concept of how the system should function. The guidance offered in this report therefore is preliminary and will be revisited in our final report, to be released on 31 May 2005. The final report will contain recommendations that address all items in the committee's Statement of Task (Box A.1).

HISTORICAL CONTEXT

Dismantling of Quarantine Station System

More than 500 people staffed the 55 federal quarantine stations at U.S. seaports, airports, land-border crossings, consulates, territories, and territorial waters in the late 1960s (Cetron, 2004; DGMQ, 2003a), a period when the medical community generally believed it was "time to close the book on infectious diseases, declare the war against pestilence won, and shift national resources to such chronic problems as cancer and heart disease." This statement, attributed by legend to U.S. Surgeon General William Stewart (Office of the Public Health Service Historian, 2002), reflected

TABLE A.1 Number of Employees and Contractors at Each
CDC Quarantine Station at U.S. Ports of Entry, Mid-2004

Quarantine Station	No. of Full-Time Equivalents
Atlanta	3
Chicago	5
Honolulu	3
Los Angeles	4
Miami	7
New York City (JFK)	8
San Francisco	3
Seattle	4
TOTAL	37

SOURCE: Personal communications: D. Kim, DGMQ, October 13, 2004;
M. Remis, DGMQ, January 18, 2005.

the public's confidence in the power of antibiotics and vaccines to eradicate
such dreaded communicable diseases as yellow fever, plague, and cholera,
which the quarantine stations had worked to barricade from the U.S. population for nearly a century.

The perception that humans had effectively controlled microbial threats
led to the dismantling of most of the federal border quarantine system in the
1970s; by the end of that decade, fewer than a dozen active stations remained
(Cetron, 2004). In mid-2004 there were eight stations with 37 full-time
equivalent staff (Table A.1). Run by the Centers for Disease Control and
Prevention (CDC), their responsibilities and capabilities have consisted of:

1. Responding to ill passengers (international travelers, immigrants,
and refugees) with suspected infectious disease.
    a. If the passenger arrives at a port with a quarantine station,
station staff evaluate the individual for signs, symptoms, and travel
history consistent with a quarantinable disease (Box A.2). If the index
of suspicion is high, the individual is sent to a health care facility for
medical evaluation and diagnosis.
    b. If the passenger arrives at port of entry lacking a quarantine
station, the station with jurisdiction[2] over the port consults the physi-

_____

[2]Each quarantine station is responsible for many ports of entry without a quarantine
station located within a specific geographic area. For example, Hartsfield International Airport in Atlanta has jurisdiction over all ports in Georgia, Alabama, Arkansas, Louisiana,
Oklahoma, Mississippi, North Carolina, South Carolina, and Tennessee. The United States
has more than 295 ports of entry (Personal communication, S. Maloney, DGMQ, January 18,
2005).

BOX A.2   Quarantinable Communicable Diseases

By executive order of the President of the United States, federal isolation and quarantine are authorized for the following communicable diseases:

1. Cholera
2. Diphtheria
3. Infectious Tuberculosis
4. Plague
5. Smallpox
6. Yellow Fever
7. Viral Hemorrhagic Fevers (Lassa, Marburg, Ebola, Crimean-Congo, South American, and others not yet isolated or named)
8. Severe Acute Respiratory Syndrome (SARS)

SOURCE: Executive Order 13,295 of April 4, 2003: Revised List of Quarantinable Communicable Diseases. 3 C.F.R. (2003)

---

cian on call at DGMQ headquarters or alerts the local health department to evaluate the individual for signs and symptoms of a quarantinable disease. If the index of suspicion is high, the individual is sent to a health care facility for diagnosis.

2. Meeting arriving refugees and parolees, visually screening them for signs and symptoms of illness, reviewing the results of their overseas medical examinations, giving local health departments notification of their arrival and the results of their oversees exams, and alerting the health departments to arrivals with Class A or B conditions (Box A.3).

3. Identifying immigrants with Class A or B diseases who arrive at a station's port or whose overseas medical examinations are forwarded to the station by the U.S. Immigration and Naturalization office at the port of arrival. The station then then sends information to relevant state and local health departments about the immigrants' final destinations, suspect diseases, and the results of their overseas medical exams.

4. Inspecting plants and animals imported legally or illegally that may pose a public health threat.

5. Inspecting cargo identified as a potential public health threat.

(Personal communications: J. Barrow and M. Remis, DGMQ, December 28, 2004; S. Maloney, DGMQ, January 18, 2005).

BOX A.3   Class A and Class B Conditions

In the context of medical examinations of individuals who seek refuge in the United States or want to immigrate to this country:
Class A conditions generally render an alien ineligible for entry into the United States; they include:

1. Communicable diseases of public health significance, including chancroid, gonorrhea, granuloma inguinale, human immunodeficiency virus (HIV) infection, leprosy (infectious), lymphogranuloma venereum, syphilis (infectious stage), and tuberculosis (active).
2. A physical or mental disorder and behavior associated with the disorder that may pose, or has posed, a threat to the property, safety, or welfare of the alien or others.
3. A history of such a disorder and behavior which is likely to recur or lead to other harmful behavior.
4. Drug abuse or addiction.

In certain cases, a waiver may be issued to an individual with a Class A condition for entry into the United States. When this occurs, immediate medical follow-up is required.
Class B conditions comprise a "physical or mental abnormality, disease or disability serious in degree or permanent in nature amounting to a substantial departure from normal well-being" (Medical Examination of Aliens. 42 C.F.R. §34.4 [2004]).
Individuals with Class B conditions may enter the United States, but must receive medical follow-up soon after arrival.

SOURCES: Medical Examination of Aliens. 42 C.F.R. §34.1–34.8 (2004); Refugee and Immigrant Health Program, Massachusetts Department of Public Health (2000).

Emergence of Infectious Diseases and the Threat of Bioterrorism

Once the border quarantine system had been largely dismantled, new and long-absent infectious diseases emerged, reemerged, and spread in humans; nearly 40 newly emerging infectious diseases were identified during the 30 years between 1973 and 2003 (GAO, 2004). The convergence of multiple interrelated factors is responsible for this phenomenon (IOM, 2003); they include:

• rapid, high-volume international and transcontinental travel, commerce, and human migration;

- mass relocation of rural populations to cities and the prevalence of overcrowded, unsanitary conditions there;
- exponential growth of population and the number of individuals susceptible to infectious disease;
- widespread changes in climate, ecology, and land use;
- more frequent contact between people and wildlife;
- reduced global investment in public health infrastructure;
- development of antimicrobial resistance.

Numerous scientists, physicians, and public health officers in national and international organizations have voiced concern about these trends and their relationship to such naturally occurring public-health threats as West Nile Virus, SARS, pandemic influenza, and HIV/AIDS. Also within the past two decades, terrorism in general and bioterrorism in particular have become grave concerns to the United States government and its citizens. Consequently, in the late 1990s, DGMQ began to explore ways that the quarantine stations at U.S. ports of entry might help protect U.S. citizens from the unintentional or intentional importation of dangerous infectious agents (Personal communication, D. Kim, DGMQ, October 13, 2004).

The outbreak of SARS in 2002 dramatically demonstrated the need for strong, well-coordinated national and international systems for disease surveillance, detection, and response. In the short term, the outbreak led to a modest but significant change at the CDC quarantine stations: the addition of nine contractors who have master's degrees in public health.

U.S. Government Invests in Biosecurity

Coupled with the microbial threats described above, SARS generated enough political will for the U.S. federal government to commit funding to biosecurity initiatives. A portion of the fiscal year 2004 budget appropriation went to DGMQ for the construction of three new CDC quarantine stations at U.S. ports of entry: Houston Intercontinental Airport; the Mexico–U.S. land border crossing in El Paso, Texas; and Dulles International Airport, located 26 miles from Washington, D.C. These three new stations are not fully staffed as of this writing.

President George W. Bush proposed further expansion of the quarantine station system under the biosecurity umbrella of his fiscal 2005 budget request to Congress[3] by calling for another 14 CDC quarantine stations at U.S. ports of entry (Figure A.1) (Office of Management and Budget, 2004).

---

[3]On December 8, 2004, Congress allocated $80 million to the Department of Health and Human Services, Office of the Secretary, "to support and expand biosurveillance activities" in fiscal year 2005 (U.S. Congress, 2004). As of this writing, it is unclear what portion of the total will go to DGMQ for expanding the quarantine station system.

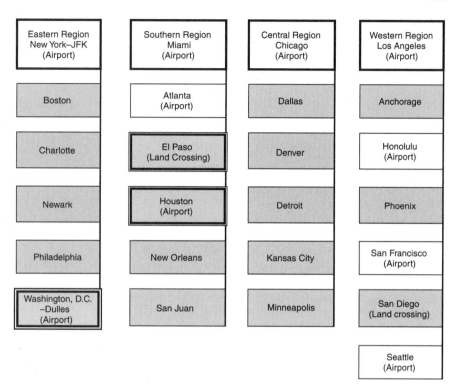

FIGURE A.1 DGMQ's proposed geographic distribution of the 25 quarantine stations in the expanded system. The New York, Miami, Chicago, and Los Angeles quarantine stations would serve as regional headquarters. The white boxes denote the eight cities where quarantine stations existed prior to 2004. The shaded boxes with a double border identify the three cities where quarantine stations opened in 2004. The shaded boxes with a single border represent the 14 cities where DGMQ plans to establish more stations beginning in 2005. The existing quarantine stations are located at airports and a land crossing, as indicated in parentheses under the name of each of those cities. Each of the next 14 stations will be located at either a seaport, airport, or land crossing, but most of this information has not been communicated to the committee as of the date of this letter.
SOURCE: Adapted from personal communication, M. Remis, DGMQ, October 22, 2004.

VISION FOR THE EXPANDED QUARANTINE STATION SYSTEM

With its new mandate, DGMQ wants the quarantine stations to do more than respond to and evaluate travelers with suspect or probable illness. It envisions playing an active, anticipatory role in nationwide biosurveillance (DGMQ, 2003b). This move may be broadly viewed as a significant step back to the robustness of the U.S. border quarantine station system before 1970, as well as a step forward toward national biosecurity based on today's technology and knowledge of microbial threats to human heath.

"CDC Quarantine Stations are gearing up to make the transition from the current focus on federal inspection services at airports to become a full partner in public health response," DGMQ states in a 2003 proposal (DGMQ, 2003b, p.1). "The transformed CDC Quarantine Stations will go beyond evaluating ill passengers to encompass a wide range of responses to infectious disease threats, whether intentional—as in the case of bioterrorism—or related to emerging pathogens. . . . [They] will bring new expertise to bridge gaps in public health and clinical practice,[4] emergency services, and response management. . . . Improved communications networks will enable passengers to be notified promptly of potential exposures to infectious diseases. These expanded services will be integrated into bioterrorism and emergency preparation and response plans and will be grounded in strengthened collaboration [with state and local health departments, the travel industry, and the health care community, as well as other federal agencies]."

DGMQ also would like the CDC quarantine stations to provide a stronger continuum of health support for refugees, whom the division helps prepare for migration to the United States. Refugees primarily enter the United States through a port with a quarantine station,[5] so the stations may be well positioned to monitor the health status of arriving refugees and collaborate with state and local officials on follow-up health evaluations and treatment.

Guidance Sought from IOM

The pace of the quarantine-station expansion at U.S. ports of entry and the potential for a functional revamping of the sytem led DGMQ to seek guidance from the Institute of Medicine (IOM) on how best to strengthen, improve, and modernize public health responses and disease surveillance in

---

[4]As of January 18, 2005, seven Quarantine Medical Officers (physicians) are on duty or have accepted offers of employment. Offers of employment have been made to two additional Quarantine Medical Officers. Offers of employment for other staff positions are also pending (Personal communication, M. Remis, DGMQ, January 18, 2005).

[5]A large number of refugees enter the United States at Newark Liberty International Airport, which lacks a quarantine station at present. The International Office for Migration does the initial processing of these refugees and provides their documentation to quarantine station staff at John F. Kennedy International Airport in New York City, who notify appropriate health departments. Newark is one of the 14 cities designated for a quarantine station.

BOX A.4   Priority Functions

1. Conduct historic* functions.
2. Plan for public health threats.
3. Conduct surveillance for public health threats.
4. Assess and respond to public health threats.
5. Communicate the nature of diseases, risks, and responses.
6. Create linkages across sectors and jurisdictions.

---

*Historic functions are the activities, including inspections, that have been carried out by the stations for at least the past decade in accordance with federal regulations.

---

its quarantine station system. The pace of the expansion also led DGMQ to request preliminary guidance early in the course of the IOM study on the types of health professionals and competences needed to meet the stations' new public health mission and traditional statutory responsibilities. We provide this preliminary guidance below.

FUNCTIONS AND COMPETENCES

The committee has preliminarily developed priority functions (Box A.4) and core competences necessary for surveillance, detection, and response to public health threats at U.S. ports of entry. The guidance in this report is based primarily on the expert judgment of the committee. As noted above, we will revisit the question of function in depth in the final report.

Guiding Framework

The competences should be considered within the following framework:

• Every station should have access to individuals who posess all the competences. These individuals could be located either on-site or off-site. Potential off-site human resources could be based at the regional stations, DGMQ headquarters, the private sector, partner agencies, or elsewhere. In general, using partners as a resource for some of the competences could help the stations build collaborative relationships that enhance the stations' overall effectiveness.

• The competences in each functional area do not necessarily comprise a job description.

- Qualified individuals may have competences in more than one functional area.
- Many different mixes of professionals could, as a team, have all the requisite competences.
- A regional station might need staff on site who collectively posess all the competences necessary to execute all of the priority functions.
- All staff who conduct the priority functions should be able to demonstrate basic familiarity with infectious diseases of public health concern.
- All staff of the quarantine station system should have access to and abilities in basic information technology, including the abilities to use e-mail, word-processing software, and the Internet.

Specialized Competences in Information Technology

At least some of the technical staff should have more advanced computer skills that enable them to use standard, off-the-shelf software for creating spreadsheets, databases, and communication products. These staff also should be capable of using software for conducting analyses and for exchanging data with partner organizations. For instance, relevant staff should be able to obtain and use airlines' electronic passenger manifests, when available, to conduct contact tracing. In addition, the stations may need access to technical support should any of their systems fail, especially during a public health emergency.

Capacities in Foreign Languages and Cultures

The quarantine stations should have access to translators in the languages of the travelers and crew who typically arrive at their port. Staff who conduct any of the priority functions should be able to identify and contact appropriate translators at any time. This competence is critical to individuals who conduct assessment and response, health communication, and risk communication.

In addition, the quarantine station staff should be able to demonstrate knowledge of and sensitivity to the cultural norms in interpersonal communication and health care of travelers and crew who typically arrive at their port.

I. Conduct Historic Functions

Historic functions are the routine activities that the quarantine stations have conducted for the past decade or more in accordance with federal regulations. The committee has placed these activities at the top of the list of priority functions to highlight the importance of maintaining them and their associated competences and human resources during this transitional period and into the future. Today's quarantine inspectors and officers collectively have nearly three centuries worth of knowledge and experience (Personal communication, D. Kim, DGMQ, October 13, 2004). To preserve this wealth of expertise, these individuals should be involved in the development of training modules for new staff who will carry out historic functions at new stations as the expansion progresses.

Historic quarantine station activities include the processing of immigrants, refugees, asylees, and parolees; and the inspection of plant items, animal items, and cargo that could pose a potential public health threat. In addition, the stations have a long history of clinically evaluating new arrivals to the United States. As described on pages 2 and 3 of this letter, today's inspectors carry out that important function in several ways: by responding to ill passengers with suspected infectious disease to determine if the individuals have symptoms and travel history consistent with a quarantinable disease (Box A.2); by visually screening refugees and parolees for signs and symptoms of illness; by identifying immigrants with Class A or B conditions (Box A.3); and by conveying the results of overseas medical examinations and other relevant information to state and local health departments (Personal communications: J. Barrow and M. Remis, DGMQ, December 28, 2004; S. Maloney, DGMQ, January 18, 2005). During its deliberations, the committee decided to consolidate all clinical competences—including those associated with the historic screening described above—under the priority function, "Assess and respond to public health threats" in part IV below; this placement is reflected in Table A.2, which is presented at the end of this letter report.

Although the stations' regulatory authority for historic functions is longstanding, the ability of the station staff to carry out these functions has greatly diminished due to the tremendous, round-the-clock volume of travelers and imported cargo and the global spread of infectious disease. For instance, the stations have a regulatory responsibility to restrict the importation of items that may pose a human health risk, including but not restricted to dogs, cats, nonhuman primates, turtles and tortoises, human remains, and etiologic agents of various kinds (42 CFR §71.51–55). However, the way these regulations are carried out varies from station to station and from port to port. In some instances, the quarantine station staff sees a significant number of imported animals or the paperwork documenting them; indeed, the staff relies on paper documentation for much of the inspection it conducts. Some imports are cleared by telephone and some by fax. In other instances, the staff relies on Customs and Border Protection (CBP) officials to perform these duties on their behalf. Even at the ports with quarantine stations, however, some of the at-risk cargo enters the

United States without being inspected or cleared by DGMQ field staff (Personal communication, J. Barrow and M. Remis, DGMQ, November 9, 2004).

The Trade Act of 2002, slowly being implemented at the ports of entry, is converting to a paperless system. DGMQ is pursuing the possibility of accessing the International Trade Data System with the goal of reviewing incoming cargo at all ports and identifying those items that might need further scrutiny (Personal communication, J. Barrow and M. Remis, DGMQ, November 9, 2004).

At any given time, specialized restrictions can be put in place when a risk is perceived. Two contemporary examples are the bans on the importation of civet cats, an important potential source of the SARS coronavirus (Zhong, 2004), and Gambian rats, the probable source of human monkeypox virus that emerged in the United States in 2003 (Di Giulio and Eckburg, 2004).

Competences Needed to Conduct Historic Functions[6]

Relevant staff members should have the ability to:

1.   Understand and carry out federal regulations applicable to the quarantine stations regarding the importation of plants, animals, and biological specimens (Foreign Quarantine. 42 C.F.R. §71.51–71.56 [2004]).

2.   Inspect plant and animal items that may pose a potential public health threat.

3.   Collaborate with staff from other federal and state agencies that also have responsibility for the inspection of imported plants and animals, including the USDA Animal and Plant Health Inspection Service, the U.S. Food and Drug Administration, state fish and wildlife agencies, and the Department of Homeland Security.

4.   Inspect cargo identified as a potential public health threat.

5.   Develop knowledge of cargo operations at airports and seaports and keep apprised of changes.

6.   Develop and maintain relationships with key individuals at private-sector transport companies that routinely use the port where the quarantine station is based.

7.   Develop relationships and maintain frequent communication with key port personnel and with employees of U.S. ports located in offices at major foreign points of origin.

8.   Process arriving refugees, immigrants, asylees, and parolees.

---

[6]Excluding the clinical aspects of historic functions; these are described in part IV.

II. Plan for Public Health Threats

Each quarantine station should be prepared to screen for and respond to the detection of microbial threats to health in arriving passengers and crew. For purposes of this report, a microbial threat of public health significance causes serious or lethal human disease and is transmissible from person to person, from animal to person, or has the potential to be transmitted either of these ways; it also may be transmissible from food or water to people. Concern is greatest for those microbes that spread readily from person to person due to their potential for wide dispersal.

The stations should develop protocols for responding to possible, probable, and definite diagnostic results, including the identification or construction of isolation units at or near ports of entry. Protocols for screening and response should be updated as new rapid diagnostics become available. Likewise, staff should periodically participate in continuing education courses. In addition, the stations should create emergency-response plans for their personnel in concordance with established emergency-response plans that cover the port where each station is located and other ports in its area of jurisdiction.[7] These plans should be developed in coordination with relevant partners.

The competences developed by the committee in this section are not inconsistent with the elaborate work done by the Center for Health Policy at Columbia University School of Nursing (Center for Health Policy, 2001, 2002). They are, however, specifically tailored to the immediate needs of quarantine stations at U.S. ports of entry in the context of the planned expansion.

Competences Needed to Plan for Public Health Threats

Relevant staff should have the ability to (National Response Team, 2001; Center for Health Policy, 2001):

1. Coordinate (with DGMQ headquarters) the station's procedures for the monitoring of global health threats.
2. Develop and maintain emergency response plans consistent with local, state, and regional plans for biological, chemical, radiological, and conventional threats.
3. If called upon, collaborate with port personnel, private-sector part-

---

[7]Each quarantine station has responsibility for ports of entry without a quarantine station within a specific geographic area. For example, Hartsfield International Airport in Atlanta has jurisdiction over all ports in Georgia, Alabama, Arkansas, Louisiana, Oklahoma, Mississippi, North Carolina, South Carolina, and Tennessee.

ners, and public-sector partners in the development of emergency response plans for biological, chemical, or radiological incidents at the port.

4. Develop and maintain routine protocols for the identification of suspect cases, probable cases, and asymptomatically infected individuals.

5. Define and articulate the station's role in emergency response within the area's jurisdictional parameters.

6. Work within an incident command structure and the National Incident Management System.

7. Maintain relationships and regular communication with relevant public health and emergency partners.[8]

8. Implement notification systems.

9. Conduct emergency preparedness training procedures, including tabletop exercises and regular drills, for station staff and—if requested— port personnel.

10. Participate in practice sessions and drills with local emergency preparedness groups.

11. Evaluate training and incident response results to ensure that all parts of the emergency plan are followed.

12. Develop plans and procedures for educating arriving passengers and crews about the health risks posed by suspected or detected microbial threats in a human traveler or in imported animals, plants, biological specimens, and other substances for which the stations have statutory responsibility.

13. Coordinate and maintain protocols for assessing and responding to the importation of biological specimens from abroad for their potential threat to public health; these include bodily fluids and human and animal tissues.

14. Manage the station's emergency resources, including contacts, equipment, materials, and facilities.

15. Effectively manage fellow staff members in the coordination and implementation of response plans and routine protocols.

16. Work comfortably with quarantine station staff, DGMQ colleagues, and all relevant partners to coordinate and implement response plans.

---

[8]These partners include area hospitals and emergency responders; community organizations; officials from public health agencies and other branches of state, local, and tribal government; area transportation safety officials; representatives and officers of transportation companies and industry organizations; port and border security personnel; law enforcement agencies; officials from such federal agencies as the Department of Homeland Security, U.S. Department of Agriculture, and U.S. Fish and Wildlife Service; international public health agencies; international transportation organizations; the media; and suppliers of critical products.

III. Conduct Surveillance for Public Heath Threats

The station system should conduct surveillance for microbial threats of public health significance as defined above. The stations and DGMQ headquarters should anticipate the arrival of infectious disease threats from abroad to the best of their ability by mining the multiple electronic disease-reporting networks and databases at their disposal. These data should be monitored, interpreted, and assessed for situations that call for the screening of at-risk inbound travelers. Since an estimated 75 percent of newly emergent infectious diseases are zoonotic in origin (Taylor et al., 2001), staff should track outbreaks of disease in animals as well as humans. The routine review and analysis of disease diagnoses in travelers and their points of origin could help local public health authorities contain community-level outbreaks of imported diseases and could stimulate the introduction of disease-specific diagnostics and interventions at the ports of entry likely to receive infected passengers. Such new technologies as thermal scans and rapid diagnostic assays may need to be adapted, implemented, and evaluated for surveillance purposes.

Competences Needed to Conduct Surveillance for Public Health Threats

Relevant staff should have the ability to:

1. Design surveillance protocols.
2. Adapt surveillance protocols to the type and severity of perceived threat.
3. Operate newly developed surveillance technology as it becomes available.
4. Follow CDC guidelines for the evaluation of surveillance systems to examine the effectiveness of new surveillance technologies in conjuction with other stations and DGMQ headquarters.
5. Collect, analyze, and interpret relevant data.
6. Use standard epidemiological and statistical software such as Epi-Info and SAS.
7. Undertake outbreak investigations.
8. Report findings to regional stations and DGMQ headquarters.
9. Participate in large-scale contact tracing.
10. Collaborate with public health officials at local, state, tribal, and international levels, with state epidemiologists, CBP partners, private-sector partners (especially transportation companies), and DGMQ staff at headquarters and other stations.
11. Respond to information about outbreaks of infectious diseases of public health concern by conducting disease surveillance and response on appropriate arrivals.

IV. Assess and Respond to Public Health Threats

At this stage of the study, the committee has approached the dual functions of assessment and response almost entirely from a clinical standpoint. The clinical aspects of the stations' historic functions are incorporated here for thematic cohesion; all other historic functions are discussed in section I.

The quarantine stations need access to a clinician who can diagnose infectious diseases of public health concern, including those that are uncommon or absent in the United States but common in or endemic to other parts of the world. The stations also need access to clinicians who can assess patients exposed to chemical, radiological, or biological agents and who can recommend prophylaxes or treatment. At times, the clinician might need to perform triage; it is unclear whether state medical licensing laws would apply to the quarantine stations in these cases. In addition, the need may arise for mass diagnostic screening of inbound (and potentially outboud) passengers, such as during an influenza pandemic. Quarantine station personnel who do direct clinical evaluation or triage are at risk for infection, so these individuals should have baseline skills in infection control and the use of such personal protective equipment as masks, protective eyewear, gloves, gowns, and containment suits (IOM, 2004), which should be available on-site. Strong relationships between the clinician and local hospitals, emergency-room physicians, clinical laboratories, and first responders will facilitate the response to public health threats.

Competences Needed to Assess and Respond to Public Health Threats

Relevant staff should have the ability to:

1. Recognize the signs, symptoms, and transmission patterns of infectious diseases of public health concern, especially those that are transmissible from person to person, rapidly progressive, and lethal. This includes diseases rarely seen in the United States but common or endemic to other parts of the world.
2. Perform triage.[9]
3. Interview patients and contacts to obtain case histories.
4. Physically examine patients and assess them, report findings to physicians with specialized expertise, make diagnoses when possible, and make decisions regarding patient referral and the need for isolation during transport to a referral facility.

---

[9]Triage: The sorting of individuals who are too well to need treatment, too ill to be saved, and those in the middle who would benefit from treatment.

5. Develop comprehensive knowledge of local resources for patient referral.

6. Develop relationships with local hospitals, physicians, first responders, and public health laboratories.

7. Collect specimens for laboratory analysis.

8. Follow appropriate protocols for infection control during direct clinical evaluations, triage, and the collection and transport of laboratory specimens. Such protocols include the use of personal protective equipment and the implementation of isolation precautions.

9. Perform rapid diagnostic tests to screen large numbers of passengers for potential exposure to infectious agents of public health concern.

10. Interpret results of diagnostic tests.

11. By telephone or equivalent, conduct pre-arrival assessments of suspect or probable cases who are aboard airplanes and ships; coordinate responses by instructing crews and deploying personnel and equipment on the ground.

12. Track patients, passengers, crews, and so on.

13. Conduct post-arrival follow-up on the health status of refugees, immigrants, and asylees.

14. Assess biological specimens for their potential to introduce a microbial threat to the public.

15. Recognize epidemiologic and other emergency indicators; interpret and understand related data.

V. Communicate the Nature of Diseases, Risks, and Responses

We have subdivided the communication function into four categories—general communication, risk communication, health education, and media relations—because the last three areas require specialized knowledge and skills. In practice, however, we expect that two or more of these functions will be integrated. For instance, communicating with the media about travelers diagnosed with an infectious disease would require some discussion of risk and some health education. In all cases, the stations, DGMQ headquarters, or both should coordinate public communications with state and local partners.

A) General Communication

The quarantine stations routinely interact with multiple partners: port officials, representatives of airlines and cruise ships, federal officials from other agencies, state and local public health officials, hospital officials, emergency responders, and so on. At least one individual at every station should be capable of communicating with these partners in a way that fosters credibility, respect, understanding, collaboration and trust (ATSDR,

1994). Individuals responsible for risk communication, health education, and media relations should also have these capabilities.

Competences needed to conduct general communication

Relevant staff members should have the ability to:

1. Communicate verbally in an articulate, poised manner with both individuals and groups.
2. Quickly build trust and rapport.
3. Distill complex information into clear, succinct messages.
4. Listen to, comprehend, and respond to diverse audiences.
5. Communicate effectively with individuals in positions of authority among partner organizations. Such individuals include pilots, captains, and officials of transport companies, hospitals, and port authorities.
6. Communicate effectively in writing and through graphics.
7. Create printed and electronic communication products for staff and stakeholders with the goal of helping the stations function more efficiently and effectively.
8. Create and give presentations to stakeholders.
9. Routinely evaluate whether messages achieve their intended outcome.
10. Collaborate effectively with communications officers at partner organizations (e.g., by developing consistent messages about a particular incident).

B) Risk Communication

Many of the public health threats that the quarantine stations encounter will be characterized at the outset by uncertainty. As the nature of the threat becomes clearer, the facts that emerge will have the potential to cause panic and distress. The stations should all have rapid access to individuals trained to discuss health-related uncertainties, risks, and concerns with individuals and groups (ATSDR, 1994).

Competences needed to communicate the nature of health risks

Relevant staff should have the ability to:

1. Understand quantitative and qualitative data on the health risks posed by suspect, probable, and confirmed cases of disease and by exposure to biological, chemical, and radiological weapons.

2. Translate quantitative measurements of risk into language that helps affected individuals develop a realistic level of concern and take appropriate actions.

3. Decrease the potential for alarm.

C) Health Education

The diagnosis of an infectious disease in a passenger or crew member often will require that a member of the quarantine station staff discuss the health implications of the diagnosis with the patient, his or her contacts, representatives of the airline or shipping company, and others. In some cases, a staff member of the quarantine station may need to explain a public health matter to a large group of passengers or others.

Competences needed to communicate the nature of diseases and appropriate responses

Relevant staff members should have the ability to:

1. Understand the signs, symptoms, prophylaxis, treatment, and infection control measures pertinent to infectious diseases of global health concern, especially those rare or absent in the United States.

2. Understand clinical information communicated by physicians and epidemiologists.

3. Explain medical conditions and provide instructions for self–care in language that is understandable to individuals at all levels of health literacy.

4. Respond to patients' questions and concerns.

5. Explain risks and proposed responses to governing legal authorities and other individuals in positions of authority (e.g., pilots, captains).

D) Media and Public Relations

From time to time, the media and the general public may express an interest in an incident managed by a quarantine station, or the station may want to alert the public in response to an incident. An individual representing the individual station, the station system, or DGMQ will need to communicate with reporters or public leaders with accuracy, good judgment, consistency, and media savvy in close coordination with partners such as local and state jurisdictions and transportation companies.

Competences needed to communicate with the media and general public

Relevant staff members should have the ability to:

1. Perform well under pressure in a fast-paced environment.
2. Demonstrate good judgment and trustworthiness in all interactions with the public and the media.
3. Understand the news cycle, the meaning and appropriate usage of such terms as "off the record" and "on background," and the general perspective of reporters, editors, and producers.
4. Formulate messages consistent with the mission of the CDC quarantine station system.
5. Coach senior staff in preparation for interviews with individual reporters and for press conferences.

VI. Create Linkages Across Sectors and Jurisdictions

The quarantine stations should develop collaborative relationships with all members of their communities and jurisdictions who respond to public health threats, as well as with relevant private-sector organizations. One example of such a linkage is the development of protocols and agreements with emergency medical services and area hospitals for the transport, care, and isolation of potentially infectious travelers, as well as reporting guidelines and jurisdictions among city, county, tribal, and state officials. Another example is the development of collaborative relationships with employees of U.S. ports who are based at major points of origin of the port's clients. (For instance, the Port of Seattle maintains permanent offices, staffed by Port employees, at major ports of origin in the Pacific.) In certain situations, it may be appropriate for quarantine station staff to take the lead in collaborative planning and responses based on the applicable incident command structure as well as on state, local, tribal, and regional laws, regulations, and practices.

When creating linkages, the station staff must follow privacy laws and practices to protect the confidentiality of patients' information.

Competences Needed to Create Linkages Across Sectors and Jurisdictions

The senior staff of each station should have the ability to:

1. Establish credibility, foster relationships, and promote information sharing with state and local officials in public health and emergency preparedness.
2. Notify state and local public health authorities of clinical, diagnostic, epidemiological, or other investigations that indicate a possible public health threat.

3. Protect the confidentiality of patients' information.

4. Be conversant in the overlapping and harmonizing functions of traditional public health agencies and other partners in all-hazards preparedness, including law enforcement, fire departments, and emergency medical technicians.

5. Describe how the quarantine station fits into the preexisting incident command structure (Center for Health Policy, 2001) and operate within that structure.

6. Take the lead, when appropriate, in coordinating public health responses within the applicable incident command structure.

7. Understand the legal authorities in public health emergency response and work within those boundaries.

8. Develop and maintain relationships with private-sector partners.

TYPES OF HEALTH PROFESSIONALS

As noted above, many combinations of health professionals and others could, as a team, have all the competences necessary to meet the priority functions. To identify the types of professionals who would likely have one or more sets of the competences outlined above, the committee brought to bear its combined knowledge on workforce issues in public health, medicine, nursing, emergency preparedness and response, epidemiology, and travelers' health. The results are presented in Table A.2 below. The selected job titles are common parlance within the U.S. public health community.

In addition to the types of professionals listed in Table A.2, the stations will need clerical workers who perform structured work in support of station operations (Center for Health Policy, 2001).

CONCLUDING REMARKS

The committee has identified six sets of core competences and 11 types of professionals that could help prevent microbial threats of public health significance from breaching U.S. borders and contain those that are imported either by accident or intentionally. We derived these competences and professionals from the six functions that we identified as priorities for the CDC quarantine station system (Box A.4). As noted above, the guidance offered in this interim letter report is preliminary and will be revisited as we continue to assess the role of the CDC quarantine station system in the context of our task (Box A.1). We encourage the reader to refer to the Statement of Task as a reminder of the breadth of subject matter to be addressed in the committee's final report.

During the next few months, we will visit several quarantine stations to personally see how they function. We will also learn how multiple private-

TABLE A.2 Types of Workers Who Could Conduct the Priority Functions Necessary for the Surveillance for, Detection of, and Response to Microbial Threats at U.S. Ports of Entry

	Priority Functions			
Type of Worker	Historic Functions[a]	Planning	Surveillance (Epidemiological)	Assessment & Response (Clinical)
Physician				x
Physician with public health background		x	x	x
Nurse practitioner		x		x
Physician's assistant				x
Nurse				x
Public health nurse		x	x	x
Public health advisor				
Baccalaureate or equivalent	x	x		
Master's or doctoral				
Trained in epidemiology	x	x	x	
Not trained in epidemiology	x	x		
Infectious disease epidemiologist		x	x	
Communication specialist				
Master's or equivalent		x		

NOTE: Any of these individuals could have the ability to manage a quarantine station. No correlation necessarily exists between level of education and rank.

and public-sector organizations presently interact with the stations and what role they envision the quarantine stations playing in the future. These information-gathering activities will likely include a discussion of the role of the quarantine stations within the National Incident Management System and relevant incident command structures. The committee's deliberations may include consideration of such issues as the degree of centralization or autonomy that the individual stations should have. We look forward to providing DGMQ with recommendations for the development of a quarantine station system capable of meeting current and projected public health needs at U.S. ports of entry.

Georges C. Benjamin, *Chair*
IOM Committee on Measures to Enhance the Effectiveness of the CDC Quarantine Station Expansion Plan for U.S. Ports of Entry

Communication[b]

Health Education	Risk Communi-cation	Media & Public Relations	Creating Linkages
x	x		x
x	x	x	x
x			x
x	x		x
x	x		x
x	x	x	x
x			x
x	x		x
x	x		x
			x
	x	x	x

[a]For purposes of this report, the historic clinical capacities of the quarantine stations are encompassed by the priority function of assessment and response.
[b]General communication competences were intentionally left out of this table.

REFERENCES

ATSDR (Agency for Toxic Substances and Disease Registry). 1994. *A Primer on Health Risk Communication Principles and Practices*. [Online]. Available: http://www.atsdr.cdc.gov/ HEC/primer.html [accessed November 11, 2004].

Center for Health Policy, Columbia University School of Nursing. 2001. *Local Public Health Competency for Emergency Response*. [Online]. Available: http://cpmcnet.columbia.edu/ dept/nursing/institute-centers/chphsr/COMPETENCIES.pdf [accessed November 22, 2004].

Center for Health Policy, Columbia University School of Nursing. 2002. *Bioterrorism & Emergency Readiness: Competencies for All Public Health Workers*. [Online]. Available: http://cpmcnet.columbia.edu/dept/nursing/institute-centers/chphsr/btcomps.html [accessed December 28, 2004].

Cetron M. 2004. *CDC Division of Global Migration and Quarantine*. Presentation at the October 21, 2004, Meeting of the IOM Committee on Measures to Enhance the Effectiveness of the CDC Quarantine Station Expansion Plan for U.S. Ports of Entry. Washington, D.C.

DGMQ (Division of Global Migration and Quarantine, National Center for Infectious Disease, Centers for Disease Control and Prevention). 2003a. *CDC—History of Quarantine—DQ*. [Online]. Available: http://www.cdc.gov/ncidod/dq/history.htm [accessed September 20, 2004].

DGMQ. 2003b. *Reinventing CDC Quarantine Stations: Proposal for CDC Quarantine Station Distribution*. Atlanta, GA: DGMQ.

Di Giulio DB, Eckburg, PB. 2004. Human monkeypox: an emerging zoonosis. *The Lancet Infectious Diseases*. 4(1):15-25.

GAO (United States Government Accountability Office). 2004. *Emerging Infectious Diseases: Review of State and Federal Disease Surveillance Efforts*. Washington, D.C.: GAO.

IOM (Institute of Medicine). 2003. *Microbial Threats to Health: Emergence, Detection, and Response*. Washington, D.C.: The National Academies Press.

IOM. 2004. *Learning from SARS: Preparing for the Next Disease Outbreak*. Washington, D.C.: The National Academies Press.

National Response Team. 2001. *Hazardous Materials Emergency Planning Guide (NRT-1)*. [Online]. Available: http://www.nrt.org/Production/NRT/NRTWeb.nsf/AllAttachments ByTitle/SA-27NRT1Update/$File/NRT-1%20update.pdf?OpenElement [accessed January 12, 2005].

Office of Management and Budget, the Executive Office of the President of the United States. 2004. *Budget of the U.S. Government, Fiscal Year 2005*. [Online]. Available: http://www.whitehouse.gov/omb/budget/fy2005/budget.html [accessed December 9, 2004].

Office of the Public Health Service Historian. 2002. *FAQ's*. [Online]. Available: http://lhncbc.nlm.nih.gov/apdb/phsHistory/faqs.html [accessed January 10, 2005].

Refugee and Immigrant Health Program, Massachusetts Department of Public Health. 2000. *Refugee Health Assessment: A Guide for Health Care Clinicians*. [Online]. Available: http://www.mass.gov/dph/cdc/rhip/rha/ [accessed January 3, 2005].

Taylor LH, Latham SM, Woolhouse ME. 2001. Risk factors for human disease emergence. *Philosophical Transactions of the Royal Society of London. Series B, Biological Sciences*. 356(1411):983–989.

U.S. Congress, House of Representatives, Committee of Conference. 2004. *Making Appropriations for Foreign Operations, Export Financing, and Related Programs for the Fiscal Year Ending September 30, 2005, and for Other Purposes: Conference Report* [to accompany H.R. 4818]. 108th Cong., 2nd Sess. Report 108-792. November 20, 2004.

Zhong N. 2004. Management and prevention of SARS in China: one contribution of 15 to a Discussion Meeting Issue "Emerging infections: what have we learnt from SARS?" *Philosophical Transactions of the Royal Society of London. Series B, Biological Sciences*. 359(1447):1115–1116.

B

Agendas of Open Sessions of Committee Meetings

From October 2004 to March 2005, the committee gathered information relevant to this study from journal articles, reports, and news articles collected by staff; from presentations and commentary by constituencies relevant to the study; from material provided by the sponsor at the committee's request; from reports by select committee and staff members of visits to five quarantine stations; and from the commissioned papers contained in the appendixes to this report.

This appendix contains the agendas of the open sessions of committee meetings, at which representatives of relevant constituencies made presentations to the group and participated in question-and-answer sessions.

Meeting 1
October 21-22, 2004
800 Eye Street, NW, Conference Room A, Washington, DC

Open Session: Thursday, October 21, 2004

10:00am	Open Session Commences Charge to the Committee, Plans for Expansion, and Workforce Issues	*Martin Cetron, Director, Division of Global Migration and Quarantine, CDC*
	A Day in the Life of a CDC Quarantine Station Manager	*Martha Remis, Officer in Charge, CDC Quarantine Station, Chicago-O'Hare Airport*

12:00pm	Partners' Perspectives on the CDC Quarantine Station System and Its Plans for Expansion	*Katherine B. Andrus, Assistant General Council, Air Transport Association of America Inc.*
		John F. Lopinto, D.V.M., Veterinary Medical Officer, USDA APHIS Animal Care
1:00pm	Open Session Adjourns	

<h3 style="text-align:center">Meeting 2
January 20-21, 2005
Mt. Washington Conference Center, 5801 Smith Avenue, Suite 1100, Baltimore, MD</h3>

Open Session, Thursday, January 20, 2005

8:00am	Open Session Commences	
8:30am	Future of Quarantine Stations	*Bill Rowley, MD, Institute for Alternative Futures*

9:30am	State and Local Partners	*ASTHO*
		  Guthrie Birkhead, MD, MPH
		  New York State Department of Health
		NACCHO
		  Pat Checko, DrPH
		  Bristol-Burlington Health District
		CSTE
		  Gilberto Chavez, MD,MPH
		  California State Epidemiologist and Chair, CSTE Working Group on Border and International Health
		TB Controllers
		  Sarah Royce, MD, MPH
		  Tuberculosis Control Branch, California Department of Health Services

10:45am   Panel Discussion

11:30am   Lunch Break

12:30pm   Quarantine Stations in   *Susan Courage, RN BScN*
            Canada: Structure   *National Coordinator,*
                                             Quarantine Services
                                             Centre for Emergency
                                             Preparedness and Response
                                             Public Health Agency of
                                             Canada

            Quarantine Stations in   *Susan Courage, RN BScN*
            Canada: Response to SARS   *National Coordinator,*
                                             Quarantine Services
                                             Centre for Emergency
                                             Preparedness and Response
                                             Public Health Agency of
                                             Canada

1:45pm   Potential Use of Modeling in   *Donald Burke, MD*
            Quarantine Stations   *Johns Hopkins University*
                                             Bloomberg School of Public
                                             Health

3:30   U.S. Customs and Border   *Anne Lombardi, Director*
            Protection (by teleconference)   *Penny Gaddini*
                                             Chicago Field Office,
                                             Department of Homeland
                                             Security

4:00   Final Questions and Discussion

4:15   Open Session Adjourns

C

Methodology Used by the Division of Global Migration and Quarantine to Select Sites for New Quarantine Stations

PROPOSAL FOR CDC QUARANTINE STATION DISTRIBUTION

Division of Global Migration and Quarantine (DGMQ)
Centers for Disease Control and Prevention (CDC)

September 16, 2003

Overview

DGMQ used the following criteria to select cities to receive new quarantine stations:

A. Volume of international human travelers
- Airports with >500,000 arriving international air travelers per year.
- Seaports in major cities with >150,000 arriving international maritime travelers per year.
- Land crossings in major cities with >10 million arriving international travelers.

B. Total volume of human travelers
- Airports with >25 million arriving international and domestic air travelers per year.

C. Volume of imported wildlife
- Major cities that serve as designated or nondesignated ports of

124

entry by the U.S. Fish and Wildlife Service to receive international shipments of wildlife.
D. National security concerns

Analysis

1. By volume of arriving international air travelers:
    a. Ports of highest priority by this criterion are New York JFK, Miami, Los Angeles, Chicago O'Hare, Newark, San Francisco, Atlanta, Houston Intercontinental, Honolulu, Washington Dulles, Dallas-Ft. Worth, Boston, Detroit, San Juan (PR), Philadelphia, Seattle, Minneapolis, and Orlando International.
    b. 75.2% direct-arriving international air traveler coverage if CDC is present in the ports described in 1.a. that have >500,000 arriving international air travelers per year.
    c. 77.3% coverage if ports near the above international airports (indirect coverage)—that is, Ft. Lauderdale (Miami), Chicago Midway (Chicago O'Hare), Sanford Orlando (Orlando International), Oakland and San Jose (San Francisco), and Baltimore (Washington Dulles)—are considered.
    d. 17.4% of arriving international air travelers are precleared in Canada (13.0%), Bahamas (2.1 %), U.S. Virgin Islands (1.1 %), Aruba (0.7%), and Bermuda (0.5%)

2. By volume of total (international and domestic) air travelers:
    a. Ports of priority (>25 million air travelers per year) by this criterion not already listed in 1.a. are Phoenix, Denver, and Las Vegas.
    b. 78.8% arriving international air traveler coverage if Phoenix (0.7%), Denver (0.4%), and Las Vegas (0.4%)—which rank 5, 6, and 7, respectively, in traveler volume in North America—are added to those listed in 1.b. and 1.c.
    c. All ports identified in 1.a. are included in the top 30 ranked airports in traveler volume in North America.
    d. Nine of 10 DHHS regional offices (that is, all but Region VII office in Kansas City, MO) located in the ports identified in 1.a. and 2.a.

3. By volume of arriving international maritime travelers:
    a. Ports of priority (> 150,000 maritime travelers per year) in major U.S. cities not already listed in 1.a. and 2.a. are San Diego and New Orleans.
    b. Anchorage, AK . . . serves as the major city through which

400,000 travelers, many of whom are international, cruise (source: International Council of Cruise Lines) and participate in land tours in Alaska and the Yukon Territory; therefore, Anchorage is listed as a port of high priority.

   c. 80.1% arriving international air traveler coverage if San Diego (0.2%), New Orleans (number of international air travelers, 58,093 or 0.1%; source: New Orleans International Airport, 2002), and Anchorage (data not available from Anchorage International Airport but estimated to be less than 0.1%) are added to ports already listed.

4. By volume of arriving international travelers by land crossings:
   a. Ports of priority (>10 million land crossing travelers per year) in major U.S. cities between the United States and Mexico are San Diego and El Paso; San Diego is already described in 3.a.
   b. El Paso has international air traffic that contributes negligibly to the coverage of arriving international air travelers.
   c. Ports of U.S.–Canada land crossings are not considered.

5. By volume of arriving international wildlife shipments:
   a. Eleven (85%) of 13 ports of entry designated by the U.S. Fish and Wildlife Service for international shipments of wildlife are covered by the ports described in 1–4; Baltimore is indirectly covered as described in 1.c., but Portland, OR, is not covered.
   b. Six (38%) of 16 nondesignated ports of entry are covered by the ports described in 1–4; of the ports not covered, only Buffalo, NY, and Tampa, FL, are major cities.

6. Summary table

Port	Int'l Air >500,000/yr	Total Air >25 million/yr	Maritime >150,000/yr	Land > 10 million/yr	Wildlife*
Anchorage			X		X
Atlanta	X	X			X
Boston	X		X		X
Chicago	X	X			X
Dallas	X	X			X
Denver		X			
Detroit	X	X		X	X
El Paso				X	X
Honolulu	X		X		X
Houston	X	X	X		X
Las Vegas		X			
Los Angeles	X	X	X		X
Miami	X	X	X		X
Minneapolis	X	X			X
New Orleans			X		X
New York					
JFK	X	X	X		X
Newark	X	X			X
Orlando	X	X	X		
Philadelphia	X		X		
Phoenix		X			
San Diego			X	X	X
San Francisco	X	X	X		X
San Juan	X		X		
Seattle	X	X	X		X
Washington,					
D.C. (Dulles)	X				

*Designated and nondesignated ports of entry used by the U.S. Fish and Wildlife Service to receive international shipments of wildlife.

D

Commissioned Paper on U.S. Seaports and the CDC Quarantine Station System

Prepared by
Rex J. Edwards
April 4, 2005

SUMMARY AND CONCLUSIONS

The Centers for Disease Control and Prevention (CDC) has contracted with the Institute of Medicine (IOM) to conduct a study assessing the role of U.S. federal quarantine stations as a public health intervention at U.S. ports of entry. The assessment, titled Measures to Enhance the Effectiveness of the CDC Quarantine Station Expansion Plan for U.S. Ports of Entry, is being conducted in the context of numerous partners across sectors, jurisdictions, and national borders.

This paper examines the CDC quarantine station system (QSS) in the context of how it operates at U.S. seaports,[1] with emphasis on identifying differences from operations at U.S. airports where all the existing stations are. The information in this paper was gathered mostly through phone and e-mail interviews of personnel at individual QSS stations, federal regulatory or inspection agencies, the local port sector, and local or state health agencies, a summary of which is included in Table D.1.[2] This information was

---

[1]The term "seaport" applies to ports which handle ocean-going vessels, including those on the U.S. Great Lakes and ports on rivers (e.g., Portland on the Columbia River).

[2]The original statement of work anticipated interviewing a standard cross-section of QSS "partners" at a specified list of ports. The initial interviews indicated that knowledge of the QSS at the local level was very limited, as shown by the difficulty of finding port-level contacts that could comment on the system. This is probably a result of the relatively low frequency of incidents requiring QSS notification or response. Subsequently, the interview process was reoriented toward getting input at a national level for federal agencies and from as many local sources as possible without regard to port.

TABLE D.1 Organizations/Agencies Providing Information for Study

	CDC	CBP	Other Federal Agencies	Local/State Health	Port Industry
Atlanta	QS*	-Savannah -Atlanta (HDQ)		-GA Office of Public Health (State Epidemiologist)	-Port of Charleston (Port Director) -New Orleans Steamship Assn. -Maritime Endeavors Shipping
Chicago	QS	-Chicago*			
Los Angeles	QS	-Los Angeles	-USCG (Los Angeles)		
Miami	QS*				
New York	QS*		-USCG-New York (Marine Safety Office)	-City of New York (Health Dept.)	-Port of NY/NJ (Port of Commerce Dept.)
San Francisco	QS	-San Francisco (Agricultural Inspector)	-USCG (San Francisco)		
Seattle	QS	-Seattle		-King Co. Health Dept (Infectious Disease, Environmental Health Services)*	-Port of Portland
National	Vessel Sanitation Program		-USCG (National Vessel Movement Center) -USDA (Foreign Agricultural Service)		

Acronyms: QS = CDC Quarantine Station; CBP = DHS U.S. Customs and Border Protection, Department of Homeland Security (including legacy customs, immigration, and USDA inspection services); HDQ = Headquaters; USCG = DHS, U.S. Coast Guard
*Multiple contacts

supplemented with general information concerning the QSS and other federal agencies, information previously gathered by the IOM committee, and other secondary sources.

Overview of Results

The QSS was a significant presence at U.S. seaports until the 1960s, when foreign passenger travel shifted from sea to air transportation. The current system is oriented toward airports on the basis of priority of perceived threats (i.e., foreign visitors by air), the physical location of all stations at airports, the limited resources available to handle even the airport responsibilities, and most important, the infrequency of incidents at seaports. The current system at seaports is incident-driven and, in some cases, based on informal, ad hoc relationships; it is restricted by the lack of a physical presence and a lack of ability to train and interact with system "partners" over an array of ports that vary geographically and by type of activity. In some of the interviews, there was a perception that the QSS (or, more likely, "public health"), rather than a regulatory or inspection entity, was a resource to be called if there was a concern for the health of port personnel (public and private). In most respects, the scope of threats and the procedures for dealing with them are common to all ports of entry.

Similarities and Differences from Airport Environments

The primary differences between the airport and seaport systems are based on the following:

- Source of threats. The primary "human" threats at airports are foreign-origin travelers (and crew) with infectious diseases, mostly arriving from countries with specific disease outbreaks. At seaports, there is a limited level of international visiting passengers, so the human threats derive from returning U.S.-origin cruise passengers and the crews of both cruise and cargo vessels; the latter pose a greater threat because there is less scrutiny of ship sanitation and arrivals are from more distant ports of call. The number of cargo-related incidents at seaports is very limited in both number and scale, primarily since live animals and the other primary threats are more likely to move in small shipments via air.

- Operating environment. A seaport is a much more open environment than an airport and has higher levels and variety of international cargo and vessel activities. While cruise activity is concentrated at a limited number of U.S. ports and foreign ports of call, the market is expanding to secondary embarkation ports, many seasonal, and to more exotic foreign points (e.g., ecotourism). Over 100 U.S. ports handle import cargo, each with a unique combination of commodities, vessel types, and foreign trade routes. Cargo vessels may operate on a nonscheduled basis, spend weeks at sea, and call at a wide variety of foreign ports. Cargo vessel crews are typically non-English-speaking, their nationalities may be unrelated to the vessel's trade route, and crew members may be from countries susceptible to disease outbreaks. Unlike airplanes, vessels are typically boarded before they reach the dock and often before federal inspection.

• Federal agency partners. For the most part, the same federal agency partners apply to both the airport and port systems with the notable exception of the U.S. Coast Guard (USCG), which has primary responsibility for vessel safety within port areas, covering a range of areas (e.g., adequacy of manning and safety equipment). The USCG receives the "notice of arrival" required for all foreign-origin vessels. This document contains information related to vessel itinerary, crew, passengers, and hazardous cargoes that is provided to USCG and other federal personnel at local ports (although not regularly to the QSS). The QSS also works cooperatively with another CDC agency, the Vessel Sanitation Program (VSP), which has primary responsibility for dealing with gastrointestinal illness aboard cruise vessels. With no stations at ports, the QSS relies on agency partners for surveillance and immediate response activities at ports, although they are no different from those at airport "subports" (i.e., those without a station). This is particularly so for "complementary" agencies, such as the U.S. Department of Agriculture (USDA) and the Food and Drug Administration (FDA) that have similar regulatory responsibilities but may have a greater presence at seaports.

• Health sector partners. QSS relationships with local and state health agencies at seaports are basically the same and may be common to all CDC relationships, e.g., operating under memoranda of agreement (MOAs) with local hospitals. The infrequency of incidents at seaports results in little contact other than for (and sometimes including) the primary ports, many of which are those nearest the airport stations. The limited number of on-site medical staff (until recently, some airport stations had no medical officers) forces dependence on local medical personnel for immediate response for both airport and seaport subports.

• Private sector partners. Perhaps the greatest differences are based on a private sector that is more decentralized and varied than airports (which are dominated by the airlines and the airport authority, albeit with a limited number of supporting contractors). Most ocean carriers will not have any personnel in most ports of call, especially for the noncontainerized cargo industry. Local port activities are typically managed by a ship agent who may deal with a particular vessel or carrier only infrequently. Responsibility for cargo unloading and certain vessel services may fall to third parties with limited contact with or relationship to the vessel operator. The much wider variety and variability of activities, particularly on the cargo side, make it difficult to ensure that vessel captains and ship agents are aware of reporting requirements for sick or dead persons.

• Port authority partners. Like airport authorities, the port authorities vary similarly with airport authorities in jurisdictional control (e.g., local, state, and county) and structure (e.g., multiairport), although ports are more likely to have private terminals that are primarily controlled by single carriers or industrial users. (Airports often have third-party-operated cargo and other facilities, but mostly all within the airport "fence" with access controlled by the airport.) In some cases, ports are structured as "landlord ports" (as opposed to "operating ports"), and the port authority itself has few if any facilities but rather leases the land to private operators. These ports have less direct contact with vessel and cargo activities and hence less control and ability to act as a "clearinghouse" for information and cooperation.

General System

On the basis of interviews with QSS and its partner agencies, several general observations can be made regarding the existing system at U.S. seaports, including:

• The overall impression gained from the interviews was that the QSS has a very limited profile at individual seaports, even those where the station is at the local airport. Very few chronic incidents have had to be dealt with in recent years (as reported by QSS staff), so there has been little direct contact with QSS by port-level partners, and even less by the general port and health sectors.[3] The system could benefit from more "face time" between the QSS staff and the public and private sectors, particularly as the partner agencies are typically much larger and undergo frequent turnover and rotations (exacerbated by significant internal reorganization by these agencies after 9/11).

• A primary conclusion that resulted from the interviews was that the current system is ad hoc and incident-driven, mostly because there have been few notable incidents at just a few seaports and none of a chronic nature.

• A general impression was that the stations were stretched just to cover airport responsibilities, and much more to expand their port activities, particularly without any evident threats. The stations have operated

---

[3]The level of contact varied by station; higher levels of contact were seemingly driven by contacts related to airport activities that also apply to local seaports.

with as few as one full-time person in the past, and it is difficult to provide adequate training to agency partners unless there is a specific threat of high interest (e.g., SARS).

- Since the system is oriented toward airport threats, the assignment of seaports to the airport systems is geographically based, and individual stations cover wide ranges of both primary and "niche" ports, each with unique profiles of vessel, cruise, and cargo activity.

- A general impression was that the ad hoc identification system for infrequent incidents leads to inconsistent responses. Most communication was said to occur by telephone, probably because of the infrequency of incidents. The current QSS system mostly depends on a "referral" system whereby partners identify a threat and then communicate it to QSS, possibly through secondary means. There are a variety of ways that a threat could be communicated to QSS, but not necessarily a standard one, particularly in regard to USCG or postvoyage threats identified by local health officials.

- A general problem is that physical access to the vast array of ports and terminals is difficult in the post-9/11 environment. Different ports having different access standards and private terminals may have different rules for getting on-site when necessary.

- A response to an incident is based on various factors, including level of threat, timing, location, and involved partners. The level of a threat dictates the type of response, and other factors will determine the extent to which a "joint response" is used, as opposed to a primarily CDC response. Timing and the location of the threat (relative to the station location) are constraints that must be dealt with. A station might also have a postincident diagnostic or policy role. One respondent noted that a key role of the QSS is (or could be) a familiarity with seaport operations (not available to general health personnel) that may useful in handling postcontact situations or response strategies.[4]

Passenger and Crew Threats

- The primary source of information on possibly infectious passengers or crew members is the vessel itself, either directly or, more likely, via a ship agent, a cruise line's medical consultant, or even a partner agency. Ship captains and, by extension, the ocean carriers and their local agents are required by law and international regulations to notify the QSS of "quarantinable" illness on board, but it is unclear whether there is a stan-

---

[4]For example, one station noted that familiarity with the role of various crew members on a cruise ship would be useful in identifying possible on-board contacts.

dard notification procedure. There were various opinions on how this system works in practice; many stations thought it worked well, while others thought that many agents and captains were unaware of the requirements. Again, this may be a result of the infrequency of incidents, but in any case the vessel personnel must know what to look for, and there is no ability to inform them other than during crisis situations (e.g., SARS). In general, it was thought that the vessel crew have an interest in identifying infectious persons and do a good job of on-board isolation, but the responsibility for dealing with specific on-board situations will differ significantly by type of ship and trade route (beyond its being ultimately the captain's responsibility).

• Cruise vessels are much more scrutinized than cargo vessels in terms of on-board sanitation, particularly by CDC's VSP. Cargo crews are more likely to be on longer voyages from more disease-prone areas and living in cramped conditions.

• In general, it was thought unlikely that partner agencies would visually identify sick persons, although there were a variety of opinions as to whether partner agencies routinely checked for illness (as opposed to reporting self-identified disease). In particular, the USCG's vessel tracking system may collect sick crew or passenger information, but this information is not routinely processed by them at the national or local level. Training of partner agencies at subports is ad hoc and differs by port region.

• Port personnel in both the private and public sectors are concerned about infectious conditions with respect to their own health and may identify sick persons. During the period when SARS was of high concern, some pilots and longshoremen refused to board vessels. The QSS should have a public communication role in these situations, particularly as port safety may be affected, and there is the potential for a widespread shutdown of foreign trade if an outbreak were to occur.

• The stations' capability to make medical assessments at seaports is very limited, mostly because of the distance between airports and the covered seaports and the lack of 24-hour medical staffing. The stations rely primarily on local health agencies (including paramedics), although state agencies may have jurisdiction or be better able to deal with situations at smaller ports. The protocols for handling specific situations at all ports seemed to vary, again on the basis of the infrequency of occurrences. Some stations maintained direct contacts with local agencies or a database of health contacts and mentioned MOAs with quarantine-certified hospitals, although this may be a general CDC function. It may be possible to utilize medical staff available through federal partners (e.g., USCG).

• In terms of possible gaps or shortfalls in the system, no contact provided any high level of concern. The main concern involved the ability to train partner agencies and the shipping community.

Cargo Threats

- The scope of incidents from cargo at seaports is extremely limited and includes (1) the prohibition of certain live animals (e.g., African rodents, which are more likely to move by air) and (2) some cargo contamination (e.g., mosquito larvae in shipments of "Lucky" bamboo and used tires shipped exposed to standing water) and disease-carrying vessels (e.g., ships from South America with disease in their ballast water), each of which was diagnosed and dealt with on ad hoc basis. Some of the interviewees (including QSS personnel) could not recall a local incident related to cargo.
- The Department of Homeland Security (DHS) U.S. Customs and Border Protection (CBP) has primary responsibility for clearing all foreign-origin cargo entering the United States (through its legacy U.S. customs function) by all ports of entry. As with airports, the CBP may have authority to clear cargo for the CDC unless a shipment is suspicious, some on a routine basis (e.g., for frequent shipments of medical samples to local hospitals). This supporting role is greatest at ports with no local airport station.
- A potential source of contacts would be other agencies with responsibility for inspecting and holding cargo at the ports, most important the USDA (for live animals and "unprocessed" foods) and FDA (for food and drugs). These agencies typically have a much larger port presence, and USDA has their inspection personnel within CBP. The QSS or, more likely, the partner agency may identify a threat covered by another agency and then directly contact it. In the case of USDA, this may occur after CBP has referred an issue to its agricultural specialist, who then might contact the QSS.
- As in an airport situation, the QSS is responsible for dealing with any cargo that is refused entry under its jurisdiction, which may include destroying or reexporting the shipment or ensuring that the cargo is not hazardous.
- Most of the stations noted that they do not have access to CBP's Automated Manifest System (AMS), which contains all the relevant information necessary to clear the cargo (origin/destination, shipper/consignee, and commodity). Access would enable them to monitor certain commodities and perhaps identify patterns creating new threats, but there is also concern as to whether they would have the capability to use the system at the local level.
- One concern was that the protocols for contacting the QSS on the basis of AMS identifications of covered imports may not be clear. Another concern was that CBP requirements for documentation may not meet CDC's requirements when CBP is responsible for clearing shipments.
- There were no gaps or shortfalls that were otherwise identified regarding cargo transportation, although logically the greatest threat would

be cargoes that are unrelated to the responsibilities of complementary federal agencies (i.e., other than agricultural materials, live animals, food, and drugs).

In conclusion, the QSS has developed primarily as an airport system, most important in terms of where the stations are. The relative infrequency and limited severity of seaport incidents have resulted in an incident-driven ad hoc system that is almost entirely dependent on local port partners and, with respect to person-borne illnesses, mostly on a self-identified and referral basis.

A more expanded seaport role or the requirement to deal with new more expansive threats would require an increased local port presence at all subports, each of which may present a high level of risk. In particular, the QSS would need to develop better relationships with (1) the local port sector (port authority, carriers, and port service firms), (2) USCG because of its primary role for port safety, and (3) the relevant DHS partner agencies. Most important, the QSS would have to change the perception that it is merely a "public health" response option when there is a concern about infection (mostly as it applies to port personnel), rather than a partner agency for surveillance of and response to foreign-origin threats to the U.S. population.

The following section provides an overview of the QSS in terms of the general scope of the system's responsibilities relative to the seaport environment, contrasting activities with those at U.S. airports. The QSS at seaports is described in general terms relative to the overall sources of threats, activities for surveillance of and response to threats, current protocols and communication patterns, and potential gaps or areas for improvement. The general system is then described in detail for the three primary areas of coverage: (1) cruise passengers, (2) vessel crews, and (3) cargo imports.

GENERAL DESCRIPTION OF THE CDC QUARANTINE STATION SYSTEM (QSS) AT SEAPORTS

The CDC QSS aims to minimize the risk that microbial threats[5] of public health significance originating abroad will enter the United States through official ports of entry. Because of a dramatic reduction in the size and resources of the QSS in the 1970s and 1980s, the stations now rely heavily on partner agencies, especially CBP, to carry out their regulatory

---

[5]A microbial threat of public health significance causes serious or lethal human disease and is transmissible from person to person, from animal to person, or potentially either way; it also may be transmissible from food or water to people. Because of their potential for wide dispersal, concern is greatest for those microbes that spread readily from person to person.

responsibilities at the more than 280 ports of entry where CDC quarantine stations do not exist.

The QSS has the same jurisdiction over the persons and cargo on vessels as on aircraft:

> Whenever the Director has reason to believe that any arriving person is infected with or has been exposed to any of the communicable diseases . . . , he/she may detain, isolate, or place the person under surveillance and may order disinfection or disinfestation as he/she considers necessary to prevent the introduction, transmission, or spread of the listed communicable diseases. (per 42 CFR Part 71.32). The communicable diseases include cholera, diphtheria, infectious TB, plague, smallpox, yellow fever, viral hemorrhagic fevers and SARS (per Executive Order 13295).

In general terms, the QSS (including both CDC and its federal partner agencies) is responsible for the surveillance of and response to communicable disease threats that could enter via U.S. seaports. Surveillance activities include specifying the scope of existing and emerging threats and identifying specific threats that might enter via a seaport. Response activities include isolating and assessing specific threats, preventing threats from entering the country (until safe), and taking (or stimulating) actions to eliminate threats (including hospitalization or quarantine of persons or re-export of cargo) and mitigate the impact of threats (identifying contacts).

In most respects, the scope of threats and the procedures for dealing with them are common to all ports of entry. The primary differences between the airport and seaport systems are related to the sources of threats, the operating environment, and the roles of and communication with various public and private partners.

Source of Threats

The QSS covers any person or cargo item arriving on a vessel from a foreign port, including cruise and other passengers, imported cargoes and personal items, crew members on cruise or cargo vessels, and illegal aliens (including stowaways).

Cruise Passengers

The majority of foreign-origin passengers that enter U.S. seaports arrive via cruise vessels, most of them originating and terminating at a U.S. port on voyages ranging from a few hours ("day cruises") to 2 weeks or more. Some passengers arrive on cargo vessels, but there are no substantial differences from cruise passengers. Similarly, passengers who arrive from

Canada or Mexico on passenger ferries receive the same coverage by the QSS. The multiday-cruise industry (which is the highest priority in terms of infectious disease) is defined by a combination of:

- Vessel type as determined by technology and passengers' comfort wishes (e.g., luxury or sailing).
- Destination market(s)—mostly foreign ports of call that are of interest to cruise visitors and can be reached within standard voyage lengths (mostly 7 days).
- U.S. embarkation port—based on location relative to large population bases and ability to access via air, as well as the ability to accommodate the vessels.

There were 184 vessels serving the U.S. cruise market in 2003.[6] Cruise vessels can vary from relatively small specialty vessels (e.g., Windjammer sailing vessels) to enormous vessels carrying almost 4,000 persons (e.g., the *Queen Mary* with 2,620 passengers and a crew of 1,253). The typical vessel carries 2,000 passengers and a crew of 950, creating a large processing problem at U.S. ports on the return voyages.

The U.S. cruise industry is oriented mostly toward the Caribbean and Southern California markets, which allow year-round sailing as shown in Table D.2. Vessels from Florida ports—led by Miami, Port Everglades, and Port Canaveral—sail primarily to Caribbean and Mexican Gulf Coast points. These three ports accounted for nearly two-thirds of total U.S cruise passengers in 2003. The Southern California ports serve both the west coast of Mexico and Hawaii (which is not covered by the QSS). Other cruise markets include summer sailings to Alaska, New England, and Great Lakes points and multiweek itineraries (e.g., Panama Canal or trans-Atlantic).

In recent years, the originating ports for Caribbean and Gulf of Mexico cruises have expanded to include Galveston, New Orleans, and New York. This trend is expected to continue as the primary ports become more congested and new ports expand or emerge to handle local passengers or new itineraries.

Of potential interest for this study is the emergence of nontraditional foreign ports of call (particularly oriented toward ecotourism) that might create exposure to more remote areas.

---

[6]Source: International Council of Cruise Lines.

TABLE D.2   2002-2003 Cruise Passengers at U.S. Ports

Ports	2002	2003	% of Total	Annual Growth
Florida (MIA)				
Miami	1,804,000	1,965,000	26%	9%
Port Everglades	1,202,000	1,213,000	16%	1%
Port Canaveral	1,028,000	1,089,000	15%	6%
Tampa	317,000	409,000	6%	29%
San Juan	298,000	325,000	4%	9%
	4,649,000	*5,001,000*	*67%*	*8%*
Southern California/Texas (LAX)				
Los Angeles	538,000	403,000	5%	-25%
Galveston	267,000	377,000	5%	41%
Long Beach	n/a	272,000	0%	n/a
San Diego	138,000	81,000	1%	-41%
Houston	6,500	15,000	0%	131%
	949,500	*1,148,000*	*15%*	*21%*
North Atlantic (JFK)				
New York	326,000	438,000	6%	34%
Boston	69,000	69,000	1%	0%
Baltimore	57,000	57,000	1%	0%
Philadelphia	1,500	24,000	0%	1500%
	453,000	*588,000*	*8%*	*30%*
Pacific Northwest (SEA)				
Seattle	118,000	158,000	2%	34%
Seward	151,000	147,000	2%	-3%
	269,000	*305,000*	*4%*	*13%*
Other U.S.				
New Orleans (ATL)	245,000	288,000	4%	18%
San Francisco (SFO)	32,000	51,000	1%	59%
All Other	32,000	51,000	1%	59%
United States	6,630,000	7,432,000	100%	12%

SOURCE: The Cruise Industry (2003 Economic Summary), International Council of Cruise Lines.

Cargo Imports

The United States is the world's largest import market, accepting a wide variety of basic commodities, agricultural products, and consumer goods from almost every country in the world. A vast majority of the import trade (as measured by weight) from overseas origins (excluding transborder NAFTA trade) arrives on oceangoing vessels.

The key characteristics associated with oceanborne import trade include:

• Vessel type. Includes large vessels carrying single commodities in bulk (e.g., petroleum, grains, and ores), general cargo vessels carrying mixed commodities either loose or on pallets, and container vessels with mixed commodities carried in standard marine containers that are sealed at origin and delivered unopened to the consignee (unless inspected). Most vessels have crews of about 20, with more on older vessels and vessels with more onboard equipment and fewer on vessels with expensive U.S. crews.

• Service type. The majority of liquid and dry bulk vessels operate on irregular schedules and have itineraries between a single origin and destination port, often on a voyage charter basis (i.e., a vessel is leased for a limited number of voyages). Liner services (including most container services and some single-commodity trades, such as fruit) serve multiple shippers and use a rotation of vessels on a fixed-day schedule between selected ports in the United States and a single world area.[7] Nonliner services, mostly limited to minor U.S. trade routes or certain commodity types, offer service between a general range of ports on a variable schedule, often calling on an inducement basis (i.e., based on a single shipper).

• Cargo handling. Port activities are determined by the type of vessel and commodity. Vessels typically must use a designated terminal, often waiting at anchorage until a berth is available. Tankers and dry bulk vessels use bulk terminals that have free-flow equipment to quickly discharge cargoes into large tanks, grain elevators, or even open areas. These are often private terminals owned and operated by a single company and may be part of an industrial facility (e.g., a petrochemical plant). Most container vessels, particularly on the major East-West trades, use container terminals with large cranes for transferring containers to storage yards or directly to rail or truck. These terminals may be operated by an ocean carrier or a third party, possibly the port itself. General cargo vessels (including automobile vessels) use general cargo terminals that have cranes and ramps to lift or roll cargo to a warehouse or storage area. These terminals may be designated for a

---

[7]The exceptions are round-the-world services that combine multiple trade routes in a single voyage, typically to avoid operating both ways in an imbalanced trade.

particular commodity (e.g., coffee or bananas) and are often owned by the port because of the diversity of carriers and commodities.

The key factors relevant to the QSS include:

- Commodities handled (in terms of being a threat).
- Foreign ports of call (in terms of period of incubation during the voyage, contagious crew, or possible introduction of illegal substances).
- Length and location of U.S. port of call (in terms of ability to inspect and identify threats).

Foreign-Origin Vessel Activity

All vessels entering a port require crew to operate at sea and in port, typically designated as officers, engine room, deck, and steward. Cargo vessels carry crew only for en route operations, using stevedores and longshoremen for cargo handling in port. Most cargo vessel crews are foreign; European or even American officers are usually coupled with crews from Third World countries. Cruise vessels require substantially larger crews, primarily for passenger services, and can average one crew member for every two passengers.

Seaports may also have foreign-origin vessels that are unrelated to either passenger or cargo transportation, including:

- Fishing vessels.
- Vessels calling for repairs, supplies, or inspection.
- Foreign military and other government vessels.
- Offshore oil-rig transfer vessels.
- Illegal alien or refugee vessels.

To the extent that individuals disembark these vessels, they interact with the QSS in ways similar to those of persons from cargo or passenger vessels. Any significant issues specific to these vessel types will be discussed in later sections.

The key factors relative to the QSS are the size and composition of the crew, the living conditions, the voyage length, and the location of origin ports. In addition to possible threats associated with vessel crews, there is a threat associated with the vessel itself. In an example provided below, cholera was arriving from South America in vessels' ballast water (water carried in the vessel hold).

Similarities to and Differences from Airport Environments

A primary objective of this paper is to explore how the seaport environment for the QSS differs from the airport or land port environment. In many respects, there are common elements that would apply regardless of how a particular person or commodity enters the country. No particular difference in the scope of infectious diseases is based on the type of port, other than that each type (or a specific port) deals with a unique mix of foreign origins and types of passengers or cargo, which thereby determines a port's "sources" and level of threats.

The general procedures for identifying and responding to particular threats should be common to all situations regardless of whether they are of foreign origin and regardless of which type of port is involved. The primary differences are based on the physical environment in which activities occur and the entities that must be dealt with. One difference is that there are no QSS stations at seaports; each seaport is covered by an airport facility as a subport. In reality, this is of minor significance to this study because there is little difference between handling a remote airport and handling a remote seaport. The problems of distance and access do not differ by environment.

The following contrasts in general terms the seaport environment with the airport environment, where all the current stations are:

- The number of seaports that handle significant amounts of import cargo is significantly higher than the number of airports that do so. In the case of airports, the top international gateways (New York, Chicago, Los Angeles, and Miami) handle the vast majority of inbound activity; secondary gateways have few daily flights. The QSS stations must handle a wider geographic range of ports, each with a unique profile.

- Seaports handle much more diversified import cargo activities than airports, which mostly handle containerized cargoes on a small number of passenger aircraft and all cargo aircraft. Major ports handle a variety of bulk, container, and general cargo vessels at public and private terminals on either a scheduled or irregular basis. Even small ports can handle a wide range of vessels and cargoes, often on a single-voyage or irregular basis.

- Most air cargoes have high value and are treated as such; many ocean cargoes are of low value and are moving to fill backhaul capacity (e.g., used tires or waste paper). Vessel crews, the majority of which in U.S. trades are now foreign, typically include low-paid deck crew from Third World countries who don't speak English. The living conditions (and points of origin) of vessel crews can't match those of an airplane and must be experienced for many weeks. Crew changes can occur en route during an ocean voyage.

- The volume of persons and cargo discharged from a vessel greatly surpasses that of a single airplane. Cruise vessels can disembark up to 4,000 persons at a time compared with over 400 for the largest airplane. A cruise vessel's crew can exceed 1,000, whereas a cargo vessel's typically is 20 or more. Cargo vessels discharge hundreds of thousands of tons compared with hundreds of thousands of pounds for all-cargo aircraft. The new megacontainerships will discharge several thousand containers at a port compared with dozens of much smaller containers at an airport. A refrigerated ship will discharge several hundred truckloads of bananas compared with a single pallet of fruit (if that) at an airport.

- Ports are much more "open" environments than airports, which have a distinct area "within the fence." Many ports cover large waterfront areas, some of which may have private facilities on private property, often covered by the owner's security and having private gates. There is no fence protecting the wharves on the waterfront side and there may be harbor access by personal and other noncommercial vessels.[8]
- The nature of an ocean voyage results in some unique sources of threats, including stowaways and illegal aliens or refugees. In terms of the QSS, the relatively long sea trips (10-20 days from China to New York) allow for more preparation and evaluation, but they can also result in en route contamination of cargo or the incubation of disease in crews. Vessels can stop at a number of foreign ports during a voyage, including some that are unscheduled. While vessels are required to give notice of arrival, arrival times can vary widely (compared with those of airlines), affecting the ability to schedule inspections. And vessels are often detained for several days for a variety of reasons.
- A vessel may be held outside a port for some time, during which interactions with shore-based personnel can occur.

In terms of the specific environment for the QSS, the most significant differences involve the entities that must be dealt with in surveillance and response. Whereas the Federal Aviation Administration (FAA) is responsible for aircraft landing at airports, inbound vessels are regulated and controlled mostly by USCG, which deals with the vast array of vessels and operating patterns. In terms of federal "partners" for surveillance, the agencies operating at airports (e.g., DHS) have the same responsibilities at seaports and additional responsibilities for vessel inspection and safety handled by CDC and USCG. The role of local and state health agencies in responding to (or even identifying) threats is basically the same, other than the location and hence the jurisdictional coverage.

A primary difference involves the authorities that own or operate ports and airports and the industries or public entities involved in port opera-

---

[8]Since 9/11, there has been a significant increase in port security, including policing of private terminal gates and designation of harbor and port areas that are off limits to the public.

tions. Like airports, port authorities are typically public or quasipublic (e.g., an independent nongovernment group appointed by public officials). Public ports can be run by cities, countries, states, or regional groups, sometimes combining multiple ports under a single authority. (Some port authorities combine airports and ports under a single authority, although each is managed separately.) Although airports often have private facilities, the scope of private and public activities at ports affects their operations more significantly. Some ports are "landlord" ports that only administer the port and lease land to private operations, as opposed to "operating" ports that own and operate public terminals and hence are more involved with port operations. This affects the ability of the QSS to design standard systems to deal with widely divergent port structures, particularly in gaining access to port facilities and wharf areas and interacting with the "port industry" through the port authority.

Most port activities involve a more diverse set of private firms than does an airport, where international air carriers will have staff at the airport to handle most functions. Except at primary ports for large liner operators, most carriers do not have local employees but rather use ship agents to manage their port calls and other local activities.[9] Most vessel-related activities are contracted out to a variety of local companies or port agencies, including ship pilotage, vessel supply, inspection, and repairs. Cargo handling (and other services) may occur at a public or private terminal, the latter are operated by a major carrier or a third party. Cruise lines follow patterns similar to those of cargo vessels but may conduct more activities in house wherever a vessel is "home-ported" (e.g., its primary port of U.S. embarkation), particularly when multiple vessels or day cruises are involved.

Again, the general functions of port operations for persons and cargo are not significantly different from those of an airport, but the vast variety and irregularity affect the ability to design standard systems to monitor and interact with them. The next section describes the general structure of the QSS as it applies as seaports.

CURRENT OPERATING ENVIRONMENT OF CDC QSS AT SEAPORTS

Coverage of U.S. Seaports by QSS

The QSS stations are all at airports but have seaport responsibilities that can span multiple coasts (including offshore) and combine a vast vari-

---

[9]Some operations by international airlines may be contracted to a third party at some airports, but operations are generally limited to one or two fixed based operators and single daily flights.

ety of activities. A port's activity profile is dictated primarily by its location relative to domestic and international markets. Cruise ports provide good access to both desirable destination markets (i.e., they are reachable within limited voyage time) and U.S. population centers; some variation is based on seasonal markets and the desire to have embarkation points closer to major U.S. cities. Cargo ports for imports provide efficient links between foreign-origin markets and U.S. consumption points, which include major metropolitan areas for consumer products or industrial facilities for base or intermediate commodities. The QSS must cover over a 100 U.S. ports that handle import cargo, including 50 that handled containerized cargo in 2003 and over 20 with cruise line operations. The U.S. seaport coverage by quarantine stations is summarized in Table D.3.

The general role of the ports in each port range can summarized as follows:

• Atlanta (South Atlantic and East Gulf): Gulf ports typically involve industrial bulk cargo activity in support of petroleum and chemical production and transfer of bulk commodities to the Mississippi River barge system. Charleston and Savannah are the top container ports for the southeastern United States and are excellent gateways to the U.S. Southeast for East-West trade (e.g., U.S.-Europe and U.S.-Asia). New Orleans is the primary East Gulf container port for general cargoes, and Gulfport is a regional import center for containerized bananas and other fruit. Wilmington (NC), Mobile, and Lake Charles handle containers mostly for local markets. New Orleans is the only significant cruise port.

• Chicago (Great Lakes): Because of long travel distances required to reach ocean trade lanes, the U.S. Great Lakes ports are mostly limited to bulk commodities destined for local industrial facilities. (The Port of Montreal does handle containers for the U.S. Midwest, based on good rail connections.) There are 20 Great Lakes ports in the top 100 U.S. import ports (as measured by weight), many of which are dedicated to a single commodity or terminal. Cruise lines operate on the Great Lakes during the summer, but they mostly call at other Great Lakes ports if at all (beyond the origin port).

• Honolulu (Hawaii): Hawaiian ports serve the local Hawaii market including U.S. domestic and foreign cargo and cruise services. (The Hawaii station was not covered in the interviews because of the difficulty of telephone contact.)

• Los Angeles (Southern California and Texas Gulf): The station located at LAX airport covers both Southern California and Texas Gulf ports. The Ports of Los Angeles and Long Beach are the largest U.S. container ports, serving both the large local market and inland markets via rail and truck intermodal services. The Port of Houston is the largest West Gulf

TABLE D.3 Seaport Coverage by CDC Quarantine Station

Station Location	Geographic Coverage	Cruise	Container	General Cargo
Atlanta	South Atlantic (excluding Florida) East Gulf (to Texas)	New Orleans (9)	Charleston (6) Savannah (9)	So. Louisiana Pt. (7) Lake Charles (9)
Chicago	Great Lakes	Minor seasonal	Minor via U.S. ports	Toledo (38) Detroit (42)
Honolulu	Hawaii	Not originating location	Honolulu (13) Kahului (26)	Honolulu (34) Barbers Pt. (51)
Los Angeles	Southern California Texas	Los Angeles (6) Galveston (7) Long Beach (9)	Los Angeles (1) Long Beach (2) Houston (11)	Houston (1) Beaumont (2) Long Beach (6)
Miami	Florida, Puerto Rico, U.S. Virgin Islands	Miami (1) Port Everglades (2)	San Juan (7) Miami (12)	Jacksonville (26) Tampa (27)
New York	North Atlantic (to Virginia)	New York (4) Boston (14)	New York (3) Hampton Rds. (8)	Port of New York/New Jersey (2) Portland, Maine (10)
San Francisco	Northern California	San Francisco (16)	Oakland (4) San Francisco (38)	Richmond (25) Oakland (39)
Seattle	Pacific Northwest Alaska	Seattle (11) Seward (12)	Tacoma (5) Seattle (10)	Seattle (30) Tacoma (32)

SOURCES: Tables D.2, D.5, and D.6.

container port serving the Texas and Oklahoma markets. Houston is the world's largest petrochemical center and generates a significant amount of foreign bulk cargo in both directions. Other West Gulf ports generate similar flows of industrial stock commodities, as do Los Angeles and Long Beach. San Diego and Port Hueneme are "niche" ports in Southern California, specializing in fruit and automobile imports. Los Angeles is the largest West Coast cruise port serving both Mexican and Hawaiian destinations, although Galveston, Long Beach, and San Diego- have emerged as new embarkation points.

- Miami (Florida, Puerto Rico, and U.S. Virgin Islands): The Port of Miami, like Miami Airport, is the cargo gateway to Latin America for both containerized and general cargo. Miami has also been the leading cruise port for many years, although other ports have worked to attract this market. Port Everglades is a competing port for both container and cruise business, and Jacksonville and Tampa are the top bulk ports. Port Manatee is a niche port for inbound and outbound fruit, and Palm Beach serves the Caribbean cruise and cargo markets. San Juan is a large cruise and container port in the Caribbean that is also covered by the Miami station, as are the U.S. Virgin Islands.

- New York (North Atlantic): The station at JFK international airport covers an area reaching from Maine to North Carolina, including ports of many sizes and activities. The Port of New York and New Jersey encompasses six terminal locations serving a wide range of cruise and cargo needs for the large New York metropolitan markets and inland destinations. Philadelphia, Baltimore, and Hampton Roads are all large international container ports and also serve other local needs, and smaller container operations are at Boston (based on barge transfers from New York), Wilmington (bananas and other fruit), Richmond, Portland (ME), and Albany. New York is the top cruise port offering seasonal voyages (mostly to Bermuda), and Boston, Philadelphia, Baltimore, and even Alexandria (VA) also offer some summer departures. The New York harbor includes a number of petroleum and chemical terminals that attract bulk commodities, as do 20 other ports in the station's range.

- San Francisco (Northern California): The San Francisco station covers the Ports of San Francisco and Oakland and other ports of San Francisco Bay and on the waterway all the way to Sacramento, which serves the central California agricultural markets, mostly outbound. Oakland is the primary container port serving both local and inland intermodal markets. San Francisco is the only cruise port providing U.S. and Canadian coastal services and serving as a port of call for cruises originating elsewhere. The San Francisco harbor contains a number of bulk terminals.

- Seattle (Pacific Northwest and Alaska): The Ports of Seattle and Tacoma are major U.S. container ports serving both the local and inland intermodal markets; they are the U.S. North American ports closest to Asia. Portland is also a major container port, and Anchorage handles U.S. origin and destination containers for the local market. Seattle and Seward are the top originating cruise ports for U.S.-Alaska services, but other ports, such as Bellingham, provide ferry services to Canada. The primary bulk terminals are at Seattle, Tacoma, and Portland, but a number of terminals are at smaller ports on the Oregon coast, the Columbia River, and Puget Sound.

General Overview of QSS Operations at Seaports

The QSS stations are responsible for surveillance of and response to infectious disease threats that might enter U.S. seaports via persons, cargo, or related transportation equipment or packaging (e.g., pallets). The following general information about the current system was developed from interviews with QSS personnel and members of their "partner" agencies and a review of secondary sources describing the agencies. The location of all QSS stations at airports and the manpower available to cover a wide geographic region require that most seaport activity must be conducted with surrogate agencies that have an active presence at the "subports" (i.e., airports or ports that don't have colocated stations). These partners are summarized in Table D.4.

The general activities required by the QSS include surveillance of and response to threats. Surveillance involves identifying what the threats are (or may be) and then identifying specific threats by inspection or other means. Response activities include analyzing and isolating a threat, devising a strategy to deal with a specific incident (including possible exposure of other persons), monitoring the threat, and possibly devising a long-term strategy or policy.

The following summarizes the general role of each partner in the QSS:

• CDC: The primary responsibility for keeping the specified threats from entering via a specific U.S. port resides with the QSS stations. The QSS headquarters in Atlanta is responsible for assisting the individual stations; facilitating the flow of information to, from, and between stations; specifying and analyzing threats; and training CBP personnel (according to one respondent). The VSP is responsible for dealing with gastrointestinal illness on cruise vessels calling at the U.S. ports. The VSP cooperates with and assists QSS with cruise-related incidents (and vice versa).

• DHS: DHS now incorporates most of the inspection functions related to foreign-origin persons, cargoes, and vessels. Processing and inspection of persons are carried out by U.S. Citizenship and Immigration Services, clearance of cargo by CBP, agriculture-related review by the Animal and Plant Health Inspection Service (APHIS) (formerly in USDA), and ves-

TABLE D.4 Partners in CDC Quarantine Station System at Seaports

	Persons	Cargo
CDC		
Quarantine Station System	S, R[a]	S, R
Vessel Sanitation Program	S	
Headquarters	S, R	S, R
Department of Homeland Security		
U.S. Customs and Border Protection		S
U.S. Citizenship and Immigration Services	S, R	
Animal and Plant Health Inspection Service		S, R
U.S. Coast Guard	S, R	
Other federal agencies		
U.S. Department of Agriculture		S, R
U.S. Fish and Wildlife Service		S
Food and Drug Administration		S, R
National Marines Fisheries		S, R
Port sector		
Port authority	S, R	S, R
Ocean carrier	S, R	S, R
Port services	S, R	S, R
Health sector		
Local and regional hospitals	S, R	
Local and state health agencies	S, R	

[a]S = Surveillance; R = Response

sels entering U.S. ports by USCG. In the interviews, most people generally referred to all the agencies as "CBP" except for USCG—a convention that will be used in the discussion.

• Other federal agencies: In their various regulatory roles, certain agencies operate at seaports and may identify situations requiring QSS intervention and act cooperatively or provide support. USDA, in its general role of protecting U.S. agriculture, operates quarantine and veterinary services at ports, as well as maintaining overseas surveillance. FDA is responsible for protecting the U.S. food and drug supply from foreign threats, and U.S. Fish and Wildlife and National Marine Fisheries operate at ports mostly to prevent importation of restricted wildlife or marine animals.

• Port sector: The primary role that the port sector has in this system is in identifying threats (particularly sick passengers or crew) and cooperating to deal with them.

• Health sector: The primary role of the health sector is to provide support in evaluating, analyzing, and treating incidents where QSS personnel are not available; working with QSS to prevent exposure; and identifying postvoyage threats that become manifest through contacts with local hospitals or doctors.

General Comments on Overall System

As stated above, the general scope of threats covered by seaports is very similar to that of airports, although on a more limited scale for passenger operations (because volumes from problem countries are lower), and for cargo activity (because levels of live "problem" animals are lower). The overall impression gained from the interviews was that the QSS has a very limited profile at individual seaports, even where the station is at a local airport. Very few chronic incidents have had to be dealt with in recent years (as reported by QSS staff), so there has been little direct contact with port-level partners by QSS and much less with the general port and health sectors. The main exceptions appear to result from areas where interaction on airport issues also covers nearby seaports.

In recent times, the only exception was the SARS crisis, which resulted in some training and local concerns over possible infection of ship pilots, longshoremen, and federal partner personnel. A higher level of interaction between the QSS and the ports was reported, but it was not uniform. (A CBP officer at a West Coast port that would have had substantial traffic from problem areas reported that not much happened at that port.)

A primary conclusion that resulted from the interviews was that the current system is ad hoc and incident-driven, mostly because there have been few notable incidents at just a few seaports and no chronic ones. A general impression was that the stations were stretched just to cover airport responsibilities, let alone expand their port activities, particularly without any evident threats. Low staffing affects the ability to deal with multiple or off-hour incidents, particularly in an environment with no consistent peaks. Ports or port ranges having a dominant type of activity may limit coverage of secondary activities (e.g., cruise vs. cargo, or container vs. breakbulk). A general disadvantage of not having a local presence is the inability to conduct regular training or to react faster, particularly during off hours.

General Comments on Surveillance

The current QSS system mostly depends on a "referral" system whereby partners identify a threat and then communicate it to QSS, possibly through secondary means (e.g., via headquarters). There are a variety of ways that a threat could be communicated to the QSS. Each station must notify headquarters of all incidents of significance, and they are then reported in the Daily Incident Report and reviewed by all stations. High-level threats may result in direct contact between stations. A local health agency might contact headquarters about a patient who had disembarked from a station's port, and information might be communicated to the local station.

Similarly, other federal agencies, many of which have much higher staffing at subports, may identify a situation in the course of their own duties and communicate it to the local quarantine station. Several of the respondents referred to the service as "public health" and summarized the program by saying that they would call public health if there were a suspicion of infectious disease, often because of concerns for industry or agency personnel. A primary source of information on sick or dead persons aboard ship are the vessels themselves, either directly or via a ship agent or other carrier representative. There may be multiple sources identifying threats, but the low level of incidents suggested that there may be gaps in the system; at the very least, the protocols for notification may not be standardized unless there is a specific concern.

The "general" problem most frequently mentioned by QSS personnel (and somewhat reinforced by the lack of awareness at subports) was that the lack of personnel and funds limited personal interactions ("face time") and training of partners at the subport level. There is a great imbalance between QSS's staffing and that of its agency partners. It is difficult to maintain personal relationships because of high turnover or rotations of personnel (e.g., every 1-2 years for USCG) and the sheer size of some agencies (e.g., CBP has hundreds of employees at certain ports). One QSS contact said he/she tried to visit every subport at least once per year; others indicated that they didn't have the time, manpower, or money to visit any. The problem is exacerbated by the significant restructuring of federal inspection services after 9/11.

Another general problem is that physical access to the vast array of ports and terminals is difficult in the post-9/11 environment. Different ports having different access standards and private terminals may have different rules for getting on-site when necessary (e.g., some require a port badge, and others require being on a list or contacting the ship agent or CBP).

There was a general sense that stations needed to become more involved with general security efforts at the port level, but again, each port has a different structure and set of players. Some of the stations maintained relationships with local port groups (e.g., security committees), but it was typically only for the port near the station or the largest covered port for a station.

General Comments on Response

A response to an incident is based on several factors: level of threat, timing, location, and involved partners. The level of threat dictates the type of response, and other factors will determine the extent to which a "joint response" is used, as opposed to a primarily CDC response. Timing and location (relative to the station location) are constraints that must be dealt with. Several contacts noted that it may take a long time just to get to various parts of a single port, let alone to a port that is far from the airport station. The QSS, often in consultation with headquarters and other partners, will evaluate, provide guidance, and resolve situations.

A station might also have a postincident diagnostic or policy role. For example, there were indications that South American cholera was entering the country via ships. In cooperation with other agencies (including vessel inspections), it was concluded that the disease was being carried in the ship's ballast (water carried for weight), which resulted in a requirement that ballast water be flushed three times before U.S. port entry. (It was unclear whether this was accomplished at the local level or at headquarters.)

The role of local and state health authorities and providers appeared no different from what would apply for nonlocal airports. The QSS mostly depends on local and state health personnel to deal directly with illness. They can't get to all points in a timely fashion, sometimes not even for a local port. Until recently, some stations did not have the expertise of medical officers. Local or state health authorities appear to respond easily when called, based on their responsibility once a threat clears the port. One respondent indicated having boarded vessels in the past with no problems.

One QSS respondent noted that a key role of the QSS is to provide an understanding of seaport operations not available to local health personnel. For example, one station noted that familiarity with crew positions may be useful in identifying on-board contact situations or in diagnosing a problem.

General Comments on Protocols and Communications and on Potential Gaps

A general impression was that the ad hoc identification procedures used for infrequent incidents leads to inconsistent responses. One QSS contact was concerned that national-level contact with CBP may not filter down to the local level. Most communication was said to occur by telephone, probably because of the infrequency of incidents. Two respondents indicated that when multiple parts of CDC (or other agencies) are involved, communication between the groups had been a problem; another noted that getting information to local health authorities was once complicated by the communications route (e.g., local QSS to state to local health). This was characterized as an unwillingness of the federal agencies to share information on a timely basis.

One respondent noted that local (or state) health agencies technically do not have jurisdiction at international ports (or airports), although they have responsibility once a person or cargo leaves the port. It has not been a problem, but the lack of formal protocols and agreements in a crisis situation might pose a problem, although there have been draft protocols in the past and one local health agency indicated it was working on a generic protocol with CDC. One concern was that it was unclear whether anyone could hold a ship thought to be a threat.

The participation in industry and multiagency forums where ideas could be exchanged varied by station, but there was a sense that this might be appropriate for an expanded system. Some stations met regularly with groups of related port agencies, first responders, and local and state health participants. It depended mostly on the location of the port, particularly if the airport had a port partner. One station suggested protocols to increase "face time" with federal and military partners.

CDC QSS AT SEAPORTS: PASSENGER AND CREW TRANSPORTATION

General Overview

The primary source of threats was thought to be vessel crews because they are more likely to get sick as a result of cramped living quarters. Cargo-vessel crews are more likely to get sick than cruise-vessel crews, which have better crew conditions and more scrutiny of sanitation and are required to have a medical officer on board. Cargo vessels are also more likely to originate in ports that have infection problems.

An associated problem is that cruise passengers often purchase restricted items overseas (knowingly or unknowingly), but that is covered under CBP clearance procedures for passengers. Similarly, illegal aliens and stowaways may present special problems or increased threats but similarly are handled with general procedures.

A central point made by many of the respondents was that the primary reason to call "public health" was not regulatory, but rather a concern by agency or industry personnel about personal exposure to infectious people. The following describes the roles, protocols, and communications for each of the partners in surveillance of and response to passenger and crew threats.

Vessel Captain, Agent, or Operator

The tradition of flying the yellow flag of quarantine on incoming vessels dates back centuries and is, in fact, the basis of the flag of the U.S. Public Health Service, which was started to deal with seaborne infectious diseases. By international health regulations, ships are responsible for contacting a port of entry with "quarantinable" illnesses, even if just sitting at anchorage (i.e., moored in a harbor). There was some dispute as to how this works; others cited USCG or CBP requirements. Some respondents thought it worked well and that the stations worked in primary ports to keep vessel operators and their agents informed; another station said only the old-timers who remember the 1960s were vigilant. One respondent noted that the shipping industry may be reluctant to accept additional security and scrutiny beyond what has occurred after 9/11.

In practice, the contact with the QSS is usually made by the ship agent unless there are local carrier personnel. The ship agents are responsible for reminding captains (via "Dear Captain" letters) of their responsibilities. A possible shortfall in this system is that it depends on captains knowing exactly what to report and to whom.

Cruise vessels are more likely to report incidents because they deal with the same set of ports over time and are more sensitive to infectious persons. Cruise ships (with 13 or more passengers) are required to have a medical officer on board and have strict guidelines for reporting gastrointestinal illnesses to the CDC's VSP, which monitors medical records and procedures very closely. An incident on a cruise vessel might be reported directly from the ship or by a ship agent but more likely by the cruise line's crew or passenger medical consultant at its home office.

There was some dispute as to whether sick crew needed to be reported in the "Notice of Arrival" that is required to be filed with USCG 96 hours before entry at a U.S. port.

In reality, vessel operators and crews are likely to be responsible with regard to possibly infectious individuals. Most operators (and their crews) don't like it when crew members are sick or take medication on board, and they are generally good at isolating crew on board. The responsibility for dealing with specific on-board situations will differ significantly by type of ship and trade route (beyond its being ultimately the captain's responsibility). Major container lines may handle medical situations at sea via corporate headquarters, and small single-voyage vessels may be the responsibility of a ship agent at a destination port. (Several stations mentioned that they have used a ship agent's doctor to respond to situations, presumably someone called by the ship agent because they did not have in-house medical staff.)

CDC

CDC's role in identifying and responding to human health risks at seaports includes the following:

- QSS: Responsible for nongastrointestinal infectious diseases on cruise vessels and all infectious diseases on other foreign-origin vessels using various port partners.

- Headquarters: Provides support to stations by identifying and communicating threat information, assisting in a response with specialists and consultation, interacting with foreign governments, providing general training to partners at a national level, and dealing with issues concerning illegals and refugees.
- VSP: Responsible for all gastrointestinal diseases on board cruise vessels and works cooperatively with QSS at the local port level.

The QSS stations, which in the past may have had only one or two people, depend on the various partners to fulfill their roles. During the SARS crisis, some ports reported a more active and visible role, particularly in training, although some did not indicate any significant difference. The role of the station varied by port as dictated by staffing and the location of problems. One station indicated that it might board vessels routinely (twice per week) to remind ship personnel about medical log requirements (although this may have been a VSP role). Others reported very little involvement with the seaports, particular if cruise activity was limited.

As with surveillance, the QSS role in responding to specific threats varies by location and circumstance. One station indicated that it might directly board vessels to evaluate a situation before other personnel, but only if at the local port.

The stations depend on local health agencies to deal with sick persons, but there seems to be no standard procedure. Some stations mentioned having formal MOAs, particularly with hospitals for quarantine cases; one respondent indicated that this was a generic CDC function. Another station said that it had no formal MOAs but maintained a database of health officers to contact at various subports. One station emphasized that the appropriate health agency to contact will vary by port (or airport) with some smaller ports covered by state agencies, while ports in large metropolitan areas might have a range of options.

It is unclear whether one of QSS's response roles is to notify other partners about infectious conditions, particularly if the information is received from another agency. This was a problem at one port where one of the partners was not informed by the agency that informed the station and was upset when they met the ship.

One station indicated that it conducts some of VSP's functions at local ports that have limited cruise operations; another indicated that it might be asked to clear crew members before they return to ship.

For diagnostic purposes or to identify previous contacts, the QSS will request itinerary and crew list information from the vessel and may also monitor a patient's status with scanned pictures. (It is unclear whether USCG provides some of this information.) One of the partners noted that there is no standard method for releasing crew and passenger information that may be deemed personal and sensitive (that is also true for airports). A formal agreement might assist in identifying past contacts.

The relative infrequency of ad hoc incidents dictates the structure of the current response system; one station said that a more widespread problem might require a more comprehensive program. With respect to protocols for a suspected or identified threat, one station reported that it keeps everyone on-board until someone can arrive on board for an evaluation and determine whether others can disembark (after providing a "locater code" for future contact). In some cases, it uses paramedics to help in the initial response (at distant ports or during off hours) and evaluation, and it might also transport an ill or dead person.

All incidents are reported to headquarters and distributed in the Daily Activity Report, although one station indicated that an imminent threat might require direct station-to-station contact. Most communications are by telephone, although fax and e-mail were also mentioned; this contrasts with USCG's report of a constant flow of e-mail for its vessel tracking system.

CDC's VSP "protects passenger and crew health by minimizing the risk of gastrointestinal illness aboard cruise ships." VSP accomplishes this mission through sanitation inspections, disease surveillance and investigations, on-site inspections of ship construction and renovation, and review of construction plans for new ships. VSP also trains crew in proper public health techniques, including food handling and preparation, drinkable-water system management, and pool and spa operation and maintenance"(source: www.cdc.gov/nceh/vsp/).

The VSP has a much larger presence in the major cruise ports (including an office in Fort Lauderdale) and much greater contact with the vessel and shore personnel. The VSP is paid for its inspection services and is self-supporting and well staffed. The primary surveillance role in regard to QSS for the VSP would be to identify nongastrointestinal cases that are reported to it (or that it is otherwise made aware of). It might also be called to respond to a vessel if QSS staff are unavailable and could cooperate in diagnosing a problem and developing a response (based on familiarity with medical officers, facilities, and recordkeeping).

CBP (Immigration Services)

In general, the immigration personnel of CBP are the "eyes and ears" of QSS at local ports. They indicated that they would be the first point of contact to identify problems with illness or death onboard in that the vessel (or its agent) must contact them to clear all passengers and crew. They have access to USCG's vessel monitoring data, but it is unclear how the data are used.

It is unclear whether sick passengers or crew have to be reported to the CBP. One shipping-industry respondent noted that CBP had a space on the "1300 or 1301 form" that requested information regarding any sick crew on-board but that it is no longer requested on the new forms. Some CBP respondents said they routinely ask about sick crew members, but it was not consistently referred to.

The likelihood that CBP personnel visually identified sick persons varied in the stations' responses. One station noted that cruise-passenger clearance was a "cattle call" and another noted that the same level of scrutiny is not applied at ports as at airports.

The primary response role of CBP is to detain and refuse entry to persons suspected of being infected, presumably at the direction of the QSS.

The level of training provided to CBP was of particular concern to the stations. Local training may be inadequate and possibly not related to the level of activity or threat (e.g., done only in low-incident or low-volume areas or for local area ports). Headquarters provides general training at CBP's national training center, but the high number of port personnel and frequent turnover make it difficult to maintain any consistent communications between CBP and the QSS at the local level.

CBP will often board vessels to do crew checks; it has access to USCG's National Vessel Movement Center (NVMC) data and may use them to see whether a vessel is eligible to enter.

USCG

USCG has a number of responsibilities in clearing a vessel to enter a port safely, including determining the adequacy and safety of manning, equipment, and the vessel itself, as well as checking whether that voyage documentation is complete and accurate. At a national level, the Ship Arrival Notification System and the NVMC together serve as a clearinghouse for the Notice of Arrival (NOA), a form that is required for all vessels arriving from a foreign port. The NOA provides information on the vessel's itinerary, any hazardous cargoes, and crew and passengers, including name, birth date, nationality, crew position, and where embarked.

The NVMC reviews the NOAs for completeness and makes them available on a USCG database that can be accessed from all ports of call by the captain of the port or CBP. Before 9/11, ships were required to notify the USCG's local Marine Safety Office (MSO) or the captain of the port within 24 hours of arrival time. Now, they must notify the NVMC within 96 hours of arrival at the first U.S. port and provide more information on crew and noncrew persons.

There was a great discrepancy in whether crew illness is reported through this system and, if so, whether it is reported to CDC or the local station. One USCG respondent referred to a "statement of no SARS" as a part of the NOA, but that might have been a temporary measure. In any case, it was indicated that USCG might make a courtesy call to CDC but had no fixed protocols. One QSS contact indicated receiving USCG vessel tracking information during the SARS crisis, but it was only temporary; others did not mention it.

The NVMC indicated that it does not "process" crew-illness information, but if it is reported (although not required), it is attached to the NOA record for the local port's use; it also noted the local MSO would not process it either.

At the local port level, the MSO conducts random inspections (under different responsibilities) of vessels guided by certain risk factors and the availability of vessel information. One MSO respondent thought that there was an item on the NOA about sick crew, although it is not on the standard form. It would be of importance to USCG only if sickness of a crew member results in substandard manning levels or if there were concern about boarding a vessel.

An MSO respondent indicated that in some cases, USCG may hold a ship at anchorage with an infectious-disease threat (perhaps under direction of the QSS) and wait out the incubation period. The respondent also indicated that the USCG has a doctor on staff that could assist with a response.[10] Most crew notifications involve injuries, not illness, and one respondent indicated that calls to CDC are infrequent.

The relationship with USCG as reported by the QSS differed significantly. One station indicated that the MSO had first responsibility for onboard illness or death, that the operations manual provides questions to ask regarding health issues, and that vessels had to make health declarations. USCG can hold a vessel at anchorage, and one station reported that during SARS, it provided on-site surveillance of symptomatic persons.

Unlike CBP, CDC does not train USCG personnel at a national level, and local contacts and knowledge are difficult with personnel rotations every 1½ -2 years. One QSS contact suggested more frequent meetings and training for USCG.

The NVMC is looking to integrate all the information reported for Immigration, Customs, and USCG; this would provide a single point of contact for vessel reporting. Perhaps CDC can get access or provide data to this expanded system.

---

[10]The USCG medical staff deal primarily with USCG personnel and port or vessel injuries, which are the primary health problems at ports.

Port Industry (Port Authority and Vessel Services)

The primary role of the general port sector, other than the vessel operator itself, is to identify any health risks encountered in the course of general business. It is more likely that it would contact CDC (or more likely USCG) to determine whether it is safe to board a vessel. When the SARS epidemic first came out there was a period of time when the pilots requested specific information from the vessels, such as whether they had been to a port that was designated as a high-risk area or whether any crew on board had been diagnosed with SARS. One QSS contact commented that the QSS had a role in communicating the true level of threats during a crisis; the shipping sector could shut down if shore-based personnel refused to assist in the safe operation of vessels entering ports.

The primary role of the port authority is providing access for the QSS (or its agents) to restricted port areas, a major concern with the SARS crisis. As noted elsewhere, policies vary by port and even by terminal, and the infrequency of visits may not dictate maintaining badges at all ports.

Local and State Health Agencies

QSS relationships with local and state health agencies at seaports are basically the same and may be generic for all CDC relationships (e.g., MOAs with hospitals). The infrequency of incidents results in little contact other than for (and sometimes including) the primary ports, many of which are those nearest to the airport stations. The small number of on-site medical staff (until recently, some airport stations had no medical officers) forces dependence on local medical personnel for immediate response for both airport and seaport subports.

A station may use designated local hospitals or physicians (often those of the ship agent) when CDC personnel are not available (in a timely manner relative to distance or during off hours). "Quarantinable" illnesses require a higher level of response—they have designated civic hospitals (certified with memo agreements) that are equipped to handle quarantine and isolation. Most contact is via telephone or e-mail, particularly for distant ports. In some cases, the station will work with local health agencies to devise a strategy (one station had a whole crew vaccinated once). The appropriate government contact depends on the port's location and size; state agencies may be appropriate for certain areas (e.g., smaller remote ports).

Passengers will often get sick only after returning home (particularly after cruises of 7 days or less), and local health officials may contact CDC (as they are supposed to) if it is known that a person visited abroad. It was thought that contact could come via headquarters or directly.

Potential Gaps or Shortfalls

No contact showed any high level of concern about gaps or shortfalls in the system. A general concern involved the ability to train partner agencies and the shipping community. One possible gap is the possibility of off-shore contact between vessel crew and shore-based personnel (e.g., port pilots) or between off-shore vessels not calling at a foreign port and other off-shore vessels. That was not considered a concern by the interviewees. It was also noted that even private vessels must process through CBP if leaving U.S. waters.

Another possible gap involves illnesses diagnosed after people leave the U.S. that would probably be identified only for ships returning to the United States. One concern offered by a QSS contact involved stowaways, who may pose a problem if infectious disease is suspected and the appropriate agency staff refuse to deal with them until the problem is diagnosed. The general problem of dealing with non-English-speaking crew was also a concern.

CDC QSS AT SEAPORTS: CARGO TRANSPORTATION[11]

General overview

Incidents related to cargo at seaports are extremely few (as reported in the interviews):

• African rodents and "bush meat": There is a prohibition on these imports, although these commodities are likely to move by air.
• Lucky bamboo: This plant commodity was shipped from Asia and was packed in a gel that somehow turned to water and contained mosquito larvae. After diagnosis, the import of this commodity was closely monitored.
• Used tires: Like lucky bamboo, some used tires imported from China were in containers with standing water that contained mosquito larvae. The problem was eventually diagnosed and eliminated.
• Cholera in South American vessels' ballast: Ships from South America were discovered to be carrying cholera in their ballast water (seawater carried on the vessel for weight and other purposes). This discovery occurred after a joint task force (including FDA) inspected incoming vessels. The result was a policy requiring vessels to flush their ballast water at least three times before arriving at a U.S. port.
• Contaminated equipment: One major port cited some repatriated

---

[11]See Tables D.5 and D.6 for data on levels of cargo traffic at U.S. seaports.

agricultural machinery that was contaminated and had to be fumigated (as its only cargo-related incident), although it was probably a USDA-related matter not involving the QSS.

Other than those incidents, some of the interviewees (including QSS personnel) could not recall a local incident related to cargo (and many of them cited the same incidents occurring in other regions). Based on the infrequency of threats, there was limited input from industry and agency partners. The following sections describe the little information that was gathered regarding cargo imports.

CDC

In the cases cited above, the QSS was mostly responsible for dealing with a problem once it was identified. No stations cited a case in which it had identified a threat and passed it on to its partners on a local basis. It is assumed that prohibited items are identified at a national level and communicated to CBP at that level. One QSS contact was concerned that this type of contact might not filter down to the local level.

As in an airport situation, the QSS is responsible for dealing with any cargo that is refused entry under its jurisdiction, which may include destroying or reexporting the shipment or ensuring that the cargo is not hazardous.

CBP (U.S. Customs and Border Protection)

CBP has primary responsibility for clearing all foreign-origin cargo entering the United States (through its legacy U.S. customs function) by all ports of entry. As with airports, CBP may have authority to clear cargo for CDC unless a shipment is suspicious, some on a routine basis (e.g., for frequent shipments of medical samples to local hospitals). This supporting role is greatest at ports with no local airport station.

The primary process involved includes a review of documentation as now filed via the AMS that contains all the relevant information necessary to clear the cargo (origin and destination, shipper and consignee, and commodity). CBP can also visually inspect or hold cargo suspected to be in violation of U.S. law. CBP contacts whichever agency has primary responsibility for a particular shipment but also has the ex-USDA unit of "agricultural specialists" to which any agricultural issue is probably referred. The general impression was that if there was a suspected problem with a shipment, CBP will contact the "logical" agency: USDA for agriculture, FDA for foods and drugs, and CDC (or "public health") if there is a perceived possibility of disease.

TABLE D.5   2003 Containerized Traffic for U.S. Ports

Quarantine Station	Port	20-Foot Equivalent Units	# of Containers	Container Weight (MT)
Los Angeles	Los Angeles (CA)	7,148,940	3,951,792	N/A
(LAX)	Long Beach (CA)	4,658,124	2,577,080	25,312,306
	Houston (TX)	1,243,706	776,403	10,812,558
	San Diego (CA)	86,136	43,068	876,669
	Freeport (TX)	67,784	N/A	469,132
	Hueneme (CA)	24,523	N/A	N/A
	Galveston (TX)	9,911	4,961	62,232
		13,239,124	7,353,304	37,532,897
New York	New York/New Jersey	4,067,812	2,382,639	N/A
(JFK)	Hampton Roads (VA)	1,646,279	947,872	12,108,920
	Baltimore (MD)	536,078	337,978	4,261,591
	Wilmington (DE)	254,191	123,378	1,379,472
	Boston (MA)	158,020	88,890	1,077,654
	Philadelphia (PA)	147,413	103,156	1,132,134
	Richmond (VA)	43,672	NA	386,765
	Portland (ME)	3,587	2,109	32,547
	Albany (NY)	892	521	4,055
		6,857,944	3,986,543	20,383,138
Miami (MIA)	San Juan (PR) (fy)	1,665,765	694,069	6,589,677
	Miami (FL) (fy)	1,028,565	363,336	7,874,579
	Jacksonville (FL) (fy)	692,422	343,568	3,405,386
	Port Everglades (FL) (fy)	569,743	324,600	3,298,591
	Palm Beach (FL) (fy)	217,558	N/A	1,007,429
	Ponce (PR) (fy)	32,497	20,718	205,605
	Fernandina (FL)	22,096	14,799	108,264
	Manatee (FL)	11,837	N/A	72,809
	Tampa (FL) (fy)	8,173	N/A	38,480
	Canaveral (FL) (fy)	678	678	N/A
		4,249,334	1,761,768	22,600,820
Seattle	Tacoma (WA)	1,738,068	906,434	11,154,908
(SEA)	Seattle (WA)	1,486,465	852,905	8,814,689
	Anchorage (AK)	521,993	208,797	1,522,418
	Portland (OR)	339,571	190,639	2,855,128
	Everett (WA)	6,815	1,338	18,682
	Vancouver (WA)	338	171	N/A
		4,093,250	2,160,284	24,365,825

TABLE D.5 Continued

Quarantine Station	Port	20-Foot Equivalent Units	# of Containers	Container Weight (MT)
Atlanta	Charleston (SC)	1,690,847	N/A	N/A
(ATL)	Savannah (GA)	1,521,728	848,502	10,045,117
	New Orleans (LA)	251,187	159,707	2,769,754
	Gulfport (MS)	199,897	107,398	1,434,571
	Wilmington (NC)	96,453	54,048	562,568
	Mobile (AL)	26,302	14,649	N/A
	Lake Charles (LA)	19,000	20,000	15,400
	Brunswick (GA)	118	59	1,469
		3,805,532	1,204,363	14,828,879
San Francisco	Oakland (CA)	1,923,104	1,079,479	N/A
(SFO)	San Francisco (CA)	20,633	13,533	501,000
		1,943,737	1,093,012	501,000
Honolulu	Honolulu (HI) (fy)	980,840	589,587	4,922,168
	Kahului (HI) (fy)	115,556	70,626	777,286
	Hilo (HI) (fy)	60,942	37,113	377,594
	Kawaihae (HI) (fy)	55,345	32,924	346,675
	Nawiliwili (HI) (fy)	42,700	26,430	228,343
	Kaunakakai (HI) (fy)	2,152	1,796	12,394
	Barbers Point (HI) (fy)	18	18	196
		1,257,553	758,494	6,664,656
Overseas	Apra (GU) (fy)	144,541	82,310	2,050,951
		144,541	82,310	2,050,951
Grand Total		35,591,015	18,400,078	128,928,166

SOURCE: American Association of Port Authorities.

Most of the stations noted that they do not have access to the AMS. Access would enable them to monitor certain commodities and perhaps identify patterns creating new threats, but there is also concern about whether they would have the capability to use the system at the local level.

One concern was that the protocols within the AMS for contacting the QSS may not be clear. It was very unclear to what extent there are CDC-flagged items in the AMS and what occurs in such a case. One QSS contact indicated that regulations limit the information that can be passed on to CDC and that the AMS protocols may need to be reviewed. (The example

TABLE D.6   U.S. Waterborne Imports—Top 100 Ports by Weight and Customs District (2003)

Quarantine Station	Port	Import Weight (Short Tons)	Rank
LAX	Houston, TX	90,335,647	1
	Beaumont, TX	63,336,752	3
	Corpus Christi,TX	44,758,661	4
	Texas City, TX	40,184,521	5
	Long Beach, CA	37,969,522	6
	Los Angeles, CA	29,962,253	8
	Freeport, TX	22,665,591	11
	Port Arthur, TX	14,259,432	21
	Matgorda Ship Channel, TX	6,451,220	31
	San Diego, CA	2,194,448	52
	Brownsville, TX	1,865,561	54
	Galveston, TX	1,064,833	66
	Port Hueneme, CA	910,801	72
LAX Total		*355,959,242*	
JFK	New York, NY and NJ	70,251,263	2
	Portland, ME	27,133,777	10
	Baltimore, MD	18,984,957	13
	Philadelphia, PA	18,615,848	15
	Paulsboro, NJ	17,908,339	16
	Marcus Hook, PA	16,077,374	19
	Boston, MA	15,634,152	20
	Hampton Roads, VA	10,155,182	24
	Providence, RI	4,402,336	36
	Portsmouth, NH	4,113,573	40
	Camden-Gloucester, NJ	3,764,289	41
	Wilmington, DE	3,400,014	43
	New Haven, CT	2,954,309	46
	Fall River, MA	1,954,888	53
	Bridgeport, CT	1,850,626	55
	Chester, PA	1,342,801	59
	New Castle, DE	1,329,415	60
	Albany, NY	1,325,761	61
	Penn Manor, PA	1,205,420	64
	Searsport, ME	996,205	69
	Richmond, VA	288,106	90
JFK Total		*223,688,635*	
ATL	South Louisiana, LA, Port of	30,857,319	7
	Lake Charles, LA	27,825,176	9
	New Orleans, LA	20,889,868	12
	Baton Rouge, LA	18,701,796	14
	Mobile, AL	17,553,389	17

TABLE D.6   Continued

Quarantine Station	Port	Import Weight (Short Tons)	Rank
	Pascagoula, MS	17,513,754	18
	Savannah, GA	13,174,550	22
	Charleston, SC	13,041,525	23
	Plaquemines, LA, Port of	8,519,740	28
	Wilmington, NC	2,739,522	48
	Georgetown, SC	2,400,943	50
	Gulfport, MS	1,228,417	63
	Brunswick, GA	1,056,658	68
	Morehead City, NC	703,318	74
ATL Total		*176,205,975*	
MIA	Jacksonville, FL	9,878,816	26
	Tampa, FL	9,230,682	27
	Port Everglades, FL	8,426,945	29
	San Juan, PR	5,008,816	33
	Miami, FL	4,915,706	35
	Ponce, PR	3,266,582	44
	Port Manatee, FL	3,189,814	45
	Port Canaveral, FL	2,950,340	47
	Palm Beach, FL	819,382	73
	Panama City, FL	663,660	78
	Pensacola, FL	292,732	88
MIA Total		*48,643,475*	
SEA	Seattle, WA	6,748,803	30
	Tacoma, WA	5,702,602	32
	Portland, OR	4,398,499	37
	Anacortes, WA	1,492,029	57
	Redwood City, CA	915,510	71
	Longview, WA	698,574	75
	Vancouver, WA	680,736	76
	Port Angeles, WA	672,165	77
	Grays Harbor, WA	323,006	84
	Everett, WA	264,683	92
	Nikishka, AK	226,934	94
	Kalama, WA	219,889	95
	Anchorage, AK	218,233	96
	Coos Bay, OR	195,189	98
	Olympia, WA	107,924	100
SEA Total		*22,864,776*	

(continued)

TABLE D.6 Continued

Quarantine Station	Port	Import Weight (Short Tons)	Rank
ORD	Toledo, OH	4,243,476	38
	Detroit, MI	3,493,535	42
	Cleveland, OH	2,708,093	49
	Burns Waterway Harbor, IN	1,269,905	62
	Milwaukee, WI	1,119,290	65
	Chicago, IL	1,057,337	67
	Ashtabula, OH	960,441	70
	Marysville, MI	584,298	79
	Duluth-Superior, MN and WI	529,060	80
	Buffalo, NY	402,376	81
	Gary, IN	393,742	82
	Lorain, OH	334,244	83
	Muskegon, MI	321,516	85
	Grand Haven, MI	318,215	86
	Indiana Harbor, IN	314,107	87
	Green Bay, WI	292,532	89
	Marquette, MI	284,738	91
	Fairport Harbor, OH	257,575	93
	Manistee, MI	196,385	97
	Conneaut, OH	177,899	99
ORD Total		*19,258,764*	
SFO	Richmond, CA	10,017,014	25
	Oakland, CA	4,203,403	39
	San Francisco, CA	1,635,880	56
	Stockton, CA	1,417,749	58
SFO Total		*17,274,046*	
HNL	Honolulu, HI	4,918,596	34
	Barbers Point, Oahu, HI	2,357,417	51
HNL Total		*7,276,013*	
Grand Total		**871,170,926**	

SOURCE: American Association of Port Authorities.

given concerned a prohibited item that was only generically described and had a "Call CDC" designation that resulted in contact of headquarters rather than the local QSS where the item was entering the United States.

Another concern was that CBP requirements for documentation may not meet CDC's requirements when CBP is responsible for clearing shipments.

USCG

As with passenger concerns, USCG is responsible for the safety of vessels entering a port. The NVMC database of NOAs contains information on "dangerous goods," but there is no apparent protocol for identifying or handling QSS-related cargoes.

Other Federal Agencies

A primary source of contacts for the QSS is other agencies with responsibility for inspecting and holding cargo at the ports, especially the USDA (for live animals and "unprocessed" foods) and FDA (for foods and drugs). These agencies typically have a much larger port presence; in the case of USDA, inspection personnel are within CBP. The QSS or more likely the partner agency may identify a threat covered by another agency and then directly contact it. In the case of USDA, that may occur after CBP has referred an issue to its agricultural specialist, who then might contact the QSS. As with other concerns at the port, the priority and awareness of QSS concerns (to the extent that there are any) depend on communications with the other agencies at the local level.

In major agricultural areas, local or state agriculture agencies might also monitor and participate in the surveillance and response process. For example, mosquito-abatement agencies in the Los Angeles area will fumigate some containers before USDA inspection, and local agencies are very vigilant about threats to local agriculture.

Port Industry (Port Authority, Terminal, Stevedore, and Vessel Services)

The port industry and port authorities did not appear to have a major role with QSS cargo threats. None of the interviewees thought it likely that a customs broker would identify a threat unless there was obvious health risk to them.

Local and State Health Agencies

There were no examples of involvement of local or state health agencies in QSS-related cargo matters. As with passengers, some problems may be identified after entry (e.g., spoiled fish not properly smoked), but it is unclear whether a comprehensive response is necessary in that most are probably another agency's responsibility (e.g., FDA for spoiled fish). A local health agency involved in one previous incident noted that it had problems in getting timely information that allowed them to prepare for incoming shipments thought to pose a risk.

Potential Gaps or Shortfalls

Other than the concerns about access to and protocols of the AMS cited above, no gaps or shortfalls regarding cargo transportation were identified. Logically, the greatest threat would be cargoes that are unrelated to the responsibilities of complementary federal agencies (i.e., other than agricultural, live animals, foods, or drugs).

E

Microbial Threats of Public Health Significance Originating in Animals or Animal Products at U.S. Ports of Entry

A Commissioned Paper
Prepared by
Nga L. Tran, Dr.P.H., M.P.H., C.I.H.
Jesse Berman, B.S.
Exponent, Inc.

April 7, 2005

INTRODUCTION

At the request of the Institute of Medicine, Exponent prepared this report describing the legal framework that established the inspection activities at U.S. ports of entry (POEs) and the roles and responsibilities of the various agencies involved in the inspection and prevention of public health threats posed by the importation of animals. In addition, day-to-day activities at port locations, communication procedures and protocols between personnel at Centers of Disease Control and Prevention (CDC) quarantine stations and other U.S. port agencies, and readily available budget and capacity information are summarized. Issues and concerns that are potential barriers to successful protection of U.S. borders from diseases in animals are also highlighted. Finally, special considerations for animal issues in the expansion plan of CDC quarantine stations are discussed.

The main sources of information that were used to develop this paper were literature posted at agency websites—those of the U.S. Department of Agriculture (USDA), CDC, and the Department of Homeland Security (DHS) U.S. Customs and Border Protection (CBP)—results of an informal survey of CDC personnel at quarantine stations, and telephone calls to the USDA Animal and Plant Health Inspection Services (APHIS) and state agriculture specialists. Names and affiliations of individuals interviewed for this report are listed in Appendix 1. Questions used in the informal survey are provided in Appendix 2.

LEGAL FRAMEWORK FOR INSPECTIONS AT
U.S. PORTS OF ENTRY

The Homeland Security Act of 2002 (HSA, P.L. 107-296) establishes DHS and its directorates. More than 22 federal agencies were consolidated into the new department, including the Immigration and Naturalization Service (INS), the Customs Service, and components of APHIS that conduct inspection and animal quarantine activities at U.S. ports (APHIS, 2003). The HSA specified which laws DHS agricultural inspectors might use to conduct inspections but it did not alter these underlying statutes (CRS, 2004). In addition, the transfer of the inspection functions of INS and Customs Service to DHS did not affect the laws that authorize these inspections. The following sections describe the underlying statutes for various types of inspections at U.S. ports.

Agriculture Inspections

Agriculture inspectors play an integral part in USDA's role in supplying a safe and affordable food supply. In part, APHIS was responsible for enforcing the laws that protect and promote U.S. agricultural health from agricultural pests and diseases by conducting inspections at various ports of entry. Under the HSA, APHIS import and entry inspection activities relating to the laws specified below were transferred to DHS. The under secretary for border and transportation security is now responsible for conducting agricultural inspections at ports of entry in accordance with the regulations, policies, and procedures issued by the secretary of agriculture for the following Acts (CRS, 2004):

- The Virus-Serum-Toxin Act (21 U.S.C. §§151 et seq.).
- The Honeybee Act (7 U.S.C. §§281 et seq.).
- Title III of the Federal Seed Act (7 U.S.C. §§1581 et seq.).
- The Plant Protection Act (7 U.S.C. §§7701 et seq.).
- The Animal Health Protection Act (7 U.S.C. §§8301 et seq.).
- The Lacey Act Amendments of 1981 (16 U.S.C. §§3371 et seq.).
- Section 11 of the Endangered Species Act of 1973 (16 U.S.C. §§1540).

In some cases, agriculture inspectors have the authority to conduct warrantless searches of any person or conveyance entering the country in furtherance of those laws. For instance, under the Plant Protection Act and the Animal Health Protection Act, agriculture inspectors have the authority to conduct warrantless searches of any person or vehicle entering the United States to determine whether the person is carrying any plant or animal in violation of the statute (7 U.S.C. §7331 (b)(1) and 7 U.S.C. §8307 (b)(1)). Agriculture inspectors also have the authority under the Lacey Act to detain for inspection any vessel, vehicle, aircraft, package, crate, or other container on the arrival of such conveyance or container in the United States from any point outside the United States (16 U.S.C. §3375). The Endangered Species Act also allows agriculture inspectors to detain for inspection any package, crate, or other container and all accompanying documents on importation (16 U.S.C. §1540).

Immigration Inspections

The former INS was responsible for enforcing and administering the Immigration and Nationality Act of 1952 (INA) (codified as amended at 8 U.S.C. §§1101 et seq.). The HSA transferred administrative authority over immigration enforcement to the Directorate of Border and Transportation Security. According to DHS regulations, all authorities and functions of the DHS to administer and enforce the immigration laws are now vested in the secretary of DHS or his delegate (8 CFR §2.1).[1] Immigration officials possess a wide variety of enforcement mechanisms to carry out their mission of enforcing the INA. Immigration enforcement activities generally include providing border security and management, conducting inspections of persons at U.S. international ports, enforcing immigration law, detaining and removing aliens found in violation of immigration and related laws, and providing immigration intelligence.

Customs Inspections

Formerly housed in the Department of the Treasury, customs inspectors enforced a number of laws to ensure all imports and exports comply with U.S. laws and regulations, collect and protect U.S. revenues, and guard against the smuggling of contraband. The HSA transferred generally all customs functions (except for certain revenue functions) to DHS in §403. Customs border activities are now conducted through the CBP and interior enforcement activities are carried out by Immigration and Customs Enforcement officers.

---

[1] 8 CFR §2.1 states, "the Secretary, in his discretion, may delegate any such authority or function to any official, officer, or employee of the DHS or any employee of the United States to the extent authorized by law." This regulation was authorized, in part, by §103 of the INA, which was amended by the HSA to charge the secretary of DHS with the administration and enforcement of the INA. There is still some question, however, as to the extent to which the attorney general has concurrent authority.

Public Health Inspection

The secretary of the Department of Health and Human Services (DHHS) has statutory responsibility for preventing the introduction, transmission, and spread of communicable diseases in the United States. Under its delegated authority, the Division of Global Migration and Quarantine (DGMQ) fulfills this responsibility through a variety of activities, including:

- Operation of quarantine stations at ports of entry.
- Establishment of standards for medical examination of persons destined for the United States.
- Administration of interstate and foreign quarantine regulations that govern the international and interstate movement of persons, animals, and cargo.

The legal foundation for these activities is found in Titles 8 and 42 of the U.S. Code and relevant supporting regulations. Interstate and foreign quarantine regulations (42 CFR70 and 71) authorize the secretary of the DHHS, through CDC, to develop and enforce regulations to prevent transmission of infectious disease from foreign countries into the United States. Under these authorities, CDC can set policy to embargo certain animals from entering the United States (DGMQ, 2004).

Title III of the Bioterrorism Act provides the secretary of DHHS with new authorities to protect the nation's food supply. The Public Health Security and Bioterrorism Preparedness Response Act requires notification and controls on the movement of agents or toxins deemed to be a threat to animal or plant health and to animal and plant products. To prevent the incursions of adverse animal health events, APHIS units are working with DHHS to implement the provisions of this act (APHIS, 2004b).

Table E.1 provides a summary of agencies that are involved in the inspection of animals and animal products at U.S. ports aimed to protect animal or public health and their legal authorities.

AGENCIES AT U.S. PORTS OF ENTRY— ROLES AND RESPONSIBILITIES

Deterrence and prevention are the first lines of defense against the introduction of animal and plant pests and pathogens from foreign sources (Personal communication, J. Annelli, APHIS, April 7, 2004). Several strategies are involved in border strategy that focuses on interdicting a threat agent at U.S. POEs (NRC, 2003). For the past several years, there have been 317 official POEs into the United States. At a given port, inspectors may be responsible for more than one mode of transportation (air, land, and sea).

TABLE E.1 Legal Authorities for Inspections at U.S. Borders

Agency	Legal and Regulatory Foundation	Authorities
DHHS-CDC	Titles 8 and 42 of the U.S Code and relevant supporting regulations, such as Interstate Quarantine (42 CFR 70) and Foreign Quarantine (42 CFR 71).	Authorizes CDC National Center for Infectious Diseases, DGMQ to make and enforce regulations necessary to prevent the introduction, transmission, or spread of communicable diseases from foreign countries into the United States.
	The Foreign Quarantine regulation (42 CFR Part 71.54, Etiologic Agents, Hosts, and Vectors)	Governs the importation of hazardous materials (etiologic agents, vectors, and materials containing etiologic agents). Importation into the United States must be accompanied by a U.S. Public Health Service importation permit. CDC regulations govern the importation of dogs, cats, turtles, monkeys, other animals, and animal products capable of causing human disease. Under these regulatory authorities, CDC has established an embargo on monkeys and other animals that could carry monkey pox virus, and birds from specified Southeast Asian countries.
DHHS-FDA	Title III of the Bioterrorism Act	Provides the DHHS secretary with new authorities to protect the nation's food supply against the threat of intentional contamination and other food-related emergencies. The Food and Drug Administration expects up to 420,000 facilities to register under this requirement.

(continued)

174

TABLE E.1 Continued

Agency	Legal and Regulatory Foundation	Authorities
DHS	The Homeland Security Act of 2002	Establishes DHS and its directorates.
U.S. Customs and Border Protection	Subtitle A, Title IV, of the Homeland Security Act of 2002 (6 U.S.C 201 et seq.)	Establishes Border and Transportation Security (CBP resides in this directorate). CBP is responsible for controlling all U.S. land, sea, and air borders; protects U.S. economic security by regulating and facilitating the lawful movement of goods and persons across U.S. borders. Agricultural Quarantine Program (border inspection) (former APHIS).
APHIS	The Animal Industry Act of 1884 as amended (21 U.S.C. 117) The Cattle Contagious Diseases The Act of 1903 as amended (21 U.S.C. 111-115, 117, 120, 123, 125-127, 134), The Farm Security and Rural Investment Act of 2002, Subtitle E Animal Health Protection Act (PL 107-171), 21 U.S.C. 114 The Animal Industry Act of 1988 The Virus-Serum-Toxin Act (21 U.S.C. §§151 et seq.) The Honeybee Act (7 U.S.C. §§281 et seq.) Title III of the Federal Seed Act (7 U.S.C. §§1581 et seq.) The Plant Protection Act (7 U.S.C. §§7701 et seq.)	Provides secretary of USDA broad authority and discretion to prevent, detect, control, and eradicate diseases of pests and animals and to promulgate regulations and take measures to prevent introduction and interstate dissemination of communicable diseases of livestock within the U.S. Legal bases for APHIS monitoring and surveillance programs.

Agency	Authority	Function
	The Lacey Act Amendments of 1981 (16 U.S.C. §§3371 et seq.) Section 11 of the Endangered Species Act of 1973 (16 U.S.C. §§1540)	
	9 CFR, Part 53, amended in 1985 (21 U.S.C., Section 151 et seq.)	To respond to certain foreign animal diseases (FADs) and other communicable diseases of livestock or poultry and pay claims growing out of destruction of animals.
	9 CFR subchapter B	To establish cooperative programs to control and eradicate communicable diseases of livestock.
	The Foreign Service Act (1980) and Executive Order 12363 (1982)	APHIS International Services (IS) activities.
U.S. Fish and Wildlife Services	Migratory Bird Treaty Act (16 U.S.C. 668-668C) Lacey Act (18 U.S.C. 703-712) Endangered Species Act (16 U.S.C. 1531-1543)	Prohibits possession, purchase, or barter of migratory bird, feathers or other parts. Prohibits importation, exportation, transportation, sale, or purchase of fish and wildlife in violation of state, federal, tribal, and foreign laws. Prohibits the importation, exportation, taking, and commercialization in interstate or foreign commerce of fish, wildlife, and plants that are listed as threatened or endangered species. Implements provisions of the Convention on International Trade in Endangered Species (CITES).

SOURCES: Bush, 2002; Crawford, 2003; Creekmore, 2003; DGMQ, 2003b, 2004; Grannis, 2003; OMB, 2004b; OSH, 2004; USFWS, 2003.

Buffalo and Detroit, for example, have air, sea, and land POEs. The likelihood of inspectors having multiple responsibilities is greater at the smaller POEs. CBP currently reports there are 216 airports that are international POEs, 143 seaports, and 115 land POEs. Two locations are inland POEs (CRS, 2004). The roles and responsibilities of the various agencies involved in the inspection and prevention of animals and animal products that could pose a public health threat by entering the United States are described below.

Department of Health and Human Services (DHHS), Centers for Diseases Control and Prevention (CDC)

The foreign quarantine regulation (42 CFR Part 71.54, Etiologic Agents, Hosts, and Vectors) governs the importation of hazardous materials (etiologic agents, vectors, and materials containing etiologic agents (OSH, 2004). CDC has established regulations that govern the importation of dogs, cats, turtles, monkeys, other animals, and animal products capable of causing human disease. Under these regulatory authorities, CDC has established an embargo on monkeys and other animals that could carry the monkeypox virus and on birds from specified Southeast Asian countries (DGMQ, 2004).

CDC officials are not present at the border on a day-to-day basis, but there are quarantine stations at the international airports in Atlanta, New York, Miami, Chicago, Los Angeles, San Francisco, Seattle, and Honolulu. The quarantine operations involve coordination of numerous agencies, including (DGMQ, 2003a):

- Epidemic Intelligence Service (EIS) and other parts of CDC.
- State and local health departments.
- CBP.
- USDA.
- U.S. Fish and Wildlife Service.
- The aircraft and maritime industry.

The CDC National Center for Infectious Diseases (NCID) DGMQ trains CBP inspectors to watch for ill persons and items of public health concern, and they work with state and local health officials in jurisdictions that may be affected under particular circumstances (CRS, 2004).

DHS Border and Transportation Security (BTS), U.S. Customs and Border Protection (CBP)

On November 21, 2002, President Bush signed legislation creating DHS to unify federal forces and protect the nation from a new host of terrorist threats. Approximately 2,600 employees from the APHIS Agriculture Quarantine and Inspection (AQI) force became part of CBP on March 1, 2003 (APHIS, 2003). This network of veterinary inspectors and animal health inspectors at all U.S. POEs is the first line of defense in identifying materials entering the United States that may be introducing foreign animal diseases. DHS acquired USDA's authority to inspect passenger declarations and cargo manifests, international passengers, baggage, cargo, and conveyances and to hold suspect items for quarantine to prevent the introduction of plant or animal diseases (GAO, 2005).

A summary of the programmatic elements and functions of CBP is provided in Table E.2.

APHIS Veterinary Services

Although DHS is now responsible for protecting the nation's border and the border inspection function of APHIS has moved to DHS, APHIS retains a significant presence in border inspection activities. The nearly 1,300 AQI employees who were not transferred continue to conduct certain domestic inspection functions, such as monitoring entry to the mainland from Hawaii and Puerto Rico (CRS, 2004). Through risk assessment, pathway analysis, and rule making, APHIS continues to set agricultural policy, including specific quarantine, testing, and other conditions under which animals, animal products, and veterinary biologics can be imported. APHIS policy is then carried out by DHS (APHIS, 2003). At POEs, there are also APHIS Veterinary Services (VS) port veterinarians who inspect live animals at border ports and animals in quarantine until testing is completed. They are at 43 VS office areas and report to the veterinarian in charge of the VS area office (Personal communication, J. Annelli, APHIS, April 7, 2004). With agricultural border inspectors now being a part of DHS, VS has identified the need for developing new protocol for training and interacting with these inspectors and the need to work with DHS to implement improvements recommended in the Animal Health Safeguarding Review regarding exclusion activities in its strategic plan (APHIS, 2004b). To ensure that necessary agricultural inspections are conducted, APHIS negotiates memoranda of understanding (MOUs) with DHS.

The VS National Center for Import/Export works to facilitate international trade; monitors health of animals presented at borders; regulates import and export of animals, animal products, and biologics; and diagnoses foreign and domestic animal diseases. This center works in partnership with the Department of the Interior's (DOI) Fish and Wildlife Service (USFWS), the APHIS Plant and Protection Quarantine, and CBP (APHIS, 2004a).

TABLE E.2 DHS, Border and Transportation Security, U.S. Customs and Border Protection, and Components Addressing Animal Diseases

Agencies	Function
Border and Transportation Security (BTS)	The largest of the five DHS directorates. Includes former U.S. Customs Service, border security function and enforcement division of INS, APHIS, Federal Law Enforcement Training Center, and the Transportation Security Administration. Responsible for securing the nation's air, land, and sea borders. Responsible for securing the nation's transportation systems and enforcing the nation's immigration laws.
U.S. Customs and Border Protection (CBP)	March 1, 2003, approx. 42,000 employees were transferred from U.S. Customs Service, INS, and APHIS to the new CBP, a new agency under the BTS Directorate within DHS. Approximately 2,700 former USDA employees from the AQI program and APHIS were transferred into DHS. Former APHIS Plant Protection and Quarantine personnel at POEs who were directly involved in terminal and plane inspections (100% time) were transferred to DHS; those with 60-70% time not doing inspection at terminals or planes were not transferred. The agricultural import and entry inspection functions that were transferred include reviewing passenger declarations and cargo manifests to target high-risk agricultural passengers or cargo shipments. The new CBP also carries out the traditional missions of the predecessor agencies making up CBP (seizing illegal drugs and other contraband at the U.S. border; apprehending people who attempt to enter the United States illegally; detecting counterfeit entry documents; determining the admissibility of people and goods; protecting our agricultural interests from harmful pests or diseases; regulating and facilitating international trade; collecting duties and fees; and enforcing all laws of the United States at our borders).
Office Field Operations (OFO)	Oversees over 25,000 employees at 20 office field operations (OFOs), 317 POEs, and 14 preclearance stations in Canada and the Caribbean. Responsible for enforcing customs, immigration, and agriculture laws and regulations at U.S. borders.

	Manages core custom and border protection programs (i.e., border security and facilitation, interdiction and security, passenger operations, targeting analysis and canine enforcement, trade compliance and facilitation, trade risk management, enforcement, and seizures and penalties and examines trade operations to focus on antiterrorism. Administers Agricultural Inspection Policy and Programs, AQI at all POEs to protect the health of U.S. plant and animal resources. Administers immigrations policy programs. Annual operating budget of $1.1 billion. Each OFO is run by a director of field operations (DFO).
Associate Commissioner of Agricultural Inspection Policy and Programs	Policy adviser to the Office of the Commissioner on all agricultural issues.
CBP port director	On March 1, 2003, CBP designated one port director at each POE in charge of all federal inspection services, establishing a single, unified chain of command.
CBP agricultural specialist	Enforces USDA regulations and seizes any articles in violation of those regulations. Conducts prearrival risk analysis. Examines cargo for quarantine disease and pests. Collects and prepares pest and disease samples and submits to USDA. Handles seizures, safeguarding, destruction, or reexportation of inadmissible cargo. Negotiates compliance agreements with importers of regulated commodities. Stationed only at POEs with large volumes of cargo and only to support the CBP officers. As of 10/4/2003, there were 1,471 full-time permanent agricultural inspectors on-board. New CBP officers will be trained at the Federal Law Enforcement Training Center (FLETC) in Glynco, GA, and agricultural specialists will continue to learn their trade at PPQ Professional Development Center in Frederick, MD. Farm groups and some members of Congress have questioned whether CBP officers will receive enough agricultural training.

(continued)

TABLE E.2 Continued

Agencies	Function
CBP and FDA	In October 2003, CBP and FDA entered into an agreement to further protect U.S. food supply. At POEs, CBP inspectors now carry out special inspection and sampling of foreign food imports and make referrals to FDA for further testing and analysis. CBP and FDA work side by side in targeting efforts, making joint decisions about any food shipments that could pose a potential threat to the United States.
National Targeting Center	Part of CBP's OFO, the National Targeting Center (NTC) provides tactical targeting and analytical research support for antiterrorism efforts to DHS and its operations center. NTC has representatives from all CBP disciplines.
CBP Laboratories and Scientific Sciences Division	On Dec. 8, 2003, moved its Radiation Portal Monitor to the NTC.

SOURCES: Bonner, 2004; CBP, 2003, 2004; DHS, 2004b, 2004c; FASS, 2003; FCBF, 2003; USAHA, 2003; Personal communication, K. Ahmad, APHIS, April 6, 2005.

U.S. Fish and Wildlife Service (USFWS)

USFWS is responsible for the protection of wildlife from environmental hazards, safeguarding habitat for endangered species, and inspection of international cargo, baggage, passengers, and mail to enforce U.S. and international laws regarding trade in endangered and protected species (USFWS, 2002). Generally, all wildlife imported into or exported from the United States for any reason must be declared to USFWS and cleared before release by CBP. Some wildlife inspection requires coordination with APHIS, FDA, INS, or CDC.

Other Agencies

The USDA Food Safety and Inspection Service (FSIS) and the DHHS Food and Drug Administration (FDA) focus on protecting public health. At POEs, FSIS and FDA inspect shipments of food and food products imported into the United States from abroad to ensure that food and related products meet U.S. standards and do not present any risk to public health (CRS, 2004). As an example, AQI personnel may inspect a shipment of sausage casings to ensure that the shipment does not pose any animal health risks, while FSIS personnel may inspect the same shipment to ensure that the product was prepared in an approved processing facility.

RESOURCES AND BUDGETS

Budget information is publicly available from the Office of Management and Budget's website for all U.S. federal agencies. However, line-item budget information on programs aimed at preventing public health threats at U.S. POEs is not readily available. Limited budget data on agricultural inspections at U.S. borders and tracking of animal and animal products movement are summarized in Table E.3. Table E.4 summarizes the existing CBP human resources dedicated to agriculture, customs, and immigration inspections at U.S. borders. The Congressional Research Service indicated that there have been more customs inspectors than immigration and agricultural inspectors combined over the period of FY 2001-2004 (CRS, 2004). Table E.5 summarizes existing human resources and capacity at CDC quarantine stations.

DAY-TO-DAY REALITY OF WORK

For Routine Notification of Imports

A survey of CDC personnel at quarantine stations indicated that most CDC work concerns animals that are regulated under CDC jurisdiction,

TABLE E.3   Level of Funding

Agency- Focus Area	FY 2003	FY 2004	FY 2005	FTEs
DHS — CBP	$5.9 billion	$5.9 billion	$6.2 billion	41,001
(Proposed for Agriculture Quarantine Program)	$407 million			
USDA-APHIS-VS Import/Export program (to develop and implement an automated system to track animal and animal product movements)			$1.355 million	
USDA-APHIS Pest and disease exclusion	$351 million (Actual)	$285 million (Est.)	$315 million (Est.)	

SOURCES: Accord, 2004; DHS, 2004a; OMB, 2004a.

such as domestic animals (dogs and cats), nonhuman primates, some reptiles (turtles and tortoises), and any animals that have an embargo or are of special concern (civet cats and African rodents). Typically, CDC handles tasks related to checking vaccination certificates and shipping regulations, rather than conducting physical inspections of animals. When inspections are done, they are cursory, i.e., visual inspection for outward signs of illness. When illness is observed, a USDA veterinarian or a private veterinarian is called in at the owner's expense. Nonhuman primates, turtles, and embargoed animals are most commonly checked. CDC will frequently field calls from the other federal agencies at POEs whenever there is a question about protocol or assistance.

According to the surveyed CDC personnel, CDC is usually notified of imports from the airline carriers or any of the CBP or APHIS inspectors that are out in the field. Most of the time, CDC will examine a paper list of what is coming into a port and from this can usually determine quickly which can be immediately released and what needs further review by its inspectors. Most of the day's activities are in the office—conducting manifest reviews, approving documents, and answering telephone queries. CDC mostly delegates different parties to check out certain cargo, since it does not have sufficient staff to conduct the physical inspections.

The procedure at the CDC quarantine location in Hawaii differs from other U.S. continental locations. Hawaii has separate regulations from the continental United States and requires all foreign carriers to submit a list of

TABLE E.4 CBP's Inspection Staff for All POE Locations, FY 2001–2004

Fiscal Year	Immigration	Customs	Agriculture	CBP non-APHIS
2001	4,717	8,184	N/A	
2002	5,422	9,008	N/A	
2003	6,741	10,538	1,480	
2004	—	—	1,446	17,784

SOURCE: CRS, 2004.

cargo coming into the state. This is usually looked at by CDC, which then clears all animal cargo or allows CBP to handle it when they are not present.

According to the surveyed CDC personnel, CBP inspectors conduct the physical inspections and determine the release of importations. CDC will study lists of incoming goods and often tells CBP what has to be inspected for the day in terms of live animals and animal products. In return, CBP will notify CDC when something of special interest arises unexpectedly. It should be noted that CBP has other major inspection responsibilities and does not actively seek animal products or other items that might be of public health concern; rather, as a courtesy, CBP will notify CDC if it sees something "unusual" during its routine work.

CDC allows CBP to sign through materials and goods when the CDC office is closed (most CDC offices are open only during business hours, except for New York's, which is open all the time). CBP provides notification to CDC of importation of dogs, cats, turtles, monkeys, other animals, and animal products capable of causing human disease. CBP will also take consideration of animals of special concern, such as civets, that have been banned by CDC. CBP personnel are trained by CDC in what to look for in animals with respect to public health threats.

According to the surveyed CDC personnel, APHIS focuses its inspections on different types of animals depending on port locations, for example, horses at the New York location and dogs at the Atlanta location. The animals for which APHIS and CDC have inspection roles and responsibilities do not overlap. Nevertheless, APHIS will frequently refer items of public health concern to the CDC quarantine staff. On the other hand, since APHIS has trained veterinarians, CDC will seek APHIS's help when it needs further veterinary investigation. While APHIS and CBP work closely together in inspections, CDC mostly performs paperwork evaluation and is infrequently called in to conduct inspections. However, CDC always inspects nonhuman primates. A procedure is also in place for APHIS to notify CDC of nonhuman primate shipments, as well as the importation of hunt-

TABLE E.5 Resources at CDC Quarantine Stations at Major U.S. Airports

Location	Holding facility or laboratory	FTEs
Atlanta	None	2
Chicago	None	3 and 1 contractor
Hawaii	None	2 and 1 contractor (not being renewed)
Los Angeles	None	2
Miami	None	1 medical officer, 1 officer in charge, 2 inspectors and 1 contracted inspector
New York	No physical resources Private veterinary facility at airport where shipments of animals can be held for inspection	6 inspectors, 1 officer in charge, 1 medical officer, and 2 contract clerical staff Quarantine officers work rotating shifts 8–8, 7 days a week
San Francisco	None devoted; animals inspected where they arrive in baggage or cargo area	2 full-time inspectors, 1 officer in charge, and intermittent clerical staff
Seattle	None	4

SOURCE: Based on Survey of Personnel at CDC quarantine stations.

ing trophies and porcupine quills that have not received the proper treatment required by CDC guidelines.

In addition, USFWS inspectors are frequently found at U.S. ports of entry conducting inspection of animals and products under their regulatory jurisdiction. USFWS will primarily contact CDC when nonhuman primates are involved. USFWS will also notify CDC of goods manufactured from animal parts, for example goatskins, which potentially carry anthrax. USFWS has a good working relationship with CDC and will frequently notify CDC of issues that fall under CDC's jurisdiction.

Local law enforcement, airlines and cargo carriers, local veterinarians, and local health groups can also be involved. These groups will inform CDC when they perceive something that might be a health threat. CDC will also contact certain private groups (such as local veterinarians and law enforcement officers) when it needs assistance. According to the Miami office, since CDC has so little staff, it frequently will involve state and local partners for assistance with law enforcement responsibilities, especially when dealing with port locations other than the home office. In these cases, a product will be held until a CDC inspector can arrive or until directions about how to proceed have been given.

For Contraband

According to CDC personnel at quarantine stations, contraband occurs infrequently. At the Los Angeles location, a frequency of six times a year was noted. At the Chicago location, it was indicated that very little contraband actually comes into the United States. However, when this occurs, contraband issues could consume from 1 to 25 hours to address, depending on CDC duty officer familiarity with the product and the circumstances surrounding the contraband, according to CDC personnel in San Francisco.

When contraband is discovered, CDC staff in Hawaii work primarily with CBP and the air carriers to find someone to take care of or dispose of it. If a situation arises such that appropriate management and disposal of animal products cannot be readily determined, CDC Atlanta would be asked to handle the situation.

At the New York quarantine location, contraband discovered in cargo is handled differently from that found on passengers. A passenger who is discovered with contraband will be isolated and told to double-bag the product for incineration by the state department of agriculture or New York City health department. Contraband discovered in cargo would be handled by a combination of CDC officers and CBP inspectors, who then relay the product for disposal by either a city or federal group.

Miami has some of the largest levels of confiscated goods, mostly in the form of animal products (skins, bone, etc.), coming into the United States as manufactured goods from the Caribbean. In Miami, any contraband found must be seized and destroyed. Currently, all contraband (waste) is burned in a state department of agriculture incinerator, but this disposal is sporadic and can vary from week to week. As a result, waste will be stored in unsafe places, such as airline hangars and storage facilities. Miami CDC personnel had suggested hiring a private medical waste disposal company that could provide dumpster and daily pickup. This approach is preferred over incineration, as it would minimize the potential of releasing pathogens into the environment and exposing the general public. Airlines are another potential partner in the discovery of contraband, and they will often let CDC know when something unusual or suspicious is found.

Game and Bush Meat:
An Example of Overlapping Roles and Responsibilities

Bush meat is a term broadly applied to game meat from wild animals that are hunted for consumption, typically in the bush of Africa but also elsewhere. A wide variety of animals are associated with this practice, including primates, hoofed animals, reptiles, birds, and rodents, many of which are protected by international wildlife and trade laws, such as the Convention on International Trade in Endangered Species of Wild Fauna and Flora (CITES). Their commercial harvest and importation into the United States is often illegal and a violation of treaties. In addition, consumption of bush meat may pose a public health risk since the animals health and origin is unknown, increasing the potential spreading pathogens to both animals and humans. Human health concerns related to bush meat include Ebola, HIV/SIV, monkeypox, herpes B, Rift Valley fever, rabies, tuberculosis, anthrax, salmonellosis, and brucellosis; animal health concerns include chronic wasting disease and TSEs (e.g., bovine spongiform encephalopathy, Creutzfelt-Jacob disease, and scrapie) (Klein, 2005).

The illegal importation of and trade in bush meat have grown in recent years, along with an increased demand for farmed game meat. Much of this meat is illegally smuggled into foreign nations under unsanitary conditions. According to USFWS, USDA, and CBP, the total amount of bush meat entering the United States is unknown, but the agencies estimate that only a small fraction of it is intercepted. The United Kingdom's Department of Food and Rural Affairs estimates that about 12,000 tons of smuggled bush meat enters the U.K. each year (Klein, 2005).

Four federal agencies have regulatory authority over domestic and imported game meats: APHIS, USFWS, CDC, and FDA. APHIS has jurisdiction under the Animal Health Protection Act to inspect, detain, quarantine, seize, and destroy animals, meat, and meat products in interstate commerce or those being imported into the United States that pose a risk of introducing a pest or foreign animal disease, such as foot-and-mouth disease (FMD) or avian influenza. USFWS has authority under the Endangered Species Act, the Lacey Act, CITES, and the Wild Bird Conservation Act to prohibit the importation of any wild animals or animal products that may threaten native wildlife or violate state, federal, or local wildlife laws.

CDC has jurisdiction under the Public Health Service Act to prohibit the importation of animals and animal products and to regulate foreign quarantine to prevent introduction of communicable diseases that threaten public health. CDC bans include importation of all nonhuman primates, African rodents (42 CFR §71.56), civets, and Asian birds. These bans specifically target protecting the public against Ebola, SIV, monkeypox, SARS, and avian influenza.

Finally, FDA's role comes under the Food, Drug, and Cosmetic Act, which says that all foods not covered by standard meat and poultry inspections must meet the same safety standards applied to all domestic foods. In addition, under the Public Health Safety Act, FDA can prohibit the interstate commerce of animal products to prevent the transmission of communicable disease harmful to humans (Klein, 2005).

When multiple federal agencies have jurisdictions over a single product (such as bush meat), determining responsibility is based primarily on the particular situation at hand. Interagency communication occurs frequently, and most federal groups are kept informed about the others' responsibilities. If an importation is discovered, the heads of local agencies will contact one another and determine whose jurisdiction involves the most stringent regulation. One interviewed source provided an example in which endangered monkey meat crossed the U.S. border. Although USFWS has primary jurisdiction because the animal is endangered, because the bush meat may contain pathogens dangerous to humans CDC would have greater priority, and its responsibility would supersede that of USFWS. Since CDC has very few local inspectors and no disposal facilities, it will often rely on inspectors from other groups (usually APHIS) to notify it of confiscated bush meat. Then, CDC can either seize the product or instruct APHIS to seize and dispose of the product on its behalf, since APHIS would have access to the proper disposal facilities.

INTERAGENCY COMMUNICATION AND REFERRALS

There is no formal or written protocol for when CDC would contact APHIS and CBP. Rather, the flow of communication is at the discretion of the officers. Interviewed CDC personnel indicated that the CDC frequently trains CBP's agricultural inspectors (formerly APHIS staff) on what to look for when inspecting animals and when to contact CDC. CDC also provides them with updates on new CDC regulations. Regular meetings are scheduled between the various groups involved with inspections at POEs (usually on a monthly basis), along with luncheons and other meetings to exchange information. CDC regularly sends informational handouts to different regions so each individual inspector will have his or her own copy of protocol and new regulations. And staff are frequently shared between the various agencies whenever the need arises.

Most interviewed CDC personnel indicated that they have not had any problems with this informal communication mechanism and that the relationship between the various agencies at U.S. POEs has been very positive. In fact, most believe that the more relaxed relationship fosters better sharing of knowledge at the local level between the various agencies and hence offers better protection against public health threats. However, several acknowledged that a more formal working protocol with APHIS and CBP could help avoid overlapping of responsibilities. Further, many noted that the effectiveness of the existing informal communication is strongly tied to the established working relationship between CDC personnel and agricultural inspectors (who are experienced former APHIS staff). With the reorganization of homeland security and the changing staff within DHS, it is becoming more difficult for CDC personnel to keep track of who in CBP is working on what project and who is in charge. CDC is finding it difficult to contact the right person to make sure that proper inspection procedure is being conducted to ensure public health protection. In addition, there is some concern regarding the reassignment of CBP inspectors into new jurisdictions that are no longer in alignment with their training or expertise.

While written protocol was not found for CDC personnel, there exists a procedure manual for animal product inspection that was created by APHIS Plant Protection and Quarantine (PPQ): the *Animal Product Manual* (APM), second edition, September 2004 (PPQ, 2004). The manual describes in detail the procedures to be used by CBP agricultural inspectors and APHIS PPQ Officers to assist them in deciding regulatory issues and referral protocols. The APM spans airport, maritime, and border operations. While primarily for regulatory decisions associated with imported cargo, the manual has an appendix that deals with baggage and the mail. The APM also has sections on procedures that cover such things as disinfection, export certification of animal products, handling of pet birds, collecting of user fees, and a glossary that provides some background on the variety of animal products the CBP agricultural inspectors and PPQ officers may encounter. The manual summarizes the referral systems described below.

U.S. Fish and Wildlife Service (USFWS)

Referral to a USFWS officer or to CBP if a USFWS officer is unavailable:

- All nonfarm animals, including birds, but excepting horses, cattle, sheep, goats, swine, dogs, cats, and pet birds.
- Animal byproducts such as pelts, coats, skins, game trophies, ivory products, and tortoiseshell products; and egg importations if from an endangered or threatened bird.
- Abandoned pet birds (also contact VS, which has jurisdiction over birds).
- All amphibians, fish, and reptiles (to determine whether they are protected by CITES).

Food and Drug Administration (FDA)

Referral of the following importations to CBP for referral to an FDA inspector:

• Any drug, medication, or food intended for animals that FDA has indicated an interest in. A local FDA inspector should be consulted for specific items of interest.
• Commercial importations of food products.
• Wild fowl meat.
• Wild ruminant meat.

Food Safety and Inspection Service (FSIS)

All meat, meat products, and shell eggs for breaking (i.e., unprocessed shelled eggs for consumption) must be referred to both Customs and FSIS. Exporters should be directed to request FSIS export certification of meat and meat products. Foreign countries must have FSIS approval that the foreign inspection service is the equivalent of FSIS. The foreign country is then allowed to issue certificates for the commercial importation of meat and meat products. In addition, FSIS inspects and samples imported meat and meat products for meeting APHIS requirements and regulations designed to prevent the spread of animal diseases. Referral of importations of shell eggs for breaking to FSIS to issue FSIS Form 5200-8, Import Request Egg Products.

DHHS Public Health Service

Referral of the following importations to customs for referral to the local Public Health Service inspector:

• Dogs, cats, and monkeys (nonhuman primates).
• Lather brushes made from hair and bristles.
• Human tissues, serum, blood, secretions, and excretions.
• If it is questionable whether an importation is of animal origin and has been imported for biological use, the question should go to a supervisor or PPQ Veterinary Regulatory Support (VRS).

APHIS Veterinary Services (VS)

VS regulations control domestic and foreign commerce in live animals, live poultry, and their products. Since 1971, VS and PPQ have shared the responsibility for implementing, enforcing, and administering animal product and foreign garbage regulations and policies to prevent the introduction of foreign animal diseases.

The following should be referred to the local VS office:

- All live animals, live birds, and hatching eggs.
- Animal semen, ova, or embryo importations; empty containers are handled by PPQ.
- Dogs imported to handle livestock except dogs from Canada, Mexico, Central America, and the West Indies.
- Abandoned pet birds (USFWS should also be contacted).

ISSUES AND CONCERNS

Interviewed CDC personnel and others raised a number of issues and concerns about potential barriers to successful protection of U.S. borders from diseases in animals. These issues and concerns are summarized below. Special considerations for expansion of CDC quarantine stations are also described.

Information Access

The biggest challenge to efforts to prevent public health threats from animal diseases imported into the United States is keeping knowledge current and getting information in a timely fashion. Interviewed New York state agriculture officials indicated that while federal agencies are fairly successful in mitigating the threat of human diseases transferred by animals in most cases, they have not been so successful in some situations, such as that of monkeypox. This is a result of failure to pass information on to local inspectors as to what the "hot" diseases are.

In a recent Government Accountability Office (GAO) report (March, 2005), it is noted that CBP's agricultural inspectors do not always receive timely information about high-risk cargo that should be held for inspection (GAO, 2005). For example, after Canada confirmed a case of bovine spongiform encephalopathy in 2003, inspectors at one border crossing did not receive a warning from USDA to hold shipments of Canadian beef in time to intercept it, and they let the shipment through. In another instance, CBP's inspectors at a seaport in a major agricultural state did not receive an alert in late 2004 about an outbreak of a strain of avian influenza that can cause death in humans until a week after the warning was released. Agricultural inspectors and port officials attributed the delay in receiving information to the transfer of some inspection roles and responsibilities from USDA to DHS. This transfer has created additional layers of communication that have impeded the rapid delivery of critical information to port inspectors. USDA used to communicate critical information directly to its agricultural inspectors, but CBP's inspectors now receive information indirectly through DHS headquarters.

CDC is usually notified of imports from the airline carriers or CBP or

APHIS inspectors who are out in the field. As the lead agency at U.S. ports, CBP has access to the Automated Manifest System (AMS), which gives advance notification of any shipments that are coming into the country and allows electronic clearance of shipments. CDC does not have access to the AMS and therefore has to rely on CBP for information. Because of the lack of access to the AMS, both CDC and USFWS require hard copies from the airlines and shippers about their importation. However, under the new Trade Act, airlines and brokers are no longer required to have hard copy of importations. CDC is concerned that compliance with requests for hard copies will cease in the future. It is also concerned about complete reliance on CBP for information since CBP is regulation-driven and does not necessarily focus on animals when it reviews the AMS. Access to the AMS would enable CDC to review incoming cargo and to capture importations of public health interest.

Human Resources

Lack of adequate staff at CDC quarantine stations is the primary concern among the interviewed CDC personnel. With severely limited human resources, CDC has had to rely on other agencies to enforce most of its regulations at U.S. POEs and is not able to oversee the vast majority of the importations. Consequently, CDC has had to accept on faith that most items are being imported with the appropriate permits or are innocuous. CDC's ability to grasp the full picture of what goes on at U.S. POEs that may have public health implications is severely affected by lack of staff.

The ratio of CDC to CBP agricultural inspection staff (former APHIS staff) is about 1:50. Given this disparity, there are not enough CDC personnel and time to conduct all the necessary training, communication, and education to keep knowledge current among CBP's inspection staff.

Another problem is that the CDC is open only during regular business hours, while CBP and APHIS are open 24 hours a day. Since shipments can come in at any hour, this makes it very difficult and haphazard for animals to have to wait until morning to be looked at. It is also costly to have to keep animals fed and watered.

The lack of veterinarian expertise at CDC quarantine locations is also of concern. Although basic knowledge of how to identify animal diseases and work with animals exists among some CDC staff at most quarantine locations, the level of training and depth of knowledge are too limited and not uniform. At the New York port location, while there is a good working relationship with veterinarians at APHIS and the state Department of Agriculture (DOA), consideration for having veterinary support in the field from CDC is suggested. One of the major issues with APHIS and DOA veterinarians is that they are not assigned to the CDC and are not always available on short notice. A CDC veterinarian will not have these prior engagements and can focus on zoonotic disease. Another advantage of having a CDC veterinarian is that he or she will have a direct link with CDC headquarters (unlike APHIS veterinarians), can help keep the local inspectors apprised of new and emerging disease threats to humans, and can speed the process of moving living organisms through quarantine. CDC veterinarians would also be an important asset in the occurrence of an outbreak, since they are better educated to handle a zoonotic threat and can better identify symptoms of new illness. It is envisioned by certain ports that a CDC veterinarian would spend part of the his or her time assisting in the physical inspection of live animals while educating inspectors and other port or airline employees about identifying and preventing zoonotic threats perceived by CDC.

Specific concerns are also being raised that primary inspectors in CBP from customs and immigrations backgrounds may not have sufficient agricultural training. Some have argued that current CBP training in agriculture for new inspectors may be inadequate. Former APHIS inspectors had required science and biology backgrounds combined with extensive pest and disease training (CRS, 2004).

Regulatory and Policy Issues

Noted as an area with overlapping regulatory authority between federal agencies are birds from Asia, which are regulated by both CBP and CDC. Some species of nonhuman primates are regulated by both USFWS and CDC. However, the general feeling is that despite these overlapping regulatory authorities, things are working well at port locations. There is a concern that there may be issues with communication among the headquarters groups.

Lack of consideration for policy implementation at the local level (i.e., port locations) is an issue that was raised by several interviewed CDC personnel. Often, CDC headquarters will issue a broad embargo policy (such as those on the importation of monkeys or civets), without any specific policies and guidance on roles, responsibilities, and interactions at the local level among the various agencies, namely, CBP, APHIS, and CDC. Leaving the details to be sorted out at the local level has often led to different and inconsistent implementing policies across the different quarantine stations. Also, in situations involving rush embargoes, time is of essence; having to spend time to sort out the details often leads to frustration at the local level. There is a need to establish plans and policies at the national level that can then filter down to the local level in a more consistent and efficient manner. CDC's set of regulations on how to deal with nonhuman primates and associated paperwork was identified as a good example that should be repeated for other animals and protocols.

While specific policies are needed in roles and responsibilities, too-specific protocols can prove to be burdensome. Protocols for specific types of rodents instead of one broad rodent protocol are an example. Efficiencies can be gained with broader protocols.

Agricultural Inspection Issues

In a recent report, GAO indicated a concern that agricultural inspections at ports of entry have declined over the last 2 years while imports have increased. Data show a decline in the number of agricultural inspections at POEs nationwide from 40.9 million in FY 2002, when USDA was fully responsible for agricultural inspections, to 37.5 million in FY 2004, when DHS had primary responsibility (GAO, 2005). No clear explanation has been found as to why this drop in inspections occurred.

Another concern is that the majority of live animals coming through ports get a cursory examination based on overall appearance of health. Only for select diseases are specific examinations or tests being done (e.g., for rabies), which can be done at import locations or before importation.

Special Considerations in the Expansion of CDC Quarantine Stations

Although there is a need for additional quarantine stations, the consensus is that it is an impractical idea at this point, since there are not even enough staff for existing stations. Rather, the first priority should be to hire new workers and expand the resources and capabilities at existing stations. Only when newly hired staff have gained enough experience and background should they be moved to staff new locations. Field inspection is more or less a hands-on learning experience. Staff can function only with adequate background and familiarity on the job. This is especially true with medical officers. It is stressed that new quarantine stations should never be opened with inexperienced inspectors and officers.

There are also some suggestions that only ports with significant internationally arriving travelers be considered for the addition of a quarantine station. Further, only if additional funding is available should consideration of quarantine staff at airports with a primarily domestic traveling public be entertained. Another suggestion is that there should be differential levels of staffing for different locations depending on volume of importations. For examples, some ports might need just a single high-level person rather than several lower-level staff. There is a huge flow of freight from Canada and Mexico, and it is questioned whether these land borders are closely watched. Food, such as bush meat, may be imported through Canada to avoid the authorities. Without staff on-site, these cases would be missed. Finally, a major expansion plan must take into consideration the fact that office space is at a premium at U.S. airports.

REFERENCES

Accord B, Administrator, APHIS. 2004. *Animal and Plant Health Inspection Service.* Statement at the March 4, 2004 hearing of the Subcommittee on Agriculture, Rural Development, Food and Drug Administration, and Related Agencies, U.S. House of Representatives.

APHIS (Animal and Plant Health Inspection Service, United States Department of Agriculture). 2003. *APHIS Fact Sheet. The Animal and Plant Health Inspection Service and Department of Homeland Security: Working Together to Protect Agriculture.* [Online] Available: http://www.aphis.usda.gov/lpa/pubs/fsheet_faq_notice/fs_aphis_homeland.pdf [accessed April 7, 2005].

APHIS. 2004a. *Veterinary Services Safeguarding Animal Health: Import/Export.* [Online] Available: http://www.aphis.usda.gov/vs/ncie/ [accessed March 1, 2004].

APHIS. 2004b. *Veterinary Services Strategic Plan FY 2004 to FY 2008.* [Online] Available: http://www.aphis.usda.gov/vs/pdf_files/strat_plan.pdf [accessed April 7, 2005].

Bonner RC, Commissioner, U.S. Customs and Border Protection. 2004. *Statement of Robert C. Bonner to the National Commission on Terrorist Attacks Upon the United States.* Statement at the January 26, 2004 hearing of the National Commission on Terrorist Attacks Upon the United States.

Bush GW. 2002. *Securing the Homeland, Strengthening the Nation.* [Online] Available: http://www.whitehouse.gov/homeland/homeland_security_book.html [accessed April 7, 2005].

CBP (U.S. Customs and Border Protection, Department of Homeland Security). 2003. *Customs and Border Protection Today.* [Online] Available: http://www.cbp.gov/xp/CustomsToday/ 2003 March/ [accessed March 31, 2004].

CBP. 2004. *Preventing Animal and Plant Pests and Diseases: More than 1.7 Million Prohibited Agricultural Items Intercepted Last Year.* [Online] Available: http://www.customs. gov/xp/cgov/newsroom/press_releases/0012004/01142004_4.xml [accessed April 2, 2004].

Crawford LM, Deputy Commissioner, FDA. 2003. *Agroterrorism: The Threat to America's Breadbasket.* Statement at the November 19, 2003 hearing of the Committee on Homeland Security and Governmental Affairs, U.S. Senate.

Creekmore L. 2003. *Preventive Measures and Existing Regulations for Chronic Wasting Diseases in the U.S.* Presentation at the September 10-11, 2003 Meeting on TSE in Animal Populations: Fact and Fiction, Fort Collins, CO.

CRS (Congressional Research Service, The Library of Congress). 2004. *Border Security: Inspection Practices, Policies, and Issues.* [Online] Available: http://fpc.state.gov/ documents/organization/33856.pdf [accessed April 7, 2005].

DGMQ (Division of Global Migration and Quarantine, National Center for Infectious Diseases, Centers for Disease Control and Prevention). 2003a. *History of Quarantine.* [Online] Available: http://www.cdc.gov/ncidod/dq/history.htm [accessed April 7, 2005].

DGMQ. 2003b. *Mission.* [Online] Available: http://wwwcdc.gov/ncidod/dq/mission.htm [accessed April 6, 2004].

DGMQ. 2004. *Importation of Pets, Other Animals, and Animal Products into the United States.* [Online] Available: http://www.cdc.gov/ncidod/dq/animal.htm [accessed March 18, 2004].

DHS (U.S. Department of Homeland Security). 2004a. *Budget in Brief, Fiscal Year 2005.* [Online] Available: http://www.dhs.gov/interweb/assetlibrary/FY_2005_BIB_4.pdf [accessed April 7, 2005].

DHS. 2004b. *DHS Organization: Department Components.* [Online] Available: http://www.dhs.gov/dhspublic/display?theme=9&content=2973 [accessed March 1, 2004].

DHS. 2004c. *Protecting Against Agricultural Terrorism.* [Online] Available: http://www.dhs.gov/dhspublic/display?theme=43&content=3117 [accessed April 2, 2004].

FASS (Federation of Animal Science Societies). 2003. *No Retraining for Agricultural Inspectors in Border Agency Plan.* [Online] Available: http://www.fass.org/fasstrack/news_item.asp?news_id=1646 [accessed April 6, 2004].

FCBF (Florida Customs Brokers & Forwarders Association, Inc.). 2003. *CBP Agriculture Specialist Fact Sheet.* [Online] Available: http://www.fcbf.com/NewsFlashDetail.asp?NewsId=47 [accessed April 4, 2004].

GAO (United States Government Accountability Office). 2005. *Homeland Security: Much Is Being Done to Protect Agriculture from a Terrorist Attack, but Important Challenges Remain.* GAO-05-214. Washington, DC: GAO.

Grannis J. 2003. *Animal Disease Outbreaks: 21st Century Issues.* Presentation at the July 11, 2003 Conference on the Economic Impact of Animal Disease on the Food Marketing Sector, Denver, CO.

Klein PN. 2005. Regulatory report: Game meat: A complex food safety and animal health issue. *Food Safety Magazine* 10(96).

NRC (National Research Council). 2003. *Countering Agricultural Bioterrorism.* Washington, DC: National Academy Press.

OMB (Office of Management and Budget, the Executive Office of the President of the United States). 2004a. *Budget of the United States Government Fiscal Year 2005: Appendix.* [Online] Available: http://www.whitehouse.gov/omb/budget/fy2005/appendix.html [accessed April 7, 2005].

OMB. 2004b. *Department of Agriculture Part Assessments* [Online] Available: http://www.whitehouse.gov/omb/budget/fy2005/pma/agriculture.pdf [accessed April 12, 2004].

OSH (Office of Health and Safety, Centers for Disease Control and Prevention). 2004. *Etiologic Agent Import Permit Program.* [Online] Available: http://www.cdc.gov/od/ohs/biosfty/imprtper.htm [accessed April 6, 2004].

PPQ. 2004. (Plant Protection and Quarantine, Animal and Plant Health Inspection Service, United States Department of Agriculture). *Animal Product Manual (Second Edition).* [Online] Available: http://www.aphis.usda.gov/ppq/manuals/pdf_files/APM.pdf [accessed April 7, 2005].

USAHA (United States Animal Health Association). 2003. *USAHA 2003 Resolution No. 21.* [Online] Available: http://www.usaha.org/resolutions/reso03/res-2103.html [accessed April 6, 2004].

USFWS (Division of Law Enforcement, US Fish and Wildlife Service). 2002. *Annual Report FY 2001.* [Online] Available: http://library.fws.gov/Pubs9/LEannual01.pdf [accessed April 7, 2005].

USFWS (Office of Law Enforcement, U.S. Fish and Wildlife Service). 2003. *FY 2002 Annual Report.* [Online] Available: http://www.fws.gov/le/pdffiles/FY2002rpt.pdf [accessed April 7, 2005].

APPENDIX 1—INTERVIEWED INDIVIDUALS

Ahmad, Khawaja N.	Supervisory VMO	USDA-APHIS-VS, JFK Airport
Akey, Dr. Bruce	Acting State Veterinarian	NYS Department of Agriculture & Markets
Becker, Margaret	Officer in Charge	CDC NYC Quarantine Station
Becker, Margaret	Deputy Commissioner	NYS Department of Agriculture & Markets
Blumensaadt, Sena	Acting Officer in Charge	CDC Chicago Quarantine Station
Ehart, Robert		National Association of State Departments of Agriculture
Dailey, Terrence	Officer in Charge	CDC Atlanta Quarantine Station
Dick, Jerre	Associate Deputy	USDA, APHIS, VS
Drew, Anthony	Officer in Charge	CDC Miami Quarantine Station
Dwyer, Susan	Officer in Charge	CDC San Francisco Quarantine Station
Houck, Dr. Peter	Quarantine Medical Officer	CDC Seattle Quarantine Station
Marty, Michael	Officer in Charge	CDC Los Angeles Quarantine Station
Mitruka, Dr. Kiren	Medical Officer	CDC Miami Quarantine Station
Riley, Lucinda	Director of Agriculture	DHS U.S. Customs and Border Protection
Tapia, Dr. Robert	Officer in Charge	CDC Hawaii Quarantine Station
Thomas, Lee Ann	Director (Live Animal)	USDA, APHIS, VS, NCIE

APPENDIX 2—LINES OF INQUIRIES

Inquiries for CDC

1. Please describe the various personnel and their respective agencies involved with prevention/mitigation of public health threats **originating from animals** entering the United States through the U.S. quarantine stations. What are their specific roles and responsibilities?

- CDC's Division of Global Migration and Quarantine (DGMQ):
- USDA/Animal Plant Health Inspection Service (APHIS):
- U.S. Customs and Border Protection (CBP):
- Immigration and Customs Enforcement (ICE)
- U.S. Fish and Wildlife Service (USFWS):
- Other personnel:

2. What is the relationship between the APHIS staff with the CDC/DGMQ staff at our ports of entry?

- Is there a protocol for when Q-station CDC/DGMQ staff would call in the APHIS staff or vice versa?
- Are there challenges in implementing the above protocol?

3.   What is the relationship between the CDC/DGMG staff with other agencies such as CBP, ICE, USFWS, etc...?

- Are there protocols from communication between CDC/DGMQ staff with other agencies, i.e. CBP, ICE, USFWS, etc...?
- Are there challenges in implementing the above protocol?

4.   What is the day-to-day reality of the work?

- For routine notification of imports
- For contraband

5.   What are the resources currently devoted to animal inspection activities at quarantine stations?

- Facility size in square feet _____

- Number of animals facility can hold at any point in time_____

- Laboratory capacity: _____

- Human resources (Full Time Employees)_____

6.   Are there barriers to successful protection of our borders from diseases in animals? If yes, what are these barriers?

- Human resources?
- Legal authority—overlapping authorities?
- Location capacity—need of additional Q-Stations?
- Other?

7.   Is there anything else of note?

Additional Inquiries for the CBP and State Department of Agriculture

1.   Are there any written policies, procedures, manuals, and training given by the CDC to prevent the spread of zoonotic disease through live animals and animal products?
2.   How are responsibilities delegated among the different federal and state groups?
3.   How well mitigated are the threat of disease under current policy and do live animals or animal products pose the greater threat to the general population?

ABBREVIATIONS

AMS	Automated Manifest System
APHIS	Animal and Plant Health Inspection Service (USDA)
APM	Animal Product Manual
AQI	Agriculture Quarantine and Inspection (USDA APHIS)
BTS	Directorate of Border and Transportation Security (DHS)
CBP	U.S. Customs and Border Protection (DHS BTS)
CDC	Centers for Disease Control and Prevention
CITES	Convention on International Trade in Endangered Species of Wild Flora and Fauna
DFO	Director of Field Operations (DHS OFO)
DGMQ	Division of Global Migration and Quarantine (CDC NCID)
DHHS	U.S. Department of Health and Human Services
DHS	U.S. Department of Homeland Security
DOI	U.S. Department of the Interior
DOJ	U.S. Department of Justice
EIS	Epidemic Intelligence Service
FAD	foreign animal diseases
FDA	Food and Drug Administration
FLETC	Federal Law Enforcement Training Center
FMD	foot-and-mouth disease
FSIS	Food Safety and Inspection Service
FTE	full-time-employee
HSA	Homeland Security Act
ICE	Immigration and Customs Enforcement
INA	Immigration and Nationality Act
INS	U.S. Immigration and Naturalization Service (formerly DOJ, now DHS)
IOM	Institute of Medicine
LSS	Laboratories and Scientific Services (CBP)
MOU	Memorandum of Understanding
NCID	National Center for Infectious Diseases (CDC)
NCIE	National Center for Import and Export (USDA APHIS)
NTC	National Targeting Center (CBP OFO)
OFO	Office of Field Operations (DHS)
POE	Port of Entry
PPQ	Plant Protection and Quarantine (USDA APHIS)
SARS	severe acute respiratory syndrome
SIV	simian immunodeficiency virus
USDA	U.S. Department of Agriculture
USFWS	U.S. Fish and Wildlife Service
VRS	Veterinary Regulatory Support
VS	Veterinary Services (USDA APHIS)

F

International Legal Considerations for the Quarantine Station Expansion

Memorandum

To: Committee on Measures to Enhance the Effectiveness of the
            CDC Quarantine Station Expansion Plan for U.S. Ports of
            Entry

From: David P. Fidler (Consultant), Professor of Law and Harry T.
            Ice Faculty Fellow, Indiana University School of Law,
            Bloomington

Re: International Legal Considerations for the Quarantine Station
            Expansion Plan

Date: May 26, 2005

EXECUTIVE SUMMARY

The memorandum responds to the committee's desire to understand the international legal considerations the federal government should have in mind as it develops its plans to expand the national quarantine system (NQS). The memorandum analyzes the basic dynamics of the relationship between public health and international law (Part 2); the revised International Health Regulations (IHR) adopted by the World Health Assembly on May 23, 2005 (Resolution WHA58.3) (Part 3); international trade law (Part 4); international human rights law (Part 5); and international legal issues connected with the expanded NQS, including stationing personnel and assets in foreign countries (Part 6). Attached to the memorandum are three annexes: a table compiling the positive and negative obligations international law imposes on the United States that may be germane to the expansion of the NQS (Annex 1); provision-by-provision analyses of the revised IHR (Annex 2) and the Agreement on the Application of Sanitary and Phytosanitary Measures (SPS Agreement) of the World Trade Organization (WTO) (Annex 3) in terms of their potential implications for the expansion of the NQS.

In terms of the expansion of the NQS within the United States, none of the bodies of international law analyzed poses a significant constraint on the federal government's expansion plans. International law recognizes each state's sovereign right to take action to protect its public's health. Expanding the NQS would constitute an exercise of that sovereign right. The areas of international law applicable to the expanded NQS analyzed in this memorandum involve disciplines on how the federal government exercises its sovereign right to protect public health. These disciplines address health measures that the expanded NQS would apply to people, goods (including plants and animals), containers used in international commerce, and means of transportation. The federal government's strategy to make the NQS more comprehensive and robust in its capabilities to protect U.S. public health will bring the expanded NQS more directly and frequently into contact with these various bodies of international law.

The United States public health system is already subject to the disciplines arising in international trade law (e.g., WTO and the SPS Agreement) and international human rights law, so organizing the expanded NQS to comply with these international legal rules will constitute continued U.S. compliance with its existing obligations under trade and human rights treaties. The most comprehensive set of disciplines the expanded NQS face appear in the revised IHR. The revised IHR will not enter into force for World Health Organization (WHO) member states that accept the new Regulations until 2007 (Article 59.2); but the United States has publicly announced its support for the revised IHR, meaning that the United States is unlikely to reject the revised IHR (Statement for the Record by the Government of the United States of America Concerning the World Health Organization's Revised International Health Regulations, May 23, 2005 [hereinafter U.S. Statement for the Record]). The revised IHR are radically different from previous versions of the IHR and thus represent a historic international legal development of which the committee should be aware as part of its deliberations.

In connection with possible plans to station U.S. public health personnel and assets in foreign countries as part of the expanded NQS, the memorandum outlines a number of international legal considerations that the committee should review in thinking about the wisdom of "forward deployment" of parts of the expanded NQS. In the context of "forward deployment," international law is less accommodating to the United States because it would be operating from the sovereign territories of other states, which have superior rights and obligations under international law concerning what happens in their territories. Stationing federal public health personnel and assets in other countries as part of the expanded NQS will have to involve cooperation with foreign governments and–in all likelihood–the negotiation of formal, written agreements governing the relationship between host governments and the U.S. public health presence in those countries.

1. INTRODUCTION

The federal government of the United States plans to expand the national quarantine system (NQS), currently operated and managed by the Division of Global Migration and Quarantine of the Centers for Disease Control and Prevention (CDC). The federal government has long operated a national quarantine program to protect the United States against the introduction of communicable diseases from foreign countries and to prevent and control infectious disease spread between the states of the union. The federal government reduced the scale of the NQS in the 1970s when public health experts believed that the threat from communicable diseases had significantly diminished. Growing concerns in the last decade about emerging and reemerging infectious diseases and the threat of bioterrorism have prompted the federal government to develop plans to enhance the NQS to address the communicable disease threats posed to the United States today.

The committee's mandate is to review the federal government's plans for expanding the NQS. As part of its review, the committee commissioned the Consultant to analyze the expansion of the NQS with respect to applicable international law. The committee believes that such an analysis will inform its deliberations of the international implications of the plans to expand the NQS. The United States will operate any expanded NQS in an environment affected by international law, making some understanding of this law pertinent to the committee's overall mandate.

2. BASIC DYNAMICS OF INTERNATIONAL LAW WITH RESPECT TO PUBLIC HEALTH PROTECTION

International law comprises the set of rules states have created to regulate their interactions with each other. For purposes of the international legal rules analyzed in this memorandum, the relevant actor is the United States. Typically, international legal analysis does not enquire into how constitutionally, or as a matter of domestic law, a state organizes itself to fulfill international legal obligations it has undertaken. As a federal system, the United States' acceptance of international legal obligations is occasionally affected by federalism. The revised International Health Regulations (IHR) are a case in point because the United States has indicated that it will have "to submit a narrowly tailored reservation . . . that will clarify that the United States will implement the IHRs in a manner consistent with our federal system of government" (U.S. Statement for the Record). Absent such reservations related to federalism, the United States cannot raise federalism as a reason for non-compliance with international legal obligations it has undertaken pursuant to treaties. Nor are questions of jurisdictional responsibilities within the federal government usually relevant for purposes of international legal analysis.

Generally speaking, states have repeatedly acknowledged in international lawmaking that each state has a sovereign right to protect its territory and people from exogenous health threats moving in people, products, plants, or animals through the channels of world trade and travel. Thus, the desire of the federal government to strengthen its ability to protect the United States from communicable disease importation and spread does not, by itself, create any international legal problems because the United States has a sovereign right to engage in this governmental activity.

International legal issues arise in this area because states have created various obligations and disciplines that regulate the manner in which they can exercise their sovereignty to protect public health. The United States is, for example, party to treaties that place limits and conditions on how it addresses potential public health threats posed by the global movement of people, animals, plants, and products. The United States is a party to various international trade agreements that regulate the exercise of U.S. sovereignty in protecting Americans from health threats from imported goods. The United States will need to operate its expanded NQS in conformity with existing and future U.S. obligations under applicable bodies of international law.

The reduced scale of the NQS during that past three decades has meant that the NQS has not interfaced significantly with international law. The limited scope of international law on infectious disease control historically also contributed to the limited relationship between the NQS and international law. Expanding the scale, capabilities, and responsibilities of the NQS might bring it into more direct contact with international law, raising the profile of U.S. obligations under international law for the operation of the NQS.

The three areas of treaty law most applicable to the expansion of the NQS are: (1) the international law directly addressing infectious disease control—the revised IHR promulgated by the World Health Organization (WHO); (2) international trade law; and (3) international human rights law. Protecting U.S. public health from disease threats will require taking action concerning people, products, animals, plants, and means of transport moving in the stream of international trade and travel. Although not exhaustive in terms of the possible international legal implications of an expanded NQS, analyzing the revised IHR, international trade law, and international human rights law constitutes the best way to provide the committee with some perspective on the relationship between an expanded NQS and international law. This memorandum addresses each of these bodies of international law in turn.

The United States will also face international legal issues if the federal government contemplates placing federal quarantine resources inside the territory of other countries. The Consultant understands that the federal government may wish to "forward deploy" public health assets to foreign ports and countries as part of the strategy to prevent and control the importation of potential health threats into the United States. Such arrangements will involve the United States negotiating agreements or arrangements with foreign countries in order to allow federal public health personnel to perform functions within the territory and jurisdiction of those sovereign nations. This memorandum contains brief commentary on the international legal issues that would arise with "forward deployment" of NQS assets in foreign countries.

3. THE INTERNATIONAL HEALTH REGULATIONS

From their original promulgation by WHO as the International Sanitary Regulations in 1951, the old IHR constituted the only international legal instrument directly on infectious disease control binding on WHO member states. Prior to the revision in 2005, WHO last revised the IHR in 1981, when the organization removed smallpox from the list of the diseases subject to the Regulations. From 1981 until the present, the IHR have applied to only three diseases—cholera, plague, and yellow fever. The concerns about emerging and reemerging infectious diseases and bioterrorism behind the federal government's plans to expand the NQS also stimulated at WHO a process to revise the IHR to make them more relevant to transnational disease threats in an era of globalization. This process began in 1995 and was completed by the World Health Assembly in May 2005 when it adopted the revised IHR.

WHO's adoption of the revised IHR, and the U.S. government's declared support for the revised IHR, means that the federal government will develop the expanded NQS in an international legal environment affected by the revised IHR. The revised IHR contain an international legal regime radically different from the old IHR and their historical precursors. Most important from the perspective of an expanded NQS, the revised IHR impose more demanding international legal rules than any previous version of the IHR.

For example, the more demanding nature of the revised IHR appears in the provision that defines "disease" in such a way that includes all sources of human illness or medical conditions (Article 1.1). This provision, and others, expands the revised IHR's scope to include disease events caused by biological, chemical, and radiological agents. Historically, the IHR applied only to communicable diseases, making the revised IHR's application to public health threats from chemical and radiological sources a significant break from the past. In addition, the revised IHR's scope creates international legal obligations for the United States not entirely encompassed by an expanded NQS, which would still be focused on communicable disease threats.

The following sections summarize the key issues the revised IHR raise for the plans to expand the NQS. The length and complexity of the revised IHR means that this memorandum cannot mention each point at which the revised IHR and the expanded NQS might interface. For those members of the committee interested in more detail, Annex 2 provides a provision-by-provision analysis.

Part I–Definitions, Purpose and Scope, Principles and Responsible Authorities

Definitions

The most important definition in the revised IHR for the expanded NQS is the definition of "disease" because this definition, as noted above, determines the scope of the revised IHR's application. "Disease" is defined to mean "an illness of medical condition, irrespective of origin or source, that presents or could present significant harm to humans" (Article 1.1). Under this definition of disease, and the scope it implies for the revised IHR, the expanded NQS will not be sufficient to meet United States obligations under the revised IHR because the federal government is not expanding the NQS with chemical and radiological threats in mind.

Purpose and Scope and Principles

The purpose and scope of the revised IHR comport with the objectives of the expansion of the NQS—preventing, protecting against, controlling, and providing a public health response to the international spread of disease in ways that avoid unnecessary interference with international traffic and trade (Article 2). The principles that should guide the implementation of the revised IHR recognize that states have "the sovereign right to legislate and to implement legislation in pursuance of their health policies" (Article 3.4). The guiding principles of the revised IHR also importantly require that the IHR be implemented "with full respect for the dignity, human rights and fundamental freedoms of persons" (Article 3.1). This principle requires the expanded NQS to implement health measures against people in ways that comply with international human rights law, a requirement not previously contained in the IHR. Other principles of the revised

IHR also require states parties to the revised IHR to respect the dignity, human rights, and fundamental freedoms of persons (see Part 5 on international human rights law below).

Responsible Authorities

The revised IHR mandate that states parties designate a single, national contact point—the National IHR Focal Point—that plays an important role in the functioning of the revised IHR (Article 4.1). The expanded NQS would have to have an organizational and communication structure to facilitate U.S. compliance with the requirements of the administrative provisions of the revised IHR.

Part II–Information and Public Health Response

Core Surveillance and Response Capacities

The old IHR had requirements for states parties to maintain certain public health capabilities at points of entry and exit, but the revised IHR contains surveillance and response capacity requirements that go far beyond anything seen in the history of the IHR. The revised IHR contain obligations for states parties to develop and strengthen core surveillance and response capacities specified in the text within five years from the entry into force of the revised IHR (Articles 5.1 and 13.1 and Annex 1). The objective is to move states parties to develop and maintain core public health capacities to identify, report, and respond effectively to public health risks and events that constitute public health emergencies of international concern. The capacities of the expanded NQS would be judged, thus, against the core capacity requirements established in the revised IHR.

Notification of Disease Events

The old IHR required states parties to report outbreaks of specific infectious diseases, namely cholera, plague, and yellow fever. The revised IHR adopts a different approach to disease notification because it requires notification not only of specific diseases (smallpox, polio, new subtypes of human influenza, and SARS) but also "all events which may constitute a public health emergency of international concern within its territory" (Article 6.1). States parties must also provide WHO with all relevant public health information if they have evidence of an unexpected or unusual public health event within their respective territories, irrespective of origin or source, which may constitute a public health emergency of international concern (Article 7).

BOX F.1   The Revised IHR's Decision Instrument (Annex 2)

Any case of smallpox, polio, human influenza caused by a new sub-type, and SARS must be notified to WHO under the revised IHR.

For any event involving (1) cholera, pneumonic plague, yellow fever, viral haemorrhagic fevers (e.g., Ebola, Lassa, Marburg), West Nile fever, and other diseases that are of special national or regional concern (e.g., dengue fever, Rift Valley fever, and meningococcal disease), or (2) other incidents of potential international public health concern, including those of unknown causes or sources, States Parties shall answer the following questions, affirmative answers to at least two of which mean that the event shall be notified to WHO under the revised IHR:

1. Is the public health impact of the event serious?
2. Is the event unusual or unexpected?
3. Is there a significant risk of international spread?
4. Is there a significant risk of international travel or trade restrictions?

Annex 2 provides examples for the application of these questions to disease events that are designed to assist the assessment and notification of events that may constitute a public health emergency of international concern.

A key objective of the notification obligations is to ensure that global disease surveillance can identify, and respond to, new disease threats—of whatever origin—not captured by disease-specific reporting. Notification of disease events is to be guided by a "decision instrument" (Annex 2). See Box F.1 on how the decision instrument works. The expanded NQS would have to be able to utilize the decision instrument in order for the United States to fulfill its notification obligations under the revised IHR.

WHO Surveillance and Verification Authorities

Under the old IHR, WHO could only officially collect and disseminate epidemiological information supplied by governments. This limitation on WHO surveillance capabilities was a serious weakness of the past IHR. The revised IHR contain a number of provisions that increase WHO authority in the area of surveillance and information verification. Under the revised IHR, the WHO can collect and use epidemiological information from nongovernmental sources (Article 9.1), request verification from states parties of informed collected by WHO (Article 10.1), disseminate information it collects (Article 11), and determine whether an event constitutes a public health emergency of international concern (Article 12).

Taken together, these new authorities for WHO in the revised IHR create an environment for the expanded NQS radically different from the way in which international surveillance and WHO operated under the old IHR. The expanded NQS might have to be involved in cooperating with WHO in verifying information WHO has received about disease events in the United States, assessing a greater stream of surveillance information disseminated by WHO, and interacting with WHO when WHO makes determinations about whether an event in the United States constitutes a public health emergency of international concern.

Part III–Recommendations

Another new feature of the revised IHR is granting WHO the authority to issue temporary recommendations in connection with public health emergencies of international concern and standing recommendations with respect to health measures needed for routine or periodic application (Articles 15 and 16). The revised IHR provide examples of the kinds of measures WHO could recommend (Article 18) and the criteria that should guide the WHO in issuing recommendations (Article 17).

Recommendations issued by WHO under the revised IHR would not be legally binding on the United States, so the issuance of recommendations would not obligate the expanded NQS to act in accordance with WHO guidance. If the United States agreed to implement WHO recommendations, then the expanded NQS would be engaged in such implementation. To implement WHO recommendations effectively, the expanded NQS would need both the domestic legal authority to act as specified in the recommendations and the capacity to so act. In addition, U.S. implementation of WHO recommendations concerning goods would have to comply with U.S. obligations under international trade law.

Part IV–Points of Entry

The expansion of the NQS involves increasing federal public health capabilities at more points of entry into the United States, which makes the provisions in the revised IHR on points of entry particularly relevant. The revised IHR contain numerous obligations for states parties with respect to capacities and measures taken at points of entry. These obligations include ensuring that designated points of entry have capacities detailed in the revised IHR; identifying the competent authorities for points of entry; furnishing to WHO information on potential public health threats at points of entry; issuing health documents to ships in accordance with requirements in the revised IHR; maintaining sanitary facilities for travelers at points of entry; supervising deratting, disinfection, disinsection, or decontamination of conveyances, containers, cargo, or goods or the application of health measures for persons at points of entry; and others.

To comply with these kinds of obligations in the revised IHR, the United States would need to ensure that the expanded NQS is authorized under domestic law and actually capable of undertaking the many duties the revised IHR create for the competent authorities at points of entry. Although the revised IHR contain point-of-entry obligations that resemble duties found in the old IHR, the expansion of the NQS means that the number of places at which these obligations may have direct effect will increase.

Part V–Public Health Measures

The revised IHR contain many rules on the application of health measures to travelers; conveyances and conveyance operators; goods, containers, and container loading areas. These rules generally attempt to balance a state party's right to apply health measures to protect its public health with the objectives of minimizing interference with travelers and international traffic. The expanded NQS would be required to operate these rules, and thus these provisions of the revised IHR are important in terms of planning for the expanded NQS. The following paragraphs provide some sense of the kinds of rules on health measures that the revised IHR impose on the United States and its expanded NQS.

Health Measures for Travelers

General principles

The revised IHR allow states parties to apply health measures on the arrival or departure of travelers, but the provisions on health measures for travelers place disciplines on the content and implementation of such measures. To begin, the revised IHR state that one of their guiding principles is the implementation of the IHR with full respect for dignity, human rights, and fundamental freedoms of persons (Article 3.1). The revised IHR give this general principle more context by requiring respect for dignity, human rights, and fundamental freedoms through treating all travelers with courtesy and respect, taking into consideration gender, sociocultural, ethnic, or religious concerns of travelers, and providing adequate food, water, shelter, protection for possessions, means of communication, and medical treatment for those quarantined, isolated, or subject to other measures for public health purposes (Article 32). Other provisions of the revised IHR apply these general requirements in specific contexts that would implicate the operation of the expanded NQS. The following paragraphs describe some of these provisions.

Medical examinations

States parties to the revised IHR are allowed to require arriving or departing travelers to undergo a "non-invasive medical examination which is the least intrusive examination that would achieve the public health objective" (Article 23.1[a][iii]). As a general matter, the revised IHR prohibit states parties from requiring invasive medical examination as a condition of entry for travelers (Article 31.1). If the state party believes that an invasive medical examination is necessary on the basis of evidence of a public health risk, then it can perform such examination provided that it is "the least intrusive and invasive medical examination that would achieve the public health objective of preventing the international spread of disease" (Article 23.2; see also Article 43.1). A state party can administer no medical examination without the prior, express informed consent of the traveler (Article 23.3), except in circumstances under which the protection of public health warrants compulsory medical examination, in which case such examination must be the least intrusive and invasive examination possible to achieve the public health objective (Article 31.2). Refusal to consent to medical examination can be grounds for denying entry to the traveler (Article 31.2).

Vaccination or other prophylaxis

As a general matter, the revised IHR prohibits states parties from requiring vaccination or other prophylaxis as a condition of entry for any traveler (Article 31.1). The revised IHR create, however, some exceptions. First, states parties can create vaccination or other prophylaxis requirements for people seeking temporary or permanent residence (Article 31.1[b]). Second, proof of vaccination against yellow fever may be required for travelers as a condition of entry to a state party (Article 31.1[c] and Annex 7). Third, a state party may require vaccination or other prophylaxis as a condition of entry for a traveler if recommended by WHO as a temporary or standing recommendation under the revised IHR. Fourth, a state party may require vaccination or other prophylaxis as a condition of entry for travelers if the state party believes that such a requirement is warranted because of an imminent public health risk (Article 31.2[b]).

A state party can administer no vaccination or other prophylaxis without the prior, express informed consent of the traveler (Article 23.3), except in circumstances under which the protection of public health warrants compulsory vaccination or other prophylaxis (Article 31.2). Refusal to consent to vaccination or other prophylaxis can be grounds for a state party to deny entry to the traveler (Article 31.2). Travelers subjected to vaccination or other prophylaxis must be informed of all risks associated with these actions (Article 23.4), and the administration of the vaccination or other prophylaxis must conform to established national or international safety guidelines in order to minimize risk to the traveler (Article 23.5).

Quarantine and isolation

A state party may use quarantine and isolation as health measures against travelers arriving or departing in two circumstances: (1) if WHO recommends quarantine and isolation as health measures needed to address a public health emergency of international concern; and (2) if the state party itself determines that quarantine and isolation are health measures justified under the circumstances to address a public health risk (Articles 23.2, 31.2[c], and 43.1). A state party must obtain the prior, express informed consent of the traveler before implementing quarantine or isolation on such persons (Article 23.3), unless the state party has grounds to believe that compulsory quarantine and isolation are required to address an imminent public health risk (Article 31.2[c]). A state party that places persons in quarantine or isolation must provide persons with, or arrange for the provision of, adequate food, water, shelter, clothing, security for possessions, medical treatment, and access to communications (Article 32).

Public health observation

States parties may place suspect travelers under public health observation pursuant to their own determinations (Articles 23.2, 30, and 31.2[c]) or WHO recommendations, but this health measure also requires the prior, express informed consent of the traveler in question (Article 23.3), unless the state party believes that compulsory public health observation is required to protect public health (Article 31.2[c]). A state party may allow a suspect traveler under public health observation to continue on an international voyage if (a) the traveler does not pose an imminent threat to public health, and (b) the state party informs the competent authority of the travelers next point of entry (Article 30).

Personal information

States parties may require as a condition of entry for travelers certain information about the travelers' itinerary and destination and the opportunity to review health documents required under the revised IHR (e.g., yellow fever vaccination certificate) (Article 23.2[a][i]-[ii]). Refusal to provide this information can be grounds for the state party to deny entry to the traveler (Article 31.2). The revised IHR contain provisions imposing obligations on states parties to keep confidential health information collected or received pursuant to the implementation of the revised IHR, except in cases in which a state party must disclose or transmit personal information for the purposes of assessing and managing a public health risk (Article 45).

Health Measures for Goods and Cargo

The revised IHR's general principle concerning health measures applied against goods and cargo is that states parties should avoid unnecessary interference with international traffic and trade (Articles 2 and 43.1). States parties may inspect goods and cargo for public health purposes on arrival or departure, subject to relevant articles of the revised IHR and applicable international agreements (Article 23.1[b]). The revised IHR define "goods" to mean "tangible products, including animals and plants, transported on an international voyage, including for utilization on board a conveyance" (Article 1.1). "Cargo" is defined as "goods carried on a conveyance or in a container" (Article 1.1).

States parties may apply health measures to goods and cargo beyond inspection "in accordance with the Regulations" (Article 23.2). The revised IHR prohibit states parties applying health measures (e.g., detention, quarantine) to goods (other than live animals) in transit without transshipment (Article 33), except when (1) states parties believe that such measures are necessary to address a public health risk, in which case the measures "shall not be more restrictive of international traffic . . . than reasonably available alternatives that would achieve the appropriate level of health protection" (Article 43.1); (2) WHO recommends such measures to address a public health risk or public health emergency of international concern (Articles 15 and 16); and (3) applicable international agreements (e.g., international trade agreements) permit such measures (Article 33).

Beyond the prohibition of additional measures on goods (other than live animals) in transit without transshipment, the revised IHR contains no more special provisions for goods and cargo. For goods and cargo entering the territory of a state party, the revised IHR do not contain the kind of detailed rules present for the treatment of travelers. The revised IHR's approach to goods and cargos highlights the importance of international trade law for health measures that may affect the flow of products in international commerce (see Part 4 below).

WHO may make recommendations to states parties about the health measures they should apply to goods and cargo (Articles 15 and 16), but these recommendations are not binding on states parties. A state party may apply a health measure to goods and cargo that achieves a greater level of protection than a WHO recommendation when it believes the protection of its public health justifies such a measure (Article 43.1). Any such measure shall not be more restrictive of international traffic than reasonably available alternatives that would achieve the appropriate level of health protection (Article 43.1).

Health Measures for Conveyances

General principles

The revised IHR's general principle concerning health measures applied against conveyances is that states parties should avoid unnecessary interference with international traffic and trade (Article 2). States parties may inspect conveyances for public health purposes on arrival or departure, subject to relevant articles of the revised IHR and applicable international agreements (Article 23.1[b]). The revised IHR define "conveyance" to mean "an aircraft, ship, train, road vehicle or other means of transport, on an international voyage" (Article 1.1).

States parties may apply health measures to conveyances beyond inspection on the basis of evidence of a public health risk "in accordance with these Regulations" (Article 23.2). WHO may make recommendations to states parties about the health measures they should apply to conveyances (Articles 15 and 16), but these recommendations are not binding on states parties. A state party may apply a health measure to a conveyance that achieves a greater level of protection than a WHO recommendation when (a) it believes the protection of its public health justifies such a measure; and (b) other applicable international agreements permit it do so (Article 43.1).

Specific rules

In addition to general principles about health measures for conveyances, the revised IHR contain "special provisions" concerning conveyances and conveyance operators (Articles 24-29 and Annexes 4 and 5). These rules are too numerous and detailed to describe here, but they constitute important provisions for the expanded NQS because it will be involved in the public health management of conveyances arriving and departing the United States.

Generally, the special provisions contain rules that, among other things, (1) prohibit states parties from taking certain actions against conveyances, with specified exceptions (Articles 25 [Ships and Aircraft in Transit] and Article 28 [Ships and Aircraft at Points of Entry]; (2) provide guidance for action states parties may take (Article 27 [Affected Conveyances]); and (3) impose positive obligations on states parties with respect to health measures and conveyances (Annex 4, §B [duty not to damage conveyances during the application of health measures]; Annex 5, ¶4 [establishment of vector control programs at points of entry and exit]).

Health Measures for Containers and Container Loading Areas

The revised IHR's general principle concerning health measures applied to containers used to ships goods and cargo on conveyances is that states parties should avoid unnecessary interference with international traffic (Article 2). States parties may inspect containers for public health purposes on arrival or departure, subject to relevant articles of the revised IHR and applicable international agreements (Article 23.1[b]). States parties may apply health measures to conveyances beyond inspection on the basis of evidence of a public health threat "in accordance with these Regulations" (Article 23.2).

WHO may make recommendations to states parties about the health measures they should apply to containers (Articles 15 and 16), but these recommendations are not binding on states parties. A state party may apply a health measure to a container that achieves a higher level of protection than a WHO recommendation when (a) it believes the protection of its public health justifies such a measure; and (b) other applicable international agreements permit it do so (Article 43.1). The revised IHR also impose on states parties positive obligations to ensure that containers and container loading areas are kept free from sources of infection or contamination (Article 34 and Annex 5, ¶4).

Part VI–Health Documents

As part of the effort to avoid unnecessary interference with international traffic, the revised IHR contain rules regulating what health documents states parties can require. The general principle is that "[n]o health documents, other than those provided for under these Regulations or in recommendations issued by WHO, shall be required in international traffic" (Article 35). The revised IHR recognize the following as health documents that states parties can require: yellow fever vaccination certificate (Annex 7); vaccination or other prophylaxis certificates relating to WHO-recommended vaccinations or prophylaxis (Annex 6); Maritime Declaration of Health (Article 37 and Annex 8); Health Part of the General Aircraft Declaration (Article 38 and Annex 9); and Ship Sanitation Control Exemption Certificate and Ship Sanitation Control Certificate (Article 39 and Annex 3).

The revised IHR's prohibition on health documents other than those recognized by the revised IHR or recommended by WHO does not apply to other health document requirements (1) applied to travelers seeking temporary or permanent residence; and (2) concerning the public health status of goods or cargo in international trade pursuant to applicable international agreements (Article 35). The general provision that allows additional health measures (Article 43) does not appear to permit states parties to require additional health documents other than those recognized by the revised IHR or recommended by WHO.

Part VII–Charges

The revised IHR prohibit states parties from charging travelers for medical examinations, vaccinations, other prophylaxis, quarantine, isolation, for certificates detailing a traveler's arrival and departure dates, and any health measures applied to the traveler's baggage (Article 40.1). States parties may charge for other health measures (Article 40.2) in accordance with specific criteria (Article 40.3). The revised IHR also contain rules on charges made for applying health measures to baggage, cargo, containers, conveyances, goods, or postal parcels (Article 41).

Part VIII–General Provisions

The revised IHR contains a number of what it calls "general provisions," which comprise a host of rules that are not necessarily connected with each other in terms of their subject matter. This memorandum has already mentioned two of these general provisions (Articles 43 [Additional Health Measures] and Article 45 [Treatment of Personal Data]). The other general provisions in this part of the revised IHR respectively involve (1) a requirement to initiate and complete all health measures under the Regulations without delay and in a transparent and nondiscriminatory manner (Article 42); (2) a duty to collaborate with other states parties to facilitate the implementation of the revised IHR (Article 44); and (3) an obligation to facilitate the transport, entry, exit, processing and disposal of specimens, reagents, and other diagnostic materials for verification and response purposes under the revised IHR (Article 46).

Article 43 on additional health measures deserves some specific attention. This provision allows states parties to apply health measures that (1) achieve the same or greater level of health protection than measures recommended by WHO under the revised IHR; or (2) are otherwise prohibited by specific rules of the revised IHR (Article 43.1). For example, under Article

43.1, a state party may impose a health measure on travelers that achieves the same or greater level of health protection than WHO has recommended or that is otherwise prohibited under specific articles of the revised IHR, provided the state party satisfies the conditions laid out in the article. The provision is important because it reflects the state's sovereign right to take action to protect its public health, even in the face of different advice from WHO.

Applying additional health measures under Article 43.1 requires, however, the state party to satisfy certain disciplines on its sovereignty. First, states parties must base any such additional health measures on scientific principles and available scientific evidence of a risk to human health or, if scientific evidence is insufficient, on available information, including information from WHO and other international organizations (Article 43.2). In addition, all such additional health measures cannot be (1) more restrictive of international traffic or (2) more intrusive or invasive to persons than reasonably available alternative measures that would achieve the level of health protection sought (Article 43.1). This dynamic echoes a similar set of rules in international trade law and international human rights law (see Parts 4 and 5 below).

A state party applying additional measures pursuant to Article 43.1 that significantly interfere with international traffic is also required (1) to provide WHO the public health rationale and scientific information supporting such measures (Article 43.3); and (2) to review the measures within three months to assess whether the measures remain appropriate (Article 43.6). WHO may ask the state party to cease application of its additional health measures (Article 43.4), and states parties affected by the additional measures may seek consultations about them (Article 43.7).

Article 43 is important for the expanded NQS because (1) it allows states parties to adopt health measures that are more protective of public health than some measures provided for in the revised IHR or recommended by WHO, provided these measures have a scientific basis and are not more restrictive/intrusive than necessary to achieve the public health objective; and (2) it establishes a process of international scientific, trade, and human rights scrutiny of such additional measures. Article 43 represents yet another example of the revised IHR attempting to balance the sovereign right to protect public health with disciplines on the exercise of such public health sovereignty.

Part IX–The IHR Roster of Experts, the Emergency Committee, and the Review Committee and Part X–Final Provisions

The last two parts of the revised IHR require less attention in terms of the plans to expand the NQS. Part IX (Articles 47–53) establishes the bodies and procedures that will be needed to operate the various mechanisms of the revised IHR. For example, the Emergency and Review Committees are needed to advise the Director-General on the issuance of temporary and standing recommendations respectively (Articles 15 and 16). The Emergency Committee also advises the Director-General on whether a disease event constitutes a public health emergency of international concern (Article 12.2).

The United States would utilize input from the expanded NQS in its dealings in the Emergency and Review Committees; and the work of these committees is important to the overall functioning of the revised IHR. Participating in these bodies and processes will not, however, be a day-to-day function of the expanded NQS, nor will the federal government view these bodies and procedures as important in contemplating what capabilities the expanded NQS needs to fulfill its mandate. Therefore, neither this memorandum nor its Annex 2 analyzes these parts of the revised IHR.

The last part of the revised IHR—the "Final Provisions" (Articles 54–66)—also does not merit detailed discussion in this memorandum because it mainly contains technical international legal matters (e.g., amendments to the IHR, relationship with other international agreements, rejection and reservations, entry into force, etc.) not directly relevant to the committee's focus on the capabilities required for the expanded NQS.

Summary on the Proposed Revision of the International Health Regulations

The revised IHR is very important for the plans to expand the NQS. The seminal nature of the content of the revised IHR, combined with U.S. government support for these new rules, means that the international legal environment in which the expanded NQS will function will be shaped significantly by the revised IHR. The revised IHR's rules address, in some way, the exercise of virtually every public health function the federal government would task the expanded NQS to fulfill—disease surveillance, notification, and reporting; surveillance and response capacity building; monitoring travelers; dealing with suspect and infected passengers (vaccination, prophylaxis, quarantine, isolation, observation); inspecting goods, cargo, and conveyances; ensuring points of entry and exit are free of disease and disease vectors and reservoirs; issuing health documents to conveyances; and cooperating and collaborating with other governments and international organizations. No other body of international law will have the impact on the expanded NQS that the revised IHR will have.

4. INTERNATIONAL TRADE LAW

The second important area of treaty law applicable to the expansion of the NQS is international trade law. The United States is party to many international trade agreements at the multilateral, regional, and bilateral levels. For purposes of this memorandum, the Consultant has focused on agreements within the WTO, namely the General Agreement on Tariffs and Trade (GATT), the Agreement on the Application of Sanitary and Phytosanitary Measures (SPS Agreement), and the General Agreement on Trade in Services (GATS). Unlike the revised IHR, the United States has had obligations under these WTO agreements since 1995 and thus already has systems in place that operate U.S. trade policy in conformity with the nation's rights and duties under international trade law.

Trade in Goods: GATT, the SPS Agreement, and the Expanded NQS

GATT and the SPS Agreement apply to governmental measures that affect international trade in goods; and thus the scope of these agreements' application is narrower than the revised IHR, which have rules applying to goods, conveyances, containers, and travelers. The impact of GATT and the SPS Agreement on the expanded NQS is, as a result, more limited because these trade agreements have no relevance for public health measures taken to address disease threats presented by people and transportation technologies. Further, as explored below, the scope of the SPS Agreement is narrower than GATT in terms of trade in goods.

General Principle and Scope

Both GATT and the SPS Agreement recognize each WTO member's sovereign right to take measures necessary for the protection of human, animal, and plant life or health (GATT, Article XX[b]; SPS Agreement, Preamble and Article 2.1). Both agreements apply, however, disciplines to the exercise of this sovereign right; and the three main categories into which these disciplines fall are explored below.

A particular threat to health may fall within the scope of both GATT and the SPS Agreement, but the SPS Agreement is the controlling treaty for "sanitary and phytosanitary measures" (SPS measures). For purposes of protecting human health, which is the objective of the expanded NQS, SPS measures fall within the SPS Agreement if a WTO member applies them to protect human life or health within its territory from risks arising from (1) additives, contaminants, toxins, or disease-causing organisms in foods, beverages, or feedstuffs; or (2) diseases carried by animals, plants or products thereof, or from the entry, establishment or spread of pests (Annex A, ¶1).

Health risks from international trade in goods not encompassed by the definition of SPS measures (e.g., trade in asbestos-containing products) fall within the scope of GATT.

The expanded NQS will most likely apply health-protecting measures against goods that fall within the SPS Agreement's definition of SPS measures. The Consultant perceives that the federal government will involve the expanded NQS as part of the effort to prevent and control risks to the safety of the country's food supply and risks presented by zoonotic and vector-borne diseases. SPS measures adopted by the United States and implemented by the expanded NQS will, therefore, have to comply with the obligations the United States has accepted under the SPS Agreement. This memorandum will, thus, focus on the SPS Agreement rather than GATT as the more pertinent treaty. The memorandum will address the most important issues for the expanded NQS raised by the SPS Agreement, but Annex 2 hereto provides a provision-by-provision analysis of the SPS Agreement's implications for the expanded NQS.

Science-Based Disciplines in the SPS Agreement

The SPS measures of WTO members that affect international trade must be based on scientific principles and a risk assessment and must not be maintained without sufficient scientific evidence (Articles 2.2 and 5.10). In situations in which relevant scientific evidence and information is insufficient, WTO members may implement SPS measures but must seek to obtain additional information to develop a more objective risk assessment and review the measure within a reasonable period of time to determine whether its application is still warranted (Article 5.7).

The science-based disciplines are serious obligations of which the expanded NQS should be aware, particularly because the expanded system may more frequently implement SPS measures that affect international trade in goods. The SPS Agreement's scientific disciplines do not, however, pose significant problems for the operations of the expanded NQS because federal public health authorities typically strive to ground their policies in scientific principles, risk assessment, and evidence because such grounding proves the most effective way to protect human health.

The WTO dispute settlement process has, to date, resolved four disputes under the SPS Agreement, only one of which (EC–Hormones) involved human health. Through these disputes, the WTO dispute settlement body has interpreted the science-based disciplines in the SPS Agreement. The Consultant has not included discussion of this case law in this memorandum because such discussion would involve lengthy technical analysis, but the Consultant would be willing to provide the committee with the state of the case law upon its request.

Harmonization Disciplines

The SPS Agreement's second category of disciplines on the sovereign right to restrict trade in goods to protect human health involves obligations on WTO members to harmonize their national SPS measures. The SPS Agreement requires WTO members to base their national SPS measures on applicable international standards, guidelines, and recommendations (Article 3.1). The SPS Agreement recognizes the Codex Alimentarius Commission as the source for international guidance on food safety, the International Office of Epizootics for animal health and zoonoses, and the Secretariat of the International Plant Protection Convention for plant health (Annex A, ¶3). Conforming national SPS measures to international standards, guidelines, and recommendations means that the SPS measures are presumed to comply with both the SPS Agreement and GATT (Article 3.2).

If a WTO member wants to implement a SPS measure that achieves a higher level of protection than a relevant international standard, guideline, or recommendation, then it may—provided that the WTO member has a scientific justification for the measure and complies with the rest of the SPS Agreement in applying the measure (Article 3.3). This provision balances the sovereign right to the WTO member to protect the health of its people with the need to justify scientifically the higher level of protection sought. The revised IHR contain the same dynamic with respect to a WHO member's ability to apply a health measure that achieves the same or greater level of health protection than WHO recommendations (IHR, Article 43), as discussed earlier. The appearance of this dynamic in both the revised IHR and SPS Agreement suggests that the expanded NQS should be aware of the need to operate with it in mind.

Trade-Related Disciplines

The last set of major obligations applied by the SPS Agreement to the SPS measures of WTO members is the trade-related disciplines. These disciplines require that WTO members apply their national SPS measures in ways that (1) are not more trade restrictive than required to achieve the level of health protection desired (Article 5.6); and (2) do not arbitrarily or unjustifiably discriminate between the goods of WTO members or constitute a disguised restriction on international trade (Articles 2.3 and 5.5). The SPS Agreement's trade-related disciplines echo the purpose and objective of the revised IHR to avoid unnecessary interference with international traffic and trade (IHR, Article 2). The expanded NQS will have to bear such trade-related considerations in mind in implementing health measures that affect international trade in goods under both the revised IHR and the SPS Agreement.

The SPS Agreement also contains a number of procedural obligations designed to reduce the burden the application of SPS measures imposes on international trade. The SPS Agreement requires transparency of information concerning SPS measures (Article 7 and Annex B) and obligates WTO members to apply their control, inspection, and approval procedures in a transparent, efficient, equitable, and nondiscriminatory manner (Article 8 and Annex C). Again, these disciplines do not present an expanded NQS with significant problems; but the expanded system will have to operate according to these obligations in applying SPS measures.

Application of National SPS Measures in the Territory of Other WTO Members

The SPS Agreement contemplates at least two situations in which one WTO member may apply its SPS measures in the territory of other WTO members. First, the SPS Agreement requires a WTO member to accept the SPS measures of another WTO member as equivalent to its own (and thus to avoid the application of multiple SPS measures, all of which achieve the same level of health protection), if the exporting WTO member can objectively demonstrate to the importing WTO member that its measures achieve the importing member's desired level of health protection (Article 4.1). To achieve recognition of SPS measure equivalence, the exporting WTO member has to allow the importing WTO member into its territory for inspection, testing, and other relevant procedures (Article 4.1). The second situation concerns the application of a SPS measure that requires control at the level of the production of the good. In such a situation, the WTO member in which the relevant production takes place has to "provide the necessary assistance to facilitate such control and the work of the controlling authorities" (Annex C, ¶2).

Given the possibility that the expanded NQS may post personnel in foreign countries, these provisions in the SPS Agreement may help facilitate cooperation between the U.S. personnel and the host government with respect to SPS measures on goods exported to the United States.

Summary on the SPS Agreement and the Expanded NQS

The SPS Agreement's importance to the expanded NQS will depend on the extent to which the expanded system applies SPS measures in ways that affect international trade in goods. The comprehensive nature of the strategy to expand the NQS suggests that its mandate will involve addressing health threats that may arise through the importation of goods into the

United States. Thus, the expanded NQS will have to operate within the disciplines created by the SPS Agreement. These disciplines do not, however, appear to present serious obstacles for the effective and efficient working of an expanded NQS.

Trade in Services: GATS and the Expanded NQS

In addition to liberalizing international trade in goods, international trade law also involves the movement of people through agreements that address international trade in services. At the WTO level, GATS provides an international legal framework designed to help liberalize international trade in services. GATS covers the temporary movement of natural persons supplying a service in the territory of another WTO member (Article 2.2[d] and Annex on Movement of Natural Persons Supplying Services under the Agreement). WTO members can make commitments to allow more foreign service suppliers to provide services on a temporary basis in their territories (Articles XVI and XVII). GATS commitments on the movement of natural persons do not apply to people seeking citizenship, residence, or employment on a permanent basis (Annex on Movement of Natural Persons Supplying Services under the Agreement, ¶2).

The United States could increase the number of foreigners coming to the United States to supply services temporarily under GATS if it made binding commitments to do so. Such binding commitments would not, however, limit or directly regulate the ability of the United States to apply its public health measures to foreign service suppliers entering the United States. GATS does not govern the application of such health measures, nor does any WTO agreement. Further, the disciplines of the revised IHR on health measures relating to entry to travelers do not preclude a state party from requiring medical examination, vaccination, or other prophylaxis as a condition for entry for any travelers seeking temporary or permanent residence (IHR, Article 31.1[b]).

In short, liberalization of trade in services through the temporary movement of natural persons into the United States under GATS would not weaken the expanded NQS' authority to carry out its public health functions. The same principle and outcome appears in the provisions on cross-border trade in services in the North American Free Trade Agreement (NAFTA, Article 1201.3).

5. INTERNATIONAL HUMAN RIGHTS LAW

The revised IHR's mandates that states parties implement their health measures "with full respect for the dignity, human rights, and fundamental freedoms of persons" (Article 3.1), "with respect for their dignity, human rights and fundamental freedoms" (Article 32), and in a manner not more intrusive or invasive for persons than necessary to achieve the public health objective (Articles 23.2 and 43.1) put international human rights law on the agenda of the expansion of the NQS. This body of law would be on the agenda without the revised IHR's reference to it because the United States is party to international human rights treaties that apply to public health measures imposed against individuals in the United States. The most important of these treaties for purposes of this memorandum is the International Covenant on Civil and Political Rights (ICCPR).

Restricting Civil and Political Rights for Public Health Purposes Under International Human Rights Law

In the area of civil and political rights, international human rights law recognizes public health as a legitimate reason for interfering with the enjoyment of certain civil and political rights. The ICCPR expressly recognizes public health as a justification for restriction specific rights (Articles 12.3, 18.3, 19.3, 21, and 22.2). The ICCPR also permits states parties to restrict other rights in accordance with grounds and procedures recognized by law (Articles 9 and 17), which includes restrictions on such rights undertaken to protect public health. Table F.1 contains the rights in the ICCPR most relevant to the kinds of public health actions the expanded NQS may have to take against individuals.

One civil and political right relevant to potential activities of the expanded NQS against which no restrictions or derogations are permitted is the right not be subject to torture or cruel, inhuman, or degrading treatment or punishment and not to be subject to medical or scientific experimentation with a person's free consent (Article 7). These rights would be relevant in circumstances in which the expanded NQS might subject individuals to (1) medical examinations, vaccination, prophylaxis or other health measures that negligently or unnecessarily caused severe pain and suffering; (2) medical examination, detention, quarantine, or isolation in cruel, inhuman, or degrading conditions; and (3) the use of experimental vaccines or drugs without the individuals' free, informed consent.

Disciplines on Public Health Restrictions on Civil and Political Rights

Although the ICCPR recognizes public health as a justification for restricting certain civil and political rights, international human rights law requires that the exercise of restrictions that are necessary to protect public health satisfy other disciplines to ensure that the rights are respected to the maximum extent possible. For derogations of rights under the ICCPR, international lawyers generally recognize the Siracusa Principles on the

TABLE F.1 Public Health-Related Civil and Political Rights in the ICCPR

Article	Content of the Civil and Political Right	Express/Implicit Recognition of Public Health	Public Health Acts Affecting Right
9.1	Everyone has the right to liberty and security of person. No one shall be subjected to arbitrary arrest or detention. No one shall be deprived of his liberty except on such grounds and in accordance with such procedures as are established by law.	Implicit	-Detention for medical examination -Quarantine -Isolation
12	1. Everyone lawfully within the territory of a State shall, within that territory, have the right of liberty of movement and freedom to choose his residence. 2. Everyone shall be free to leave any country, including his own.	Express (Article 12.3)	-Detention for medical examination -Quarantine -Isolation
17.1	No one shall be subjected to arbitrary or unlawful interference with his privacy, family, home or correspondence, nor to unlawful attacks on his honour and reputation.	Implicit	-Compulsory medical examination, vaccination, prophylaxis, or other invasive or intrusive health measure -Collection and dissemination of personal information
18.1	Everyone shall have the right to freedom of thought, conscience, and religion.	Express (Article 18.3)	-Compulsory medical examination, vaccination, prophylaxis, or other invasive or intrusive health measure
19.2	Everyone shall have the right to freedom of expression	Express (Article 19.3)	-Restrictions on publishing or disseminating information necessary to protect public health
21	The right of peaceful assembly shall be recognized.	Express (Article 21, second sentence)	-Restricting public or gatherings in order to protect public health
22.1	Everyone shall have the right to freedom of association with others, including the right to form and join trade unions for the protection of their interests.	Express (Article 22.2)	-Restricting public or gatherings in order to protect public health

Limitation and Derogation of Provisions in the International Covenant on Civil and Political Rights (Siracusa Principles) as an authoritative statement of the disciplines states parties to the ICCPR must satisfy to restrict civil and political rights legitimately.

For a restriction on a civil and political right to be necessary within the meaning of the ICCPR, the restriction must (1) be based (where applicable) on one of the grounds justifying restrictions contained in the relevant article of the ICCPR; (2) respond to a pressing public or social need; (3) pursue a legitimate aim; (4) be proportionate to the legitimate aim; and (5) be no more restrictive than is required to achieve the purpose sought by restricting the right (Siracusa Principles, Article 10). In addition, the restrictive measure must be applied in a nondiscriminatory manner (ICCPR, Articles 2.1 and 26).

The revised IHR attempt to incorporate some of these disciplines, illustrating the importance of international human rights law for the expanded NQS. The revised IHR require, among other things, that health measures have a scientific basis and justification; not be applied to individuals without their consent unless in a situation of imminent public health danger; be not more intrusive or invasive than reasonably available alternatives that would achieve the same level of health protection; be applied in ways sensitive to sociocultural, gender, ethnic, and religious concerns; operate in a manner that protects personal information as confidential; and be applied in a nondiscriminatory manner.

Further, the revised IHR also echo the right of all persons deprived of their liberty to be treated with humanity and with respect for the inherent dignity of the human person (ICCPR, Article 10.1) in its provision requiring states parties to provide for the needs of people subject to health measures (IHR, Article 32[c]). Thus, international human rights law will be important in interpreting what provisions of the revised IHR mean and how states parties apply health measures to travelers.

International human rights law has, however, broader application than the revised IHR. The expanded NQS may have to implement public health measures restricting civil and political rights against individuals who are not travelers within the meaning of the revised IHR—natural persons undertaking an international voyage (IHR, Article 1.1). The expanded NQS may have to restrict the civil and political rights of persons traveling within the United States, meaning the revised IHR would not apply but the ICCPR would. In a situation involving people moving within the United States, the overlap is between the ICCPR and U.S. constitutional law, which makes preparing the expanded NQS for operating in a manner sensitive to civil and political rights an important task for the federal government.

6. INTERNATIONAL LEGAL CONSIDERATIONS CONCERNING "FORWARD DEPLOYMENT" OF THE EXPANDED NQS

The above analysis of the revised IHR, international trade law, and international human rights law assumes that the expanded NQS would be applying public health measures in U.S. territory. As noted earlier, the Consultant understands that the federal government may wish to include in the expansion of the NQS the placement of U.S. public health personnel and resources in the territories of foreign countries. This aspect of the strategy to expand the NQS raises different international considerations, which this part briefly explores.

The federal government generally, and the CDC specifically, have great experience with using public health experts and resources in international cooperation with other countries and international organizations. To the Consultant's knowledge, such cooperative ventures traditionally have not involved, however, establishing a permanent presence in other countries for purposes of minimizing exogenous threats to public health in the United States. Such a permanent presence implicates some basic principles of international law worth noting in this memorandum.

Federal government plans to expand the NQS by establishing assets overseas would require the full cooperation and permission of the foreign governments because these governments have sovereignty over their territories that the United States cannot infringe under international law. The principle prohibiting interference in the domestic affairs of other states supports the principle of sovereignty in underscoring the necessity that "forward deployment" of the expanded NQS be agreed in advance between the federal government and the foreign government.

Such agreements may be informal or formal under international law. The nature of the activities that the expanded NQS might undertake in the foreign country (e.g., inspection goods, cargo, and travelers bound for the United States) touch, however, on aspects of sovereignty and the organization of a country's domestic affairs that would make the expanded NQS' activities politically sensitive for a foreign government. A foreign government might be nervous about what kinds of information flows between the part of the expanded NQS in its territory and the rest of the system back in the United States. In all likelihood, a foreign government agreeing to host assets and personnel from the expanded NQS will require that the scope of the expanded NQS' activities in its territory be carefully delineated in a formal, written agreement.

Another reason why a foreign government may insist on clearly defining the nature of the expanded NQS' activities in its territory relates to that government's own responsibilities under international law. A foreign government will need to avoid situations in which inspections and control measures desired by the expanded NQS in its territory do not violate the government's obligations under the revised IHR, international trade law, or international human rights law. A foreign government cannot "outsource" its international legal obligations to the United States through the assets and personnel of the expanded NQS in its territory.

Other reasons pointing to the need for formal, written agreements are more practical and involve establishing the procedures through which the expanded NQS would interact with the public health authorities of the host country. Would U.S. public health personnel stationed overseas have authority to administer medical examinations, vaccination, or prophylaxis to travelers bound for the United States, or would those "hands-on" functions be managed by the host government's public health personnel? Would U.S. public health personnel incur personal liability under foreign law for engaging in expanded NQS activities in the host country? Would the United States government incur liability to foreign nationals or the foreign government for the negligence or problems caused by U.S. public health personnel stationed overseas as part of the expanded NQS.

The Consultant raises these issues and questions not to imply that a strategy of "forward deployment" would be impossible or ill-advised from an international legal perspective. The federal government engages in similar arrangements with foreign governments in connection with (1) U.S. customs officials stationed in Canada screening travelers destined for the United States at Canadian airports; (2) U.S. inspections of foreign production facilities for purposes of applying national sanitary or phytosanitary measures; and (3) homeland security efforts seeking to increase the security of U.S. ports by inspecting containers and vessels at foreign ports of departure rather than just at the U.S. ports of entry. Whether these examples could serve as models or precedents for "forward deployment" of the expanded NQS would have to be studied more comprehensively.

ANNEX 1

TABLE F.2 Summary Table of Important Positive and Negative Obligations the United States Has Under International Law Relevant to the Expansion of the National Quarantine System

Positive Obligations[a]	Negative Obligations[b]
Measures Applied Against Individuals	• No treatment of individuals that constitutes torture or cruel, inhuman, or degrading treatment or punishment (ICCPR, Art. 7).
• Measures against individuals must be implemented with full respect for the dignity, human rights, and fundamental freedoms of persons (IHR 2005, Arts. 3.1 and 32).	• No medical or scientific experimentation on individuals without their free and informed consent (ICCPR, Art. 7).
• All travelers must be treated with courtesy and respect, taking into consideration gender, sociocultural, ethnic or religious concerns of the travelers (IHR 2005, Art. 32).	• No medical examination, vaccination, prophylaxis, or other health measure can be carried out on travelers without their express informed consent, unless there is evidence of an imminent public health threat (IHR 2005, Arts. 23.3 and 31.2).
• For travelers quarantined, isolated, or subject to other public health measures, the government must provide adequate food, water, accommodation and shelter, clothing, protection of baggage and other possessions, means of communication, medical treatment, and other appropriate assistance (IHR 2005, Art. 32).	• No invasive medical examination, vaccination, or other prophylaxis shall be required as a condition of entry for any traveler except in limited circumstances (IHR 2005, Art. 31.1).
• Travelers to be vaccinated or offered prophylaxis shall be informed of any risk associated with vaccination or with nonvaccination and with the use or nonuse of prophylaxis (IHR 2005, Art. 23.4).	• No health documents, other than those provided for under the IHR or recommended by WHO, shall be required of travelers, except for travelers seeking temporary or permanent residence (IHR 2005, Art. 35).
• Any medical examination, medical procedure, vaccination or other prophylaxis that involves a risk of disease transmission shall only be performed on, or administered to, a traveler in accordance with established national or international safety guidelines and standards in order to minimize risk (IHR 2005, Art. 23.5).	• No denial of entry to a traveler in possession of a certificate of vaccination or other prophylaxis in conformity with the IHR as a consequence of the disease to which the certificate refers, unless the competent authority has indications or evidence that the vaccination or other prophylaxis was not effective (IHR 2005, Art. 36.2).
• For charges assessed under the IHR, each state party shall have only one tariff for such charge and every charge shall conform to the tariff, not exceed the actual cost of the services, be levied	• No charge shall be assessed against travelers for any medical examination, vaccination, prophylaxis, health measures applied to *(continued)*

TABLE F.2 Continued

Positive Obligations[a]	Negative Obligations[b]
in a nondiscriminatory fashion, and be published at least ten days in advance of any levy (IHR 2005, Arts. 41.3 and 41.1). • Health measures must be initiated and completed without delay, and applied in a nondiscriminatory manner (IHR 2005, Art. 42). • For health measures that differ from those otherwise recommended under the IHR or are otherwise prohibited by the IHR, states parties shall base their determinations upon scientific principles and evidence (IHR 2005, Art. 43.1); shall provide to WHO the public health rationale and scientific information for the measure (IHR 2005, Art. 43.3); and shall review such measure within three months (IHR 2005, Art. 43.6). • Personal information collected or received pursuant to the IHR shall be kept confidential, except to the extent necessary to disclose or transmit it for public health purposes (IHR 2005, Art. 45.1). • States parties shall inform WHO of health measures they implement that significantly interfere with the movement of travelers and which are applied based on an event in an area not covered by a temporary or standing recommendation (IHR 2005, Art. 43.5).	baggage, or isolation or quarantine, except for travelers seeking temporary and permanent residence (IHR 2005, Art. 40.1). • For health measures that differ from those otherwise recommended under the IHR or are otherwise prohibited by the IHR, such measures shall not be more invasive or intrusive to persons than reasonably available alternatives that would achieve the appropriate level of health protection (IHR 2005, Art. 43.1). • No infringements on the rights of liberty, freedom of movement, privacy, freedom of thought and expression, peaceful assembly, and freedom of association except for a pressing or urgent public health threat and the infringing measure pursued as legitimate aim, is proportionate to that aim, is no more restrictive than is required to achieve the public health purpose sought by restricting the right, and is applied in a nondiscriminatory manner (ICCPR and Siracusa Principles).

Measures Applied Against Goods
Science-Based Disciplines

• SPS measures must be based on scientific principles and only be maintained with sufficient scientific evidence (SPS Agreement, Art. 2.2).
• SPS measures must be based on a risk assessment, which includes consideration of scientific issues and other factors (SPS Agreement, Arts. 5-1-5.3).

- SPS measures that differ from applicable international standards, guidelines, and recommendations must have a scientific justification (SPS Agreement, Art. 3.3).
- States parties shall ensure that their SPS measures are adapted to the SPS characteristics of the area from which products come and shall recognize the concepts of pest- or disease-free areas and areas of low pest or disease prevalence (SPS Agreement, Art. 6).
- For health measures that differ from those otherwise recommended under the IHR or are otherwise prohibited by the IHR, states parties shall base their determinations upon scientific principles and evidence (IHR 2005, Art. 43.2); shall provide to WHO the public health rationale and scientific information for the measure (IHR 2005, Art. 43.3); and shall review such measure within three months (IHR 2005, Art. 43.6).

Harmonization Disciplines

- States parties shall base their SPS measures on international standards, guidelines, or recommendations, where they exist (SPS Agreement, Art. 3.1).
- States parties shall accept the SPS measures of other WTO members as equivalent if the exporting WTO member objectively demonstrates to the importing WTO member that its measures achieve the importing member's appropriate level of health protection (SPS Agreement, Art. 4.1).

Trade-Related Disciplines

- Health measures must be initiated and completed without delay, and applied in a nondiscriminatory manner (IHR 2005, Art. 42).
- For charges assessed under the IHR, each state party shall have

- For health measures that differ from those otherwise recommended under the IHR or are otherwise prohibited by the IHR, such measures shall not be more restrictive of international

(continued)

TABLE F.2 Continued

Positive Obligations[a]	Negative Obligations[b]
only one tariff for such charge and every charge shall conform to the tariff, not exceed the actual cost of the services, be levied in a nondiscriminatory fashion, and be published at least ten days in advance of any levy (IHR 2005, Arts. 40.3 and 41.1). • States parties shall inform WHO of health measures they implement that significantly interfere with international traffic and which are applied based on an event in an area not covered by a temporary or standing recommendation (IHR 2005, Art. 43.5). • Implementation and application of SPS measures shall be transparent (SPS Agreement, Art. 7 and Annex B). Annex B contains rules concerning the publication of regulations, enquiry points, and notification procedures. • States parties shall follow the obligations concerning the operation of control, inspection, and approval procedures laid out in Annex C (SPS Agreement, Art. 8). • States parties shall take account of the special needs of developing country WTO members in the preparation and application of SPS measures (SPS Agreement, Art. 10.1).	traffic than reasonably available alternatives that would achieve the appropriate level of health protection (IHR 2005, Art. 43.1). • Goods (other than live animals) in transit without transshipment shall not be subject to health measures under the IHR or detained for public health purposes, except under Article 43 or unless authorized by applicable international agreements (IHR 2005, Art. 33). • No health documents, other than those provided for under the IHR or recommended by WHO, shall be required in international traffic, except for document requirements concerning the public health status of goods pursuant to applicable international agreements (IHR 2005, Art. 35). • States parties shall not use arbitrary or unjustifiable distinctions in levels of SPS protection if such distinctions result in discrimination or a disguised restriction on international trade (SPS Agreement, Art. 5.5). • SPS measures shall not be more trade-restrictive than required to achieve the appropriate level of SPS protection, taking into account technical and economic feasibility (SPS Agreement, Art. 5.6).

Measures Applied at Points of Entry and Against Means of Transportation and Trade

• States parties shall fulfill several obligations concerning public health capacities and competent authorities at points of entry and shall provide WHO, when requested, with public health information on points of entry (IHR 2005, Art. 19). • States parties shall designate ports and airports that shall develop public health capacities identified in Annex 1 (IHR 2005, Art. 20.1).	• Unless authorized by other IHR provisions or applicable international agreements, states parties shall apply no health measure to (1) a ship not coming from an affected area that passes through a maritime canal or waterway in the territories of such states parties on its way to a port in the territory of another state (such ships shall be permitted to take on fuel, water, food, and

- States parties shall ensure that Ship Sanitation Control Exemption Certificates and Ship Sanitation Control Certificates are issued in accordance with the IHR and shall send to WHO a list of ports authorized to issue these documents and provide sanitation services to ships (IHR 2005, Art. 20.2–20.3).
- States parties shall take all practicable measures consistent with the IHR to ensure that conveyance operators undertake certain actions related to health measures (IHR 2005, Art. 24).
- States parties shall ensure that container shippers use containers that are free from sources of infection or contamination, including vectors and reservoirs, particularly during the course of packing (IHR 2005, Art.34.1).
- States parties shall ensure that container loading areas are kept free from sources of infection or contamination, including vectors or reservoirs (IHR 2005, Art. 34.2).
- When the volume of container traffic is sufficiently large, states parties shall take all practicable measures to assess the sanitary condition of container loading areas and containers (IHR 2005, Art. 34.3).
- States parties shall, as far as practicable, have facilities for inspection and isolation of containers available at container loading areas (IHR 2005, Art. 34.4).
- A Maritime Declaration of Health shall conform to the model declaration provided in Annex 8, and ship sanitation certificates shall conform to the model certificate in Annex 3 and be valid for a maximum period of six months (IHR 2005, Arts. 37.3, 39.1, 39.3).
- States parties shall inform aircraft operators or their agents of the requirements concerning the Health Part of the Aircraft General Declaration (IHR 2005, Art. 38).

supplies); (2) a ship which passes through waters within its jurisdiction without calling at a port or on the coast; and (3) an aircraft in transit at an airport within its jurisdiction (such aircraft may be restricted to a particular area of the airport with no embarking and disembarking and shall be permitted to take on fuel, water, food, and supplies (IHR 2005, Art. 25).
- Subject to other IHR provisions and applicable international agreements, a ship or aircraft shall not be prevented for public health reasons from calling at any point of entry and shall not be refused *free practique* by states parties for public health reasons (in particular ships and aircraft shall not be prevented from embarking or disembarking, discharging or loading cargo or stores, or taking on fuel, water, and supplies) (IHR 2005, Art. 28).
- No health documents, other than those provided for under the IHR or recommended by WHO, shall be required in international traffic (IHR 2005, Art. 35).

(continued)

232

TABLE F.2 Continued

Positive Obligations[a]	Negative Obligations[b]
• Whenever possible, ship sanitation control measures shall be carried out when the ship and holds are empty and, in the case of a ship in ballast, before loading (IHR 2005, Art. 39.4). • States parties shall issue Ship Sanitation Control Certificates when control measures are required and have been satisfactorily completed (IHR 2005, Art. 39.5). •States parties shall note on the Ship Sanitation Control Certificate when control measures cannot be satisfactorily completed (IHR 2005, Art. 39.7). • Charges levied for the application of health measures must conform to specific requirements (IHR 2005, Art. 40.3). • Health measures must be initiated and completed without delay, and applied in a nondiscriminatory manner (IHR 2005, Art. 42). • For health measures that differ from those otherwise recommended under the IHR or are otherwise prohibited by the IHR, states parties shall base their determinations upon scientific principles and evidence (IHR 2005, Art. 43.2); shall provide to WHO the public health rationale and scientific information for the measure (IHR 2005, Art. 43.3); and shall review such measure within three months (IHR 2005, Art. 43.6). *Measures Related to Administration, Surveillance, and Response* • States parties shall designate a National IHR Focal Point that shall be accessible at all times, and shall provide WHO with contact details of the National IHR Focal Point (IHR 2005, Arts. 4.–4.2, 4.4).	

(continued)

- States parties shall develop, strengthen, and maintain the capacity to detect, assess, notify, and report public health events in accordance with the IHR (IHR 2005, Art. 5.1).
- States parties shall notify WHO of all events which may constitute a public health emergency of international concern within their territories as well as any health measure implemented in response to those events, and continue to communicate with WHO about the events and their management (IHR 2005, Art. 6.1).
- States parties must provide WHO with all relevant public health information if they have evidence of an unexpected or unusual public health event within their respective territories, irrespective of origin or source, which may constitute a public health emergency of international concern (IHR 2005, Art. 7).
- States parties shall inform WHO within 24 hours of receipt of evidence of a public health threat identified outside their territories that may cause international disease spread (IHR 2005, Art. 9.2).
- When requested by WHO, states parties shall provide verification information to WHO concerning public health events in their territories (IHR 2005, Art. 10.2).
- States parties shall develop, strengthen, and maintain the capacity to respond promptly and effectively to public health threats and public health emergencies of international concern (IHR 2005, Art. 13.1).
- The competent authorities shall fulfill several responsibilities and obligations with respect to dealing with travelers, goods, cargo, conveyances, and containers at points of entry (IHR 2005, Art. 22).
- States parties undertake to collaborate with each other, to the extent possible, in the implementation of the IHR (IHR 2005, Art. 44).

TABLE F.2 Continued

Positive Obligations[a]	Negative Obligations[b]
• States parties shall facilitate the transport, entry, exit, processing, and disposal of specimens, reagents, and other diagnostic materials for verification and response purposes under the IHR (IHR 2005, Art. 46). • States parties shall report to the World Health Assembly on the implementation of the IHR as decided by the World Health Assembly (IHR 2005, Art. 54.1).	

NOTE: Areas of international law covered: Revised International Health Regulations (IHR 2005), the Agreement on the Application of Sanitary and Phytosanitary Measures (SPS Agreement) of the World Trade Organization, and the International Covenant on Civil and Political Rights (ICCPR).

[a]Positive obligations = duties under international law that require affirmative action from the United States.
[b]Negative obligations = duties under international law that require the United States not to take certain actions.

ANNEX 2

TABLE F.3 Analysis of the Revised International Health Regulations: Implications for Plans to Expand the National Quarantine System

Revised IHR	Implications for Plans to Expand the National Quarantine System (NQS)
PART 1—DEFINITIONS, PURPOSE AND SCOPE, PRINCIPLES, AND RESPONSIBLE AUTHORITIES	
Article 1 Definitions "Disease" means an illness or medical condition, irrespective of origin or source, that presents or could present significant harm to humans.	The definition of "disease" in the revised IHR is important to the expanded NQS because this definition helps establish the scope of the revised IHR and the scope of its obligations. The revised IHR define "disease" to include chemical and radiological sources as well as biological sources. Thus, the revised IHR's obligations on surveillance and response would go beyond communicable diseases. At present, the federal government appears to be designing the expanded NQS for communicable disease threats only.
Article 2 Purpose and scope The purpose and scope of these Regulations are to prevent, protect against, control and provide a public health response to the international spread of disease in ways that are commensurate with and restricted to public health risks, and which avoid unnecessary interference with international traffic and trade.	The purpose and scope of the revised IHR should not pose problems for the plans for the expanded NQS because the objectives of preventing, protecting, and controlling public health risks and providing a public health response to the spread of disease are consistent with the goals of the expanded NQS. Similarly, the United States has an interest in expanding the NQS in ways that do not unnecessarily interfere with international trade and travel.
Article 3 Principles 1. The implementation of these Regulations shall be with full respect for the dignity, human rights and fundamental freedoms of persons.	For the expanded NQS, Article 3.1 is important because it mandates that WHO member state implementation of the revised IHR shall occur with full respect for human rights and fundamental freedoms.

(continued)

TABLE F.3 Continued

Revised IHR	Implications for Plans to Expand the National Quarantine System (NQS)
2. The implementation of these Regulations shall be guided by the Charter of the United Nations and the Constitution of the World Health Organization.	The provision requires the expanded NQS to implement measures taken against people to comply with international human rights disciplines on the application of public health measures to individuals. See discussion in Memorandum on the disciplines found in international human rights law.
3. The implementation of these Regulations shall be guided by the goal of their universal application for the protection of all people of the world from the international spread of disease.	Article 3.5 is important because it recognizes the right of the United States to legislate, and implement such legislation, to protect public health through its expanded NQS.
4. States have, in accordance with the Charter of the United Nations and the principles of international law, the sovereign right to legislate and to implement legislation in pursuance of their health policies. In doing so they should uphold the purpose of these Regulations.	
Article 4 Responsible authorities	
1. Each State Party shall designate or establish a National IHR Focal Point and the authorities responsible within its respective jurisdiction for the implementation of health measures under these Regulations.	This provision of the revised IHR presents an organizational and administration challenge for the expanded NQS. First, the United States has to designate a single National IHR Focal Point that can manage the functions indicated in Article 3.2 (perhaps the CDC in Atlanta). The CDC has to network all the pieces and components of the expanded NQS together to make sure that the National IHR Focal Point can fulfill its functions under the revised IHR. Second, Article 4.1 requires states parties to designate all authorities within their jurisdictions that will implement health measures under the revised IHR. Such authorities would include the components of the expanded NQS.
2. National IHR Focal Points shall be accessible at all times for communications with the WHO IHR Contact Points provided for in paragraph 3 of this Article. The functions of National IHR Focal Points shall include: (a) sending to WHO IHR Contact Points, on behalf of the State Party concerned, urgent communications concerning the implementation of these Regulations, in particular under Articles 6 to 12; and (b) disseminating information to, and consolidating input	

from, relevant sectors of the administration of the State Party concerned, including those responsible for surveillance and reporting, points of entry, public health services, clinics and hospitals and other government departments.

3. WHO shall designate IHR Contact Points, which shall be accessible at all times for communications with National IHR Focal Points. WHO IHR Contact Points shall send urgent communications concerning the implementation of these Regulations, in particular under Articles 6 to 12, to the National IHR Focal Point of the States Parties concerned. WHO IHR Contact Points may be designated by WHO at the headquarters or at the regional level of the Organization.

4. States Parties shall provide WHO with contact details of their National IHR Focal Point and WHO shall provide States Parties with contact details of WHO IHR Contact Points. These contact details shall be continuously updated and annually confirmed. WHO shall make available to all States Parties the contact details of National IHR Focal Points it receives pursuant to this Article.

PART II—INFORMATION AND PUBLIC HEALTH RESPONSE

Article 5 Surveillance
1. Each State Party shall develop, strengthen and maintain, as soon as possible but no later than five years from the entry into force of these Regulations for that State Party, the capacity to detect, assess, notify and report events in accordance with these Regulations, as specified in Annex 1.

Article 5.1 is important for the expanded NQS because it requires the development, strengthening, and maintenance of surveillance capabilities in accordance with Annex 1 of the revised IHR as part of the revised IHR's obligations on "core capacity requirements" for surveillance and response. The plan to expand and strengthen the

(continued)

TABLE F.3 Continued

Revised IHR	Implications for Plans to Expand the National Quarantine System (NQS)
2. Following the assessment referred to in paragraph 2, Part A of Annex 1, a State Party may report to WHO on the basis of a justified need and an implementation plan and, in so doing, obtain an extension of two years in which to fulfil the obligation in paragraph 1 of this Article. In exceptional circumstances, and supported by a new implementation plan, the State Party may request a further extension not exceeding two years from the Director-General, who shall make the decision, taking into account the technical advice of the Committee established under Article 50 (hereinafter the "Review Committee"). After the period mentioned in paragraph 1 of this Article, the State Party that has obtained an extension shall report annually to WHO on progress made towards the full implementation.	NQS should constitute U.S. actions to develop and improve surveillance capacities as required by Article 5.1. The federal government would have to make sure, however, that the capabilities being included in the expanded NQS, combined with other federal and state public health assets, meet the core capacity requirement for surveillance mandated by Article 5.1 and Annex 1. For example, Annex 1 requires, at the local community level, the capacities "to detect events involving disease or death above expected levels for the particular time and place in all areas within the territory of the State Party" (Annex 1, Part A, ¶4[a]). The expanded NQS would only constitute part of such national surveillance capacities.
3. WHO shall assist States Parties, upon request, to develop, strengthen and maintain the capacities referred to in paragraph 1 of this Article.	
4. WHO shall collect information regarding events through its surveillance activities and assess their potential to cause international disease spread and possible interference with international traffic. Information received by WHO under this paragraph shall be handled in accordance with Articles 11 and 45 where appropriate.	

Article 6 Notification

1. Each State Party shall assess events occurring within its territory by using the decision instrument in Annex 2. Each State Party shall notify WHO, by the most efficient means of	The obligations in Articles 6.1 and 6.2 require close coordination and good communications between the parts of the expanded NQS and the U.S. National IHR Focal Point in order to notify WHO of events

that may constitute a public health emergency of international concern within the time limits specified in the revised IHR. Further, Article 6.1 requires each part of the expanded NQS to be able to utilize the decision instrument contained in Annex 2 of the revised IHR. Articles 6.1 and 6.2 require states parties to report other types of information to WHO, including all health measures implemented in response to events that may constitute a public health emergency of international concern and other forms of public health information available to it (as indicated in Article 6.2); and the expanded NQS would need to be able to fulfill these requirements as well.

communication available, by way of the National IHR Focal Point, and within 24 hours of assessment of public health information, of all events which may constitute a public health emergency of international concern within its territory in accordance with the decision instrument, as well as any health measure implemented in response to those events. If the notification received by WHO involves the competency of the International Atomic Energy Agency (IAEA), WHO shall immediately notify the IAEA.

2. Following a notification, a State Party shall continue to communicate to WHO timely, accurate and sufficiently detailed public health information available to it on the notified event, where possible including case definitions, laboratory results, source and type of the risk, number of cases and deaths, conditions affecting the spread of the disease and the health measures employed; and report, when necessary, the difficulties faced and support needed in responding to the potential public health emergency of international concern.

Article 7 Information-sharing during unexpected or unusual public health events

If a State Party has evidence of an unexpected or unusual public health event within its territory, irrespective of origin or source, which may constitute a public health emergency of international concern, it shall provide to WHO all relevant public health information. In such a case, the provisions of Article 6 shall apply in full.

Article 7 is what remains of a provision that, in previous negotiating texts, referred specifically to suspected intentional releases of biological, chemical, or radionuclear agents. In the revised IHR, it is difficult to see how Article 7's requirements go beyond what states parties are already bound to do under Article 6. From the U.S. perspective, Article 7 is perhaps further evidence that the revised IHR apply to intentional releases of biological, chemical, or radionuclear agents. The expanded NQS might be involved in having to address such a suspected intentional release and thus be affected by Article 7.

(continued)

TABLE F.3 Continued

Revised IHR	Implications for Plans to Expand the National Quarantine System (NQS)
Article 8 Consultation In the case of events occurring within its territory not requiring notification as provided in Article 6, in particular those events for which there is insufficient information available to complete the decision instrument, a State Party may nevertheless keep WHO advised thereof through the National IHR Focal Point and consult with WHO on appropriate health measures. Such communications shall be treated in accordance with paragraphs 2 to 4 of Article 11. The State Party in whose territory the event has occurred may request WHO assistance to assess any epidemiological evidence obtained by that State Party.	Article 8 outlines discretionary actions that states parties may take with respect to events not requiring notification to WHO under Article 6; and, thus, Article 8 would not impose any obligations or limits on the expanded NQS.
Article 9 Other reports 1. WHO may take into account reports from sources other than notifications or consultations and shall assess these reports according to established epidemiological principles and then communicate information on the event to the State Party in whose territory the event is allegedly occurring. Before taking any action based on such reports, WHO shall consult with and attempt to obtain verification from the State Party in whose territory the event is allegedly occurring in accordance with the procedure set forth in Article 10. To this end, WHO shall make the information received available to the States Parties and only where it is duly justified may WHO maintain the confidentiality of the source. This information will be used in accordance with the procedure set forth in Article 11.	Article 9.1 empowers WHO to collect and use sources of information from nongovernmental sources of information and, thus, would not impose any obligations or limits on the expanded NQS. This authority for WHO could affect the expanded NQS if WHO collects nongovernmental information concerning disease events in the United States, requiring input from the expanded NQS if WHO seeks to consult with the United States concerning verification of such reports. The obligation in Article 7.2 would affect the expanded NQS because the NQS may receive information about public health risks outside the United States that may cause international disease spread, particularly if the expanded NQS has established offices or capabilities in foreign countries. This obligation could create friction with any host government that does not want to notify WHO

2. States Parties shall, as far as practicable, inform WHO within 24 hours of receipt of evidence of a public health risk identified outside their territory that may cause international disease spread, as manifested by exported or imported:

   (a) human cases;
   (b) vectors which carry infection or contamination; or
   (c) goods that are contaminated.

Article 10 Verification

1. WHO shall request, in accordance with Article 9, verification from a State Party of reports from sources other than notifications or consultations of events which may constitute a public health emergency of international concern allegedly occurring in the State's territory. In such cases, WHO shall inform the State Party concerned regarding the reports it is seeking to verify.

2. Pursuant to the foregoing paragraph and to Article 9, each State Party, when requested by WHO, shall verify and provide:

   (a) within 24 hours, an initial reply to, or acknowledgement of, the request from WHO;
   (b) within 24 hours, available public health information on the status of events referred to in WHO's request; and
   (c) information to WHO in the context of an assessment under Article 6, including relevant information as described in that Article.

3. When WHO receives information of an event that may constitute a public health emergency of international concern, it shall offer to collaborate with the State Party concerned in assessing the potential for international disease spread, possible interference with international traffic and the

pursuant to Article 6 of the revised IHR. The United States would have to be careful in negotiating any arrangement with a foreign government not to bind itself to rules that prevent fulfillment of the obligation in Article 9.2.

The Article 10 verification process affects the expanded NQS because the nature of information required to be provided to WHO under Article 10.2 would, in all likelihood, involve various components of the expanded NQS. The expanded NQS must have, therefore, the capacity to respond to such verification requests from WHO. In the unlikely event that the United States would request assistance from WHO to manage a disease threat pursuant to Article 10.3, the collaboration with WHO in the United States would have to draw on various assets of the expanded NQS.

(continued)

TABLE F.3 Continued

Revised IHR	Implications for Plans to Expand the National Quarantine System (NQS)
adequacy of control measures. Such activities may include collaboration with other standard-setting organizations and the offer to mobilize international assistance in order to support the national authorities in conducting and coordinating on-site assessments. When requested by the State Party, WHO shall provide information supporting such an offer. 4. If the State Party does not accept the offer of collaboration, WHO may, when justified by the magnitude of the public health risk, share with other States Parties the information available to it, whilst encouraging the State Party to accept the offer of collaboration by WHO, taking into account the views of the State Party concerned. *Article 11 Provision of information by WHO* 1. Subject to paragraph 2 of this Article, WHO shall send to all States Parties and, as appropriate, to relevant intergovernmental organizations, as soon as possible and by the most efficient means available, in confidence, such public health information which it has received under Articles 5 to 10 inclusive and which is necessary to enable States Parties to respond to a public health risk. WHO should communicate information to other States Parties that might help them in preventing the occurrence of similar incidents. 2. WHO shall use information received under Articles 6 and 8 and paragraph 2 of Article 9 for verification, assessment and assistance purposes under these Regulations and, unless otherwise agreed with the States Parties referred to in those	Article 11 concerns responsibilities of WHO for the provision of information to states parties to the revised IHR. The expanded NQS will have to develop communication mechanisms to distribute information provided by WHO that is relevant for addressing public health problems and events in the United States.

provisions, shall not make this information generally available to other States Parties, until such time as:

(a) the event is determined to constitute a public health emergency of international concern in accordance with Article 12; or

(b) information evidencing the international spread of the infection or contamination has been confirmed by WHO in accordance with established epidemiological principles; or

(c) there is evidence that:

(i) control measures against the international spread are unlikely to succeed because of the nature of the contamination, disease agent, vector or reservoir; or

(ii) the State Party lacks sufficient operational capacity to carry out necessary measures to prevent further spread of disease; or

(d) the nature and scope of the international movement of travellers, baggage, cargo, containers, conveyances, goods or postal parcels that may be affected by the infection or contamination requires the immediate application of international control measures.

3. WHO shall consult with the State Party in whose territory the event is occurring as to its intent to make information available under this Article.

4. When information received by WHO under paragraph 2 of this Article is made available to States Parties in accordance with these Regulations, WHO may also make it available to the public if other information about the same event has already become publicly available and there is a need for the dissemination of authoritative and independent information.

(continued)

244

TABLE F.3 Continued

Revised IHR	Implications for Plans to Expand the National Quarantine System (NQS)
Article 12 Determination of a public health emergency of international concern 1. The Director-General shall determine, on the basis of the information received, in particular from the State Party within whose territory an event is occurring, whether an event constitutes a public health emergency of international concern in accordance with the criteria and the procedure set out in these Regulations. 2. If the Director-General considers, based on an assessment under these Regulations, that a public health emergency of international concern is occurring, the Director-General shall consult with the State Party in whose territory the event arises regarding this preliminary determination. If the Director-General and the State Party are in agreement regarding this determination, the Director-General shall, in accordance with the procedure set forth in Article 49, seek the views of the Committee established under Article 48 (hereinafter the "Emergency Committee") on appropriate temporary recommendations. 3. If, following the consultation in paragraph 2 above, the Director-General and the State Party in whose territory the event arises do not come to a consensus within 48 hours on whether the event constitutes a public health emergency of international concern, a determination shall be made in accordance with the procedure set forth in Article 49. 4. In determining whether an event constitutes a public health emergency of international concern, the Director-General shall consider:	Article 12 concerns the power in the revised IHR for the WHO Director-General to declare whether an event constitutes a public health emergency of international concern. The only obligation on the United States under Article 12 is to consult with the Director-General concerning whether an event constitutes a public health emergency of international concern. Elements of the expanded NQS could be called upon by the CDC to participate in such a consultation process and/or in the Article 49 procedure mentioned in Articles 12.2 and 12.3.

(a) information provided by the State Party;
(b) the decision instrument contained in Annex 2;
(c) the advice of the Emergency Committee;
(d) scientific principles as well as the available scientific evidence and other relevant information; and
(e) an assessment of the risk to human health, of the risk of international spread of disease and of the risk of interference with international traffic.

5. If the Director-General, following consultations with the State Party within whose territory the public health emergency of international concern has occurred, considers that a public health emergency of international concern has ended, the Director-General shall take a decision in accordance with the procedure set out in Article 49.

Article 13 Public health response
1. Each State Party shall develop, strengthen and maintain, as soon as possible but no later than five years from the entry into force of these Regulations for that State Party, the capacity to respond promptly and effectively to public health risks and public health emergencies of international concern as set out in Annex 1. WHO shall publish, in consultation with Member States, guidelines to support States Parties in the development of public health response capacities.

2. Following the assessment referred to in paragraph 2, Part A of Annex 1, a State Party may report to WHO on the basis of a justified need and an implementation plan and, in so doing, obtain an extension of two years in which to fulfil the obligation in paragraph 1 of this Article. In exceptional circumstances and supported by a new implementation plan,

Article 13.1 is important for the expanded NQS because it requires the development, strengthening, and maintenance of response capabilities in accordance with Annex 1 of the revised IHR as part of the revised IHR's obligations on "core capacity requirements" for surveillance and response. The plan to expand and strengthen the NQS should constitute U.S. actions to develop and improve response capacities as required by Article 13.1. The federal government would have to make sure, however, that the capabilities being included in the expanded NQS, combined with other federal and state public health assets, meet the core capacity requirement for surveillance mandated by Article 13.1 and Annex 1. For example, Annex 1 requires, at the national level, seven response capacities provided on a 24-hour basis (Annex 1, Part A, ¶4–6). The expanded NQS would only constitute part of such national response capacities. WHO could

(continued)

TABLE F.3 Continued

Revised IHR	Implications for Plans to Expand the National Quarantine System (NQS)
the State Party may request a further extension not exceeding two years from the Director-General, who shall make the decision, taking into account the technical advice of the Review Committee. After the period mentioned in paragraph 1 of this Article, the State Party that has obtained an extension shall report annually to WHO on progress made towards the full implementation.	also call on the resources and expertise of the expanded NQS under Article 13.4 to provide support for WHO-coordinated response activities, perhaps as WHO has historically called on the CDC for support in international response activities.
3. At the request of a State Party, WHO shall collaborate in the response to public health risks and other events by providing technical guidance and assistance and by assessing the effectiveness of the control measures in place, including the mobilization of international teams of experts for on-site assistance, when necessary.	
4. If WHO, in consultation with the States Parties concerned as provided in Article 12, determines that a public health emergency of international concern is occurring, it may offer, in addition to the support indicated in paragraph 3 of this Article, further assistance to the State Party, including an assessment of the severity of the international risk and the adequacy of control measures. Such collaboration may include the offer to mobilize international assistance in order to support the national authorities in conducting and coordinating on-site assessments. When requested by the State Party, WHO shall provide information supporting such an offer.	
5. When requested by WHO, States Parties should provide, to the extent possible, support to WHO-coordinated response activities.	

6. When requested, WHO shall provide appropriate guidance and assistance to other States Parties affected or threatened by the public health emergency of international concern.

Article 14 Cooperation of WHO with intergovernmental organizations and international bodies

1. WHO shall cooperate and coordinate its activities, as appropriate, with other competent intergovernmental organizations or international bodies in the implementation of these Regulations, including through the conclusion of agreements and other similar arrangements.

2. In cases in which notification or verification of, or response to, an event is primarily within the competence of other intergovernmental organizations or international bodies, WHO shall coordinate its activities with such organizations or bodies in order to ensure the application of adequate measures for the protection of public health.

3. Notwithstanding the foregoing, nothing in these Regulations shall preclude or limit the provision by WHO of advice, support, or technical or other assistance for public health purposes.

PART III—RECOMMENDATIONS

Article 15 Temporary recommendations

1. If it has been determined in accordance with Article 12 that a public health emergency of international concern is occurring, the Director-General shall issue temporary recommendations in accordance with the procedure set out in Article 49. Such temporary recommendations may be modified or extended as appropriate, including after it has been

This provision has little direct relevance for the expanded NQS because it addresses WHO cooperation with other intergovernmental organizations and international bodies.

Article 15 empowers the WHO Director-General to issue temporary recommendations to states parties to assist them in responding to public health emergencies of international concern. Such recommendations would not be binding on states parties to the revised IHR but represent recommended guidance from WHO. If the United States agreed to implement such temporary recommendations,

(continued)

TABLE F.3 Continued

Revised IHR	Implications for Plans to Expand the National Quarantine System (NQS)
determined that a public health emergency of international concern has ended, at which time other temporary recommendations may be issued as necessary for the purpose of preventing or promptly detecting its recurrence. 2. Temporary recommendations may include health measures to be implemented by the State Party experiencing the public health emergency of international concern, or by other States Parties, regarding persons, baggage, cargo, containers, conveyances, goods and/or postal parcels to prevent or reduce the international spread of disease and avoid unnecessary interference with international traffic. 3. Temporary recommendations may be terminated in accordance with the procedure set out in Article 49 at any time and shall automatically expire three months after their issuance. They may be modified or extended for additional periods of up to three months. Temporary recommendations may not continue beyond the second World Health Assembly after the determination of the public health emergency of international concern to which they relate. *Article 16 Standing recommendations* WHO may make standing recommendations of appropriate health measures in accordance with Article 53 for routine or periodic application. Such measures may be applied by States Parties regarding persons, baggage, cargo, containers, conveyances, goods and/or postal parcels for specific, ongoing public health risks in order to prevent or reduce the international spread of disease and avoid unnecessary	then the expanded NQS might be called on to carry out the recommendations. Article 18 (below) contains a list of the types of recommendations WHO may issue to states parties with respect to persons (Article 18.1) and conveyances, containers, goods, cargo, baggage, and postal parcels (Article 18.2). To carry out temporary recommendations, the expanded NQS would need to have sufficient national legal authority to implement such recommendations. Article 16 empowers the WHO Director-General to issue standing recommendations concerning health measures to be applied routinely or periodically. Such recommendations would not be binding on states parties to the revised IHR but represent recommended guidance from WHO. If the United States agreed to implement such standing recommendations, then the expanded NQS might be called on to carry out the recommendations. To carry out standing recommendations,

the expanded NQS would need to have sufficient national legal authority to implement such recommendations.

The revised IHR direct this provision at the WHO Director-General, and it does not create obligations for or limitations on the expanded NQS.

interference with international traffic. WHO may, in accordance with Article 53, modify or terminate such recommendations, as appropriate.

Article 17 Criteria for recommendations

When issuing, modifying or terminating temporary or standing recommendations, the Director-General shall consider:

(a) the views of the States Parties directly concerned;

(b) the advice of the Emergency Committee or the Review Committee, as the case may be;

(c) scientific principles as well as available scientific evidence and information;

(d) health measures that, on the basis of a risk assessment appropriate to the circumstances, are not more restrictive of international traffic and trade and are not more intrusive to persons than reasonably available alternatives that would achieve the appropriate level of health protection;

(e) relevant international standards and instruments;

(f) activities undertaken by other relevant intergovernmental organizations and international bodies; and

(g) other appropriate and specific information relevant to the event. With respect to temporary recommendations, the consideration by the Director-General of subparagraphs (e) and (f) of this Article may be subject to limitations imposed by urgent circumstances.

(continued)

TABLE F.3 Continued

Revised IHR	Implications for Plans to Expand the National Quarantine System (NQS)
Article 18 Recommendations with respect to persons, conveyances, containers, goods, cargo, baggage and postal parcels 1. Recommendations issued by WHO to States Parties with respect to persons may include the following advice: – no specific health measures are advised; – review travel history in affected areas; – review proof of medical examination and any laboratory analysis; – require medical examinations; – review proof of vaccination or other prophylaxis; – require vaccination or other prophylaxis; – place suspect persons under public health observation; – implement quarantine or other health measures for suspect persons; – implement isolation and treatment where necessary of affected persons; – implement tracing of contacts of suspect or affected persons; – refuse entry of suspect and affected persons; – refuse entry of unaffected persons to affected areas; and – implement exit screening and/or restrictions on persons from affected areas. 2. Recommendations issued by WHO to States Parties with respect to baggage, cargo, containers, conveyances, goods and postal parcels may include the following advice: – no specific health measures are advised; – review manifest and routing; – implement inspections;	Article 18.1 lists possible recommendations that WHO could issue with respect to persons, and Article 18.2 lists possible recommendations concerning conveyances, containers, goods, cargo, baggage, and postal parcels. As noted above, the United States would not be obligated as a matter of international law to implement any WHO recommendation issued under the revised IHR. The United States would have to have domestic legal authority to implement any recommendations it decided to follow. These recommendations could involve restrictions on entry into the United States or exit from the United States. In addition, implementing recommendations with respect to persons would have to comply with the provisions of the revised IHR that address protecting the rights and dignity of individuals and applicable international human rights law. Implementing recommendations with respect to goods would have to comply with relevant rules of international trade law.

- review proof of measures taken on departure or in transit to eliminate infection or contamination;
- implement treatment of the baggage, cargo, containers, conveyances, goods, postal parcels or human remains to remove infection or contamination, including vectors and reservoirs;
- the use of specific health measures to ensure the safe handling and transport of human remains;
- implement isolation or quarantine;
- seizure and destruction of infected or contaminated or suspect baggage, cargo, containers, conveyances, goods or postal parcels under controlled conditions if no available treatment or process will otherwise be successful; and
- refuse departure or entry.

PART IV—POINTS OF ENTRY

Article 19 General obligations
Each State Party shall, in addition to the other obligations provided for under these Regulations:
(a) ensure that the capacities set forth in Annex 1 for designated points of entry are developed within the timeframe provided in paragraph 1 of Article 5 and paragraph 1 of Article 13;
(b) identify the competent authorities at each designated point of entry in its territory; and
(c) furnish to WHO, as far as practicable, when requested in response to a specific potential public health risk, relevant data concerning sources of infection or contamination, including vectors and reservoirs, at its points of entry, which could result in international disease spread.

Article 19(a) imposes obligations on the expanded NQS. First, the provision would require the United States to develop the core capacities indicated in Annex 1, Part B of the revised IHR for designated ports of entry. Given that the expansion of the NQS focuses on points of entry into the United States, such as seaports and airports, the obligations in Article 19(a) and Annex 1, Part B would be directly relevant to the expanded NQS. The core capacity requirements for ports of entry resonate with the federal government's desire to make the expanded NQS a resource that does more than engage in narrow quarantine activities. Articles 19(b) and (c) also impose duties on the expanded NQS to identify the proper authorities for each designated point of entry and to furnish to WHO in connection with a specific public health threat information concerning sources of infection or contamination at points of entry.

(continued)

TABLE F.3 Continued

Revised IHR	Implications for Plans to Expand the National Quarantine System (NQS)

Article 20 Airports and ports
1. States Parties shall designate the airports and ports that shall develop the capacities provided in Annex 1.
2. States Parties shall ensure that Ship Sanitation Control Exemption Certificates and Ship Sanitation Control Certificates are issued in accordance with the requirements in Article 39 and the model provided in Annex 3.
3. Each State Party shall send to WHO a list of ports authorized to offer:
  (a) the issuance of Ship Sanitation Control Certificates and the provision of the services referred to in Annexes 1 and 3; or
  (b) the issuance of Ship Sanitation Control Exemption Certificates only; and
  (c) extension of the Ship Sanitation Control Exemption Certificate for a period of one month until the arrival of the ship in the port at which the Certificate may be received. Each State Party shall inform WHO of any changes which may occur to the status of the listed ports. WHO shall publish the information received under this paragraph.
4. WHO may, at the request of the State Party concerned, arrange to certify, after an appropriate investigation, that an airport or port in its territory meets the requirements referred to in paragraphs 1 and 3 of this Article. These certifications may be subject to periodic review by WHO, in consultation with the State Party.
	Article 20.1 requires states parties to designate ports and airports that will develop the core capacities found in Annex 1, Part B. The United States, thus, has to identify which ports and airports will have the core capacities required by the revised IHR.
	
	Article 20.2 imposes obligations on those parts of the expanded NQS that concern seaports because it requires states parties to ensure that specific ship sanitation documents are issued in accordance with Article 39 and Annex 3 of the revised IHR. Article 20.3 would require the United States to provide WHO with a list of seaports authorized to issue these ship sanitation documents.
	
	Under Article 20.4, the United States could request the WHO to certify that airports and seaports in its territory have the required core capacities and, in the case of seaports, can issue the ship sanitation documents in accordance with the revised IHR. Such a certification process would be entirely voluntary on the part of the United States, and thus this provision creates no obligations for the expanded NQS.

5. WHO, in collaboration with competent intergovernmental organizations and international bodies, shall develop and publish the certification guidelines for airports and ports under this Article. WHO shall also publish a list of certified airports and ports.

Article 21 Ground crossings
1. Where justified for public health reasons, a State Party may designate ground crossings that shall develop the capacities provided in Annex 1, taking into consideration:
(a) the volume and frequency of the various types of international traffic, as compared to other points of entry, at a State Party's ground crossings which might be designated; and
(b) the public health risks existing in areas in which the international traffic originates, or through which it passes, prior to arrival at a particular ground crossing.
2. States Parties sharing common borders should consider:
(a) entering into bilateral or multilateral agreements or arrangements concerning prevention or control of international transmission of disease at ground crossings in accordance with Article 57; and
(b) joint designation of adjacent ground crossings for the capacities in Annex 1 in accordance with paragraph 1 of this Article.

Article 22 Role of competent authorities
1. The competent authorities shall:
(a) be responsible for monitoring baggage, cargo, containers, conveyances, goods, postal parcels and human remains departing and arriving from affected areas, so that they

Article 21 refers to a discretionary procedure under which the United States could designate ground crossings that shall have the core capacities identified for points of entry in Annex 1, Part B. Thus, the United States could designate any ground-crossing component of the expanded NQS as a point of entry having all the core capacities recognized by the revised IHR as important. Article 21 also encourages the United States to develop agreements with Mexico and Canada concerning the prevention and control of disease at ground crossings.

Articles 22.1 and 22.3 impose numerous obligations on the various parts of the expanded NQS. The revised IHR define "competent authorities" as "the authority responsible for the implementation and application of health measures under these Regulations" (Article 1.1).

(continued)

TABLE F.3 Continued

Revised IHR	Implications for Plans to Expand the National Quarantine System (NQS)
are maintained in such a condition that they are free of sources of infection or contamination, including vectors and reservoirs; (b) ensure, as far as practicable, that facilities used by travellers at points of entry are maintained in a sanitary condition and are kept free of sources of infection or contamination, including vectors and reservoirs; (c) be responsible for the supervision of any deratting, disinfection, disinsection or decontamination of baggage, cargo, containers, conveyances, goods, postal parcels and human remains or sanitary measures for persons, as appropriate under these Regulations; (d) advise conveyance operators, as far in advance as possible, of their intent to apply control measures to a conveyance, and shall provide, where available, written information concerning the methods to be employed; (e) be responsible for the supervision of the removal and safe disposal of any contaminated water or food, human or animal dejecta, wastewater and any other contaminated matter from a conveyance; (f) take all practicable measures consistent with these Regulations to monitor and control the discharge by ships of sewage, refuse, ballast water and other potentially disease-causing matter which might contaminate the waters of a port, river, canal, strait, lake or other international waterway; (g) be responsible for supervision of service providers for services concerning travellers, baggage, cargo, containers, conveyances, goods, postal parcels and human remains at	Federal quarantine stations in the expanded NQS would fall into the definition of "competent authorities" and thus be directly subject to the mandates of Article 22.1 and 22.3 and any other obligation the revised IHR impose on competent authorities.

points of entry, including the conduct of inspections and medical examinations as necessary;

(h) have effective contingency arrangements to deal with an unexpected public health event; and

(i) communicate with the National IHR Focal Point on the relevant public health measures taken pursuant to these Regulations.

2. Health measures recommended by WHO for travellers, baggage, cargo, containers, conveyances, goods, postal parcels and human remains arriving from an affected area may be reapplied on arrival, if there are verifiable indications and/or evidence that the measures applied on departure from the affected area were unsuccessful.

3. Disinsection, deratting, disinfection, decontamination and other sanitary procedures shall be carried out so as to avoid injury and as far as possible discomfort to persons, or damage to the environment in a way which impacts on public health, or damage to baggage, cargo, containers, conveyances, goods and postal parcels.

PART V—PUBLIC HEALTH MEASURES
Chapter I—General provisions

Article 23 Health measures on arrival and departure

1. Subject to applicable international agreements and relevant articles of these Regulations, a State Party may require for public health purposes, on arrival or departure:
(a) with regard to travellers:
(i) information concerning the traveller's destination so that the traveller may be contacted;
(ii) information concerning the traveller's itinerary to ascertain if there was any travel in or near an affected

Articles 23.1 and 23.2 allow states parties to apply certain health measures to travelers, conveyances, containers, cargo, goods, postal parcels, and human remains. These provisions contain no binding duties; but Article 23.2 indicates that states parties, in applying additional health measures to suspect or affected travelers, should use the least intrusive and invasive medical examination that would achieve the public health objective.

(continued)

TABLE F.3 Continued

Revised IHR	Implications for Plans to Expand the National Quarantine System (NQS)
area or other possible contacts with infection or contamination prior to arrival, as well as review of the traveller's health documents if they are required under these Regulations; and/or (iii) a non-invasive medical examination which is the least intrusive examination that would achieve the public health objective; (b) inspection of baggage, cargo, containers, conveyances, goods, postal parcels and human remains. 2. On the basis of evidence of a public health risk obtained through the measures provided in paragraph 1 of this Article, or through other means, States Parties may apply additional health measures, in accordance with these Regulations, in particular, with regard to a suspect or affected traveller, on a case-by-case basis, the least intrusive and invasive medical examination that would achieve the public health objective of preventing the international spread of disease. 3. No medical examination, vaccination, prophylaxis or health measure under these Regulations shall be carried out on travellers without their prior express informed consent or that of their parents or guardians, except as provided in paragraph 2 of Article 31, and in accordance with the law and international obligations of the State Party. 4. Travellers to be vaccinated or offered prophylaxis pursuant to these Regulations, or their parents or guardians, shall be informed of any risk associated with vaccination or with non-vaccination and with the use or non-use of prophylaxis in accordance with the law and international obligations of the State Party. States Parties shall inform medical	Articles 23.3, 23.4, and 23.5 contain mandatory obligations that affect how the expanded NQS would operate with respect to travelers. Article 23.3 requires that states parties obtain the express consent for an individual before carrying out any health measure on the individual, except in situations provided for in Article 31.2 (see below), and carry out such measures in accordance with the states parties' domestic law and international obligations. Article 23.4 requires that states parties inform travelers to be vaccinated or offered prophylaxis of any risk associated with such measures in accordance with the states parties' domestic laws and international obligations. Article 23.5 requires states parties to perform any health measure that involves the risk of disease transmission to be performed only on a traveler in accordance with established national or international safety guidelines and standards in order to minimize the risk.

practitioners of these requirements in accordance with the law of the State Party.

5. Any medical examination, medical procedure, vaccination or other prophylaxis which involves a risk of disease transmission shall only be performed on, or administered to, a traveller in accordance with established national or international safety guidelines and standards so as to minimize such a risk.

Chapter II—Special provisions for conveyances and conveyance operators

Article 24 Conveyance operators

1. States Parties shall take all practicable measures consistent with these Regulations to ensure that conveyance operators:
   (a) comply with the health measures recommended by WHO and adopted by the State Party;
   (b) inform travellers of the health measures recommended by WHO and adopted by the State Party for application on board; and
   (c) permanently keep conveyances for which they are responsible free of sources of infection or contamination, including vectors and reservoirs. The application of measures to control sources of infection or contamination may be required if evidence is found.

2. Specific provisions pertaining to conveyances and conveyance operators under this Article are provided in Annex 4. Specific measures applicable to conveyances and conveyance operators with regard to vector-borne diseases are provided in Annex 5.

Article 24.1 requires the United States to ensure that all conveyance operators comply with, and inform travelers of, health measures recommended by WHO and adopted by the United States. In addition, Article 24.1 requires the United States to keep all conveyances for which it is responsible permanently free of infection or contamination, including vectors and reservoirs. The expanded NQS may well have to be involved in the fulfillment of these obligations.

Article 24.2 refers to specific provisions pertaining to conveyances and conveyance operates found in Annexes 4 and 5 of the revised IHR. Section A of Annex 4 contains obligations on conveyance operators (e.g., to facilitate inspections), and the United States would have to use domestic law to impose these obligations on conveyance operators as part of the expanded NQS. Section B of Annex 4 imposes obligations on states parties that apply control measures to conveyances, containers, cargo, goods, and baggage: (1) such control measures must be carried out so as to avoid as far as possible injury or discomfort to people or damage to property; and (2) states parties

(continued)

258

TABLE F.3 Continued

Revised IHR	Implications for Plans to Expand the National Quarantine System (NQS)
	must be put in writing the control measures applied and the reasons therefore. These duties would affect the operation of the expanded NQS.
	Annex 5 contains specific measures for the control of vector-borne diseases that states parties may apply or use, but Annex 5 only has three obligations on states parties: (1) requiring states parties to mandate that conveyance operators report information on the presence of vectors on board and the measures used to eradicate them; (2) requiring states parties to have programs to control disease vectors of public health concern around the boundaries of points of entry and exit in their territories; and (3) requiring competent authorities that have undertaken control measures to inform the competent authorities of the conveyance's next port or airport of call that follow-up control measures are required. Each of these obligations would affect the operation of the expanded NQS.
Article 25 Ships and aircraft in transit Subject to Articles 27 and 43 or unless authorized by applicable international agreements, no health measure shall be applied by a State Party to: (a) a ship not coming from an affected area which passes through a maritime canal or waterway in the territory of that State Party on its way to a port in the territory of another State. Any such ship shall be permitted to take on, under the supervision of the competent authority, fuel, water, food and supplies;	Article 25 prohibits states parties from applying health measures to ships and aircraft in transit and requires states parties to allow ships and aircraft in transit to take on fuel, water, food, and supplies. The provision provides three exceptions to the prohibition: (1) if the ship or aircraft is an affected conveyance (Article 27); (2) if the state party in question believes that additional health measures are scientifically justified (Article 43); and (3) if an applicable international agreement permits the state party to apply health measures. This provision would be of direct concern to the expanded NQS.

This prohibition might affect the expanded NQS, but most civilian lorries, trains or coaches entering the United States from Canada or Mexico are unlikely to pass through the United States without embarking, disembarking, loading, or discharging.

Article 27.1 requires states parties to consider a conveyance affected if evidence or indications of a public health risk are found on board and then provides options for how states parties should deal with the affected conveyance. This provision would not create difficulties for the expanded NQS because addressing evidence or indications of public health risks on board conveyances would be within its mandate. Elements of the expanded NQS would have to have capabilities to undertake dealing with the affected conveyance.

Article 27.2 addresses the procedure if the competent authorities at the point of entry are not equipped to apply adequate control measures to an affected conveyance, and this provision would only be relevant if a component of the expanded NQS did not have the appropriate capabilities. Article 27.2 requires the competent authority

(continued)

(b) a ship which passes through waters within its jurisdiction without calling at a port or on the coast; and

(c) an aircraft in transit at an airport within its jurisdiction, except that the aircraft may be restricted to a particular area of the airport with no embarking and disembarking or loading and discharging. However, any such aircraft shall be permitted to take on, under the supervision of the competent authority, fuel, water, food and supplies.

Article 26 Civilian lorries, trains and coaches in transit
Subject to Article 27 and 43 or unless authorized by applicable international agreements, no health measure shall be applied to a civilian lorry, train or coach not coming from an affected area which passes through a territory without embarking, disembarking, loading or discharging.

Article 27 Affected conveyances
1. If clinical signs or symptoms and information based on fact or evidence of a public health risk, including sources of infection and contamination, are found on board a conveyance, the competent authority shall consider the conveyance as affected and may:
(a) disinfect, decontaminate, disinsect or derat the conveyance, as appropriate, or cause these measures to be carried out under its supervision; and
(b) decide in each case the technique employed to secure an adequate level of control of the public health risk as provided in these Regulations. Where there are methods or materials advised by WHO for these procedures, these should be employed, unless the competent authority determines that other methods are as safe and reliable.

260

TABLE F.3 Continued

Revised IHR	Implications for Plans to Expand the National Quarantine System (NQS)
The competent authority may implement additional health measures, including isolation of the conveyances, as necessary, to prevent the spread of disease. Such additional measures should be reported to the National IHR Focal Point. 2. If the competent authority for the point of entry is not able to carry out the control measures required under this Article, the affected conveyance may nevertheless be allowed to depart, subject to the following conditions: (a) the competent authority shall, at the time of departure, inform the competent authority for the next known point of entry of the type of information referred to under subparagraph (b); and (b) in the case of a ship, the evidence found and the control measures required shall be noted in the Ship Sanitation Control Certificate. Any such conveyance shall be permitted to take on, under the supervision of the competent authority, fuel, water, food and supplies. 3. A conveyance that has been considered as affected shall cease to be regarded as such when the competent authority is satisfied that: (a) the measures provided in paragraph 1 of this Article have been effectively carried out; and (b) there are no conditions on board that could constitute a public health risk.	at the point of entry to notify the competent authority at the next known point of entry about the affected conveyance, to note evidence of infection and control measures needed on a ship's sanitation control certificate, and to allow any affected conveyance to take on fuel, water, and supplies.

Article 28 Ships or aircraft at points of entry

1. Subject to Article 43 or as provided in applicable international agreements, a ship or an aircraft shall not be prevented for public health reasons from calling at any point of entry. However, if the point of entry is not equipped for applying health measures under these Regulations, the ship or aircraft may be ordered to proceed at its own risk to the nearest suitable point of entry available to it, unless the ship or aircraft has an operational problem which would make this diversion unsafe.

2. Subject to Article 43 or as provided in applicable international agreements, ships or aircraft shall not be refused free pratique by States Parties for public health reasons; in particular they shall not be prevented from embarking or disembarking, discharging or loading cargo or stores, or taking on fuel, water, food and supplies. States Parties may subject the granting of free pratique to inspection and, if a source of infection or contamination is found on board, the carrying out of necessary disinfection, decontamination, disinsection or deratting, or other measures necessary to prevent the spread of the infection or contamination.

3. Whenever practicable and subject to the previous paragraph, a State Party shall authorize the granting of free pratique by radio or other communication means to a ship or an aircraft when, on the basis of information received from it prior to its arrival, the State Party is of the opinion that the arrival of the ship or aircraft will not result in the introduction or spread of disease.

Articles 28.1 and 28.2 prevent a state party from refusing for public health reasons to (1) allow a ship or an aircraft from calling any point of entry; and (2) grant a ship or aircraft free pratique. (Article 1.1 defines *free pratique* as "permission for a ship to enter a port, embark or disembark, discharge or load cargo or stores; permission for an aircraft, after landing, to embark or disembark, discharge or load stores; and permission for a train or road vehicle, upon arrival, to embark or disembark, discharge or load cargo or stores.") These prohibitions have two exceptions: (1) if the state party prevents entry or free pratique using additional health measures justified by Article 43; and (2) if prevention of entry or free pratique is justified by another applicable international agreement. The elements of the expanded NQS would be in the position of having to make the kinds of decisions referred to in Articles 28.1 and 28.2.

Articles 28.4, 28.5(a), and 28.6 require officers and pilots of ships and aircraft to communicate various types of information to the port or airport of entry concerning defined situations (e.g., indications of illness on board). The parts of the expanded NQS would have to have the capacity to receive and act on such information provided by officers and pilots of ships and aircraft. These provisions would also allow the expanded NQS to require such communications from officers and pilots of ships and aircraft.

(continued)

TABLE F.3 Continued

Revised IHR	Implications for Plans to Expand the National Quarantine System (NQS)
4. Officers in command of ships or pilots in command of aircraft, or their agents, shall make known to the port or airport control as early as possible before arrival at the port or airport of destination any cases of illness indicative of a disease of an infectious nature or evidence of a public health risk on board as soon as such illnesses or public health risks are made known to the officer or pilot. This information must be immediately relayed to the competent authority for the port or airport. In urgent circumstances, such information should be communicated directly by the officers or pilots to the relevant port or airport authority.	
5. The following shall apply if a suspect or affected aircraft or ship, for reasons beyond the control of the pilot in command of the aircraft or the officer in command of the ship, lands elsewhere than at the airport at which the aircraft was due to land or berths elsewhere than at the port at which the ship was due to berth:	
(a) the pilot in command of the aircraft or the officer in command of the ship or other person in charge shall make every effort to communicate without delay with the nearest competent authority;	
(b) as soon as the competent authority has been informed of the landing it may apply health measures recommended by WHO or other health measures provided in these Regulations;	
(c) unless required for emergency purposes or for communication with the competent authority, no traveller on board the aircraft or ship shall leave its vicinity and no	

(continued)

cargo shall be removed from that vicinity, unless authorized by the competent authority; and

(d) when all health measures required by the competent authority have been completed, the aircraft or ship may, so far as such health measures are concerned, proceed either to the airport or port at which it was due to land or berth, or, if for technical reasons it cannot do so, to a conveniently situated airport or port.

6. Notwithstanding the provisions contained in this Article, the officer in command of a ship or pilot in command of an aircraft may take such emergency measures as may be necessary for the health and safety of travellers on board. He or she shall inform the competent authority as early as possible concerning any measures taken pursuant to this paragraph.

Article 29 Civilian lorries, trains and coaches at points of entry
WHO, in consultation with States Parties, shall develop guiding principles for applying health measures to civilian lorries, trains and coaches at points of entry and passing through ground crossings.

Chapter III—Special provisions for travelers

Article 30 Travellers under public health observation
Subject to Article 43 or as authorized in applicable international agreements, a suspect traveller who on arrival is placed under public health observation may continue an international voyage, if the traveller does not pose an imminent public health risk and the State Party informs the competent authority of the

This provision requires WHO to develop guidelines on health measures applied to conveyances at ground crossings. Such guidance from WHO would not be binding on the expanded NQS.

Article 30 sets down the procedure the expanded NQS would use in connection with a suspect traveler placed under public health observation. The expanded NQS may allow such traveler to continue an international voyage, provided that the traveler does not pose an imminent public health risk. If the United States allows such a suspect

264

TABLE F.3 Continued

Revised IHR	Implications for Plans to Expand the National Quarantine System (NQS)
point of entry at destination, if known, of the traveller's expected arrival. On arrival, the traveller shall report to that authority.	traveler to continue on an international voyage, then it must inform the competent authority of the point of next entry or destination. Similarly, the United States could receive information from other IHR states parties that a suspect traveler's next port of entry or destination is the United States.
Article 31 Health measures relating to entry of travellers 1. Invasive medical examination, vaccination or other prophylaxis shall not be required as a condition of entry of any traveller to the territory of a State Party, except that, subject to Articles 32, 42 and 45, these Regulations do not preclude States Parties from requiring medical examination, vaccination or other prophylaxis or proof of vaccination or other prophylaxis: (a) when necessary to determine whether a public health risk exists; (b) as a condition of entry for any travellers seeking temporary or permanent residence; (c) as a condition of entry for any travellers pursuant to Article 43 or Annexes 6 and 7; or (d) which may be carried out pursuant to Article 23. 2. If a traveller for whom a State Party may require a medical examination, vaccination or other prophylaxis under paragraph 1 of this Article fails to consent to any such measure, or refuses to provide the information or the documents referred to in paragraph 1(a) of Article 23, the State Party concerned may, subject to Articles 32, 42 and 45, deny entry to that traveller. If there is evidence of an imminent public health risk, the State Party may, in	Article 31 contains rules on the implementation of health measures against travelers and, thus, are of importance to the expanded NQS. The basic rule prohibits requiring that travelers undergo invasive medical examination, vaccination, or other prophylaxis as a condition of entry. The expanded NQS could, thus, only implement invasive medical examination, vaccination, or other prophylaxis against a traveler under four exceptions: (1) when necessary to determine whether a public health risk exists; (2) as a condition of entry for any travelers seeking temporary or permanent residence; (3) as an additional health measure justified under Article 43 and subject to Article 43's disciplines; (4) as a condition of entry under Annexes 6 (Vaccination, Prophylaxis and Related Certificates) and 7 (Requirements Concerning Vaccination or Prophylaxis for Specific Diseases [concerning yellow fever]); and (5) examinations, vaccinations, or prophylaxis carried out under Article 23. Concerning a traveler that refuses to give his or her consent to examination, vaccination, or prophylaxis as required by Article 23, a state party may either (1) refuse entry to that traveler; or (2) if the state party has evidence that there is evidence of an imminent public health risk, compel the traveler to undergo measures necessary to control such risk (examination, vaccination, prophylaxis, isolation,

accordance with its national law and to the extent necessary to control such a risk, compel the traveller to undergo or advise the traveller, pursuant to paragraph 3 of Article 23, to undergo:

(a) the least invasive and intrusive medical examination that would achieve the public health objective;

(b) vaccination or other prophylaxis; or

(c) additional established health measures that prevent or control the spread of disease, including isolation, quarantine or placing the traveller under public health observation.

Article 32 Treatment of travellers

In implementing health measures under these Regulations, States Parties shall treat travellers with respect for their dignity, human rights and fundamental freedoms and minimize any discomfort or distress associated with such measures, including by:

(a) treating all travellers with courtesy and respect;

(b) taking into consideration the gender, sociocultural, ethnic or religious concerns of travellers; and

(c) providing or arranging for adequate food and water, appropriate accommodation and clothing, protection for baggage and other possessions, appropriate medical treatment, means of necessary communication if possible in a language that they can understand and other appropriate assistance for travellers who are quarantined, isolated or subject to medical examinations or other procedures for public health purposes.

quarantine, public health observation) (Article 31.2). Use of compulsory measures would also be subject to the disciplines found in Articles 32 (Treatment of Travellers), 42 (Implementation of Health Measures), and 45 (Treatment of Personal Data) of the revised IHR.

This provision mandates that states parties treat travelers with respect of their dignity, human rights, and fundamental freedoms and minimize any discomfort or distress associated with the implementation of health measures. This mandate specifically mentions (but is not necessarily limited to) treating all travelers with courtesy and respect, taking into consideration gender, sociocultural, ethnic, or religious concerns of travelers; and providing for various necessities (food, water, shelter, medical treatment) for travelers who are quarantined, isolated, or subject to medical examination or other public health measures. This provision would have direct implications for the expanded NQS' treatment of travelers.

(continued)

TABLE F.3 Continued

Revised IHR	Implications for Plans to Expand the National Quarantine System (NQS)
Chapter IV—Special provisions for goods, containers and container loading areas	
Article 33 Goods in transit Subject to Article 43 or unless authorized by applicable international agreements, goods, other than live animals, in transit without transshipment shall not be subject to health measures under these Regulations or detained for public health purposes.	The general rule in Article 33 is that goods (excluding live animals) in transit without transshipment (i.e., the goods are on their way to another destination without crossing through the territory of the state party in question) shall not be subject to health measures or detained for public health purposes. This rule has two exceptions: (1) a health measure issued pursuant to Article 43; or (2) a measure authorized by an applicable international agreement (e.g., an international trade agreement). This duty requires the expanded NQS to identify goods in transit without transshipment from goods being imported into the United States for purposes of applying public health measures.
Article 34 Container and container loading areas 1. States Parties shall ensure, as far as practicable, that container shippers use international traffic containers that are kept free from sources of infection or contamination, including vectors and reservoirs, particularly during the course of packing. 2. States Parties shall ensure, as far as practicable, that container loading areas are kept free from sources of infection or contamination, including vectors and reservoirs. 3. Whenever, in the opinion of a State Party, the volume of international container traffic is sufficiently large, the competent authorities shall take all practicable measures consistent with these Regulations, including carrying out	Article 34 contains various rules that impose on states parties obligations to ensure that containers and container loading areas are not, and do not become, sources of infection or contamination. These rules require the expanded NQS to have the ability to inspect containers and container loading areas within the United States and to monitor private-actor compliance with domestic legal obligations to keep containers and container loading areas free from sources of infection and contamination.

inspections, to assess the sanitary condition of container loading areas and containers in order to ensure that the obligations contained in these Regulations are implemented.

4. Facilities for the inspection and isolation of containers shall, as far as practicable, be available at container loading areas.

5. Container consignees and consignors shall make every effort to avoid cross-contamination when multiple-use loading of containers is employed.

PART VI—HEALTH DOCUMENTS

Article 35 General rule

No health documents, other than those provided for under these Regulations or in recommendations issued by WHO, shall be required in international traffic, provided however that this Article shall not apply to travellers seeking temporary or permanent residence, nor shall it apply to document requirements concerning the public health status of goods or cargo in international trade pursuant to applicable international agreements. The competent authority may request travellers to complete contact information forms and questionnaires on the health of travellers, provided that they meet the requirements set out in Article 23.

This provision regulates what kind of health documents a state party can require of travelers and traders and thus is directly relevant to the tasks the expanded NQS will be undertaking. Article 35 establishes a general rule—a state party can require no health documents concerning international traffic except documents provided for in the revised IHR (e.g., yellow fever vaccination certificate [Annex 7]) or recommended by WHO. The scope of this general rule does not include document requirements for persons seeking temporary or permanent residence or concerning the public health status of goods or cargo permitted under other applicable international agreements (e.g., international trade agreements).

Article 35 does not contain any express exceptions. Further, Article 43.1(b) on additional health measures does not mention Article 35 as one of the prohibitions that an additional health measure could

(continued)

TABLE F.3 Continued

Revised IHR	Implications for Plans to Expand the National Quarantine System (NQS)
	legitimately ignore. It is not clear whether a state party may require additional health documents besides those recommended by WHO under Article 43.1(a), which allows additional health measures that achieve the same or greater level of health protection than WHO recommendations.
	These rules on health documents directly affect the operations of the expanded NQS.
Article 36 Certificates of vaccination or other prophylaxis 1. Vaccines and prophylaxis for travellers administered pursuant to these Regulations, or to recommendations and certificates relating thereto, shall conform to the provisions of Annex 6 and, when applicable, Annex 7 with regard to specific diseases. 2. A traveller in possession of a certificate of vaccination or other prophylaxis issued in conformity with Annex 6 and, when applicable, Annex 7, shall not be denied entry as a consequence of the disease to which the certificate refers, even if coming from an affected area, unless the competent authority has verifiable indications and/or evidence that the vaccination or other prophylaxis was not effective.	The provision regulates (1) vaccines and prophylaxis administered under the revised IHR; and (2) certificates of vaccination or other prophylaxis issued under the Regulations. Vaccines or other prophylaxis administered to travelers must be of suitable quality and those vaccines or prophylaxis designated by WHO shall be subject to its approval (Annex 6, ¶1). If WHO requests, a state party must provide evidence of the suitability of the vaccines and prophylaxis administered within its territory under the IHR (Annex 6, ¶1). Annex 6 also contains rules that determine the form of certificates to be issued to travelers and how forms are completed. Annex 6, ¶2 provides that "[n]o departure shall be made from the model of the certificate specified in this Annex." The administration of vaccination or other prophylaxis by the expanded NQS to travelers implicates the United States' duty to comply with these rules.

(continued)

Article 37 Maritime Declaration of Health

1. The master of a ship, before arrival at its first port of call in the territory of a State Party, shall ascertain the state of health on board, and, except when that State Party does not require it, the master shall, on arrival, or in advance of the vessel's arrival if the vessel is so equipped and the State Party requires such advance delivery, complete and deliver to the competent authority for that port a Maritime Declaration of Health which shall be countersigned by the ship's surgeon, if one is carried.

2. The master of a ship, or the ship's surgeon if one is carried, shall supply any information required by the competent authority as to health conditions on board during an international voyage.

3. A Maritime Declaration of Health shall conform to the model provided in Annex 8.

4. A State Party may decide:
   (a) to dispense with the submission of the Maritime Declaration of Health by all arriving ships; or
   (b) to require the submission of the Maritime Declaration of Health under a recommendation concerning ships arriving from affected areas or to require it from ships which might otherwise carry infection or contamination.

The State Party shall inform shipping operators or their agents of these requirements.

This provision would allow (but does not mandate) the United States to require that the masters of ships arriving in U.S. territory ascertain the health conditions on board the vessel and deliver (at arrival or earlier) a Maritime Declaration of Health in the form provided in Annex 8. If the United States adopted such a requirement, it would be obliged to notify shipping interests about its rules on Maritime Declarations of Health. A U.S. requirement for delivery of Maritime Declarations of Health would affect the expanded NQS because this system would be receiving and, if necessary, acting upon the Maritime Declarations of Health.

TABLE F.3 Continued

Revised IHR	Implications for Plans to Expand the National Quarantine System (NQS)

Article 38 Health Part of the Aircraft General Declaration
1. The pilot in command of an aircraft or the pilot's agent, in flight or upon landing at the first airport in the territory of a State Party, shall, to the best of his or her ability, complete and deliver to the competent authority for that airport the Health Part of the Aircraft General Declaration which shall conform to the model specified in Annex 9.
2. The pilot in command of an aircraft or the pilot's agent shall supply any information required by the State Party as to health conditions on board during an international voyage and any health measure applied to the aircraft.
3. A State Party may decide:
  (a) to dispense with the submission of the Health Part of the Aircraft General Declaration by all arriving aircraft; or
  (b) to require the submission of the Health Part of the Aircraft General Declaration under a recommendation concerning aircraft arriving from affected areas or to require it from aircraft which might otherwise carry infection or contamination.
The State Party shall inform aircraft operators or their agents of these requirements.
	This provision would allow (but does not mandate) the United States to require that pilots of aircraft arriving in U.S. territory complete and deliver the Health Part of the Aircraft General Declaration in the form provided in Annex 9. If the United States adopted such a requirement, it would be obliged to notify aircraft operators about its rules on the Health Part of the General Aircraft Declaration. A U.S. requirement for delivery of the Health Part of the General Aircraft Declaration would affect the expanded NQS because this system would be receiving and, if necessary, acting upon this declaration.

Article 39 Ship sanitation certificates 1. Ship Sanitation Control Exemption Certificates and Ship Sanitation Control Certificates shall be valid for a maximum period of six months. This period may be extended by one month if the inspection or control measures required cannot be accomplished at the port.	This provision sets out the rules and procedure for the issuance and validity of ship sanitation certificates. Annex 3 of the revised IHR contains the model ship sanitation control exemption certificate and the ship sanitation control certificate, to which such certificates issued by states parties must conform. These rules, thus, apply to the

(continued)

issuance of such certificates by the expanded NQS.

2. If a valid Ship Sanitation Control Exemption Certificate or Ship Sanitation Control Certificate is not produced or evidence of a public health risk is found on board a ship, the State Party may proceed as provided in paragraph 1 of Article 27.

3. The certificates referred to in this Article shall conform to the model in Annex 3.

4. Whenever possible, control measures shall be carried out when the ship and holds are empty. In the case of a ship in ballast, they shall be carried out before loading.

5. When control measures are required and have been satisfactorily completed, the competent authority shall issue a Ship Sanitation Control Certificate, noting the evidence found and the control measures taken.

6. The competent authority may issue a Ship Sanitation Control Exemption Certificate at any port specified under Article 20 if it is satisfied that the ship is free of infection and contamination, including vectors and reservoirs. Such a certificate shall normally be issued only if the inspection of the ship has been carried out when the ship and holds are empty or when they contain only ballast or other material, of such a nature or so disposed as to make a thorough inspection of the holds possible.

7. If the conditions under which control measures are carried out are such that, in the opinion of the competent authority for the port where the operation was performed, a satisfactory result cannot be obtained, the competent authority shall make a note to that effect on the Ship Sanitation Control Certificate.

TABLE F.3 Continued

Revised IHR	Implications for Plans to Expand the National Quarantine System (NQS)
PART VII—CHARGES *Article 40 Charges for health measures regarding travellers* 1. Except for travellers seeking temporary or permanent residence, and subject to paragraph 2 of this Article, no charge shall be made by a State Party pursuant to these Regulations for the following measures for the protection of public health: (a) any medical examination provided for in these Regulations, or any supplementary examination which may be required by that State Party to ascertain the health status of the traveller examined; (b) any vaccination or other prophylaxis provided to a traveller on arrival that is not a published requirement or is a requirement published less than 10 days prior to provision of the vaccination or other prophylaxis; (c) appropriate isolation or quarantine requirements of travellers; (d) any certificate issued to the traveller specifying the measures applied and the date of application; or (e) any health measures applied to baggage accompanying the traveller. 2. State Parties may charge for health measures other than those referred to in paragraph 1 of this Article, including those primarily for the benefit of the traveller. 3. Where charges are made for applying such health measures to travellers under these Regulations, there shall be in each State Party only one tariff for such charges and every charge shall: (a) conform to this tariff; (b) not exceed the actual cost of the service rendered; and (c) be levied without distinction as to the nationality, domicile or residence of the traveller concerned.	Article 40 contains the rules on charges for the administration of health measures with respect to travelers. Article 40.1 prohibits charges for certain health measures, except with respect to travelers seeking temporary or permanent residence. Article 40.5 allows states parties to seek reimbursement for the costs of health measures listed in Article 40.1 from conveyance operators or owners or insurance sources. Article 40.2 allows charges to be made for other health measures but only under the disciplines provided for in Articles 40.3 and 40.4. These rules would affect whether and how the expanded NQS could charge for any health measures it applies to travelers.

(continued)

4. The tariff, and any amendment thereto, shall be published at least 10 days in advance of any levy thereunder.

5. Nothing in these Regulations shall preclude States Parties from seeking reimbursement for expenses incurred in providing the health measures in paragraph 1 of this Article:

   (a) from conveyance operators or owners with regard to their employees; or

   (b) from applicable insurance sources.

6. Under no circumstances shall travellers or conveyance operators be denied the ability to depart from the territory of a State Party pending payment of the charges referred to in paragraphs 1 or 2 of this Article.

Article 41 Charges for baggage, cargo, containers, conveyances, goods or postal parcels

1. Where charges are made for applying health measures to baggage, cargo, containers, conveyances, goods or postal parcels under these Regulations, there shall be in each State Party only one tariff for such charges and every charge shall:

   (a) conform to this tariff;

   (b) not exceed the actual cost of the service rendered; and

   (c) be levied without distinction as to the nationality, flag, registry or ownership of the baggage, cargo, containers, conveyances, goods or postal parcels concerned.

   In particular, there shall be no distinction made between national and foreign baggage, cargo, containers, conveyances, goods or postal parcels.

2. The tariff, and any amendment thereto, shall be published at least 10 days in advance of any levy thereunder.

Article 41 regulates how states parties can charge for health measures applied to baggage, cargo, containers, conveyances, goods, or postal parcels. The expanded NQS would have to have the capabilities to abide by these disciplines.

TABLE F.3 Continued

Revised IHR	Implications for Plans to Expand the National Quarantine System (NQS)
PART VIII—GENERAL PROVISIONS	
Article 42 Implementation of health measures Health measures taken pursuant to these Regulations shall be initiated and completed without delay, and applied in a transparent and non-discriminatory manner.	The provision imposes on the expanded NQS duties to implement health measures applied under the IHR without delay, transparently, and in a nondiscriminatory manner. Earlier provisions of the revised IHR subjected their rules to fulfillment of Article 42, so this duty is important in the overall scheme of the revised IHR.
Article 43 Additional health measures 1. These Regulations shall not preclude States Parties from implementing health measures, in accordance with their relevant national law and obligations under international law, in response to specific public health risks or public health emergencies of international concern, which: (a) achieve the same or greater level of health protection than WHO recommendations; or (b) are otherwise prohibited under Article 25, Article 26, paragraphs 1 and 2 of Article 28, Article 30, paragraph 1(c) of Article 31 and Article 33, provided such measures are otherwise consistent with these Regulations. Such measures shall not be more restrictive of international traffic and not more invasive or intrusive to persons than reasonably available alternatives that would achieve the appropriate level of health protection. 2. In determining whether to implement the health measures referred to in paragraph 1 of this Article or additional health	Article 43 is a very important provision in the revised IHR, and thus for the expanded NQS. This provision would allow the expanded NQS to apply health measures that (1) achieve the same or greater level of health protection than WHO recommendations; or (2) are otherwise prohibited by specified provisions of the revised IHR. Implementing such additional health measures has to be done in a way that is not otherwise inconsistent with the revised IHR. Further, states parties are required to base such additional health measures on scientific principles and scientific evidence of a risk to human health, or where the scientific evidence is insufficient on available information, including information from WHO and other relevant international organizations. Article 43.1 also mandates that any additional health measure not be (1) more restrictive of international traffic, and (2) not more intrusive or invasive to persons than reasonably available alternative measures that would achieve the level of health protection sought. Article 43.2 and 43.5 impose other requirements, namely providing

measures under paragraph 2 of Article 23, paragraph 1 of Article 27, paragraph 2 of Article 28 and paragraph 2(c) of Article 31, States Parties shall base their determinations upon:

(a) scientific principles;

(b) available scientific evidence of a risk to human health, or where such evidence is insufficient, the available information including from WHO and other relevant intergovernmental organizations and international bodies; and

(c) any available specific guidance or advice from WHO.

3. A State Party implementing additional health measures referred to in paragraph 1 of this Article which significantly interfere with international traffic shall provide to WHO the public health rationale and relevant scientific information for it. WHO shall share this information with other States Parties and shall share information regarding the health measures implemented. For the purpose of this Article, significant interference generally means refusal of entry or departure of international travellers, baggage, cargo, containers, conveyances, goods, and the like, or their delay, for more than 24 hours.

4. After assessing information provided pursuant to paragraph 3 and 5 of this Article and other relevant information, WHO may request that the State Party concerned reconsider the application of the measures.

5. A State Party implementing additional health measures referred to in paragraphs 1 and 2 of this Article that significantly interfere with international traffic shall inform WHO, within 48 hours of implementation, of such measures and their health rationale unless these are covered by a temporary or standing recommendation.

WHO the public health rationale and scientific information supporting the additional health measure and reviewing the additional health measure within 90 days to assess whether it should still be applied.

Implementation of additional health measures under Article 43 creates the possibility that (1) WHO may ask the state party to cease application of such measure (Article 43.4); and (2) another state party affected by the additional health measure may seek consultations about the measure (Article 43.7).

This article is important to the expanded NQS for a number of reasons, the most important being: (1) it allows states parties to adopt health measures that are more protective than specific measures provided for in the IHR or recommended by WHO; (2) it applies disciplines on the adoption of additional measures that require scientific evidence and the least restrictive/instrusive measures possible; and (3) it sets up a process through which such additional measures can be subjected to international scrutiny by WHO and other states parties.

(continued)

TABLE F.3 Continued

Revised IHR	Implications for Plans to Expand the National Quarantine System (NQS)
6. A State Party implementing a health measure pursuant to paragraph 1 or 2 of this Article shall within three months review such a measure taking into account the advice of WHO and the criteria in paragraph 2 of this Article. 7. Without prejudice to its rights under Article 56, any State Party impacted by a measure taken pursuant to paragraph 1 or 2 of this Article may request the State Party implementing such a measure to consult with it. The purpose of such consultations is to clarify the scientific information and public health rationale underlying the measure and to find a mutually acceptable solution. 8. The provisions of this Article may apply to implementation of measures concerning travellers taking part in mass congregations. *Article 44 Collaboration and assistance* 1. States Parties shall undertake to collaborate with each other, to the extent possible, in: (a) the detection and assessment of, and response to, events as provided under these Regulations; (b) the provision or facilitation of technical cooperation and logistical support, particularly in the development, strengthening and maintenance of the public health capacities required under these Regulations; (c) the mobilization of financial resources to facilitate implementation of their obligations under these Regulations; and	Article 44.1 establishes some general duties to collaborate on disease prevention, control, and response; and these duties do not raise significant concerns for plans for the expanded NQS. Perhaps the most important of these general obligations concerns making sure that domestic laws are formulated to allow the implementation of the revised IHR.

(d) the formulation of proposed laws and other legal and administrative provisions for the implementation of these Regulations.

2. WHO shall collaborate with States Parties, upon request, to the extent possible, in:
   (a) the evaluation and assessment of their public health capacities in order to facilitate the effective implementation of these Regulations;
   (b) the provision or facilitation of technical cooperation and logistical support to States Parties; and
   (c) the mobilization of financial resources to support developing countries in building, strengthening and maintaining the capacities provided for in Annex 1.

3. Collaboration under this Article may be implemented through multiple channels, including bilaterally, through regional networks and the WHO regional offices, and through intergovernmental organizations and international bodies.

Article 45 Treatment of personal data

1. Health information collected or received by a State Party pursuant to these Regulations from another State Party or from WHO which refers to an identified or identifiable person shall be kept confidential and processed anonymously as required by national law.

2. Notwithstanding paragraph 1, States Parties may disclose and process personal data where essential for the purposes of assessing and managing a public health risk, but State Parties, in accordance with national law, and WHO must ensure that the personal data are:
   (a) processed fairly and lawfully, and not further processed in a way incompatible with that purpose;

Article 45.1 concerns obligations to keep personal information gathered in implementing the IHR confidential, except where sharing of such information is essential for the purposes of assessing and managing a public health risk (Article 45.2). Overall, Article 45 raises the need for the expanded NQS to develop and implement systems of keeping personally identifiable information confidential.

(continued)

278

TABLE F.3 Continued

Revised IHR	Implications for Plans to Expand the National Quarantine System (NQS)
(b) adequate, relevant and not excessive in relation to that purpose; (c) accurate and, where necessary, kept up to date; every reasonable step must be taken to ensure that data which are inaccurate or incomplete are erased or rectified; and (d) not kept longer than necessary. 3. Upon request, WHO shall as far as practicable provide an individual with his or her personal data referred to in this Article in an intelligible form, without undue delay or expense and, when necessary, allow for correction. *Article 46 Transport and handling of biological substances, reagents and materials for diagnostic purposes* States Parties shall, subject to national law and taking into account relevant international guidelines, facilitate the transport, entry, exit, processing and disposal of biological substances and diagnostic specimens, reagents and other diagnostic materials for verification and public health response purposes under these Regulations.	This provision contains a requirement that states parties facilitate the movement of biological substances, specimens, reagents, and other materials needed for verifying and responding to public health events and risks. This obligation might be particularly important for the expanded NQS because of the CDC's role of participating in international disease verification and response activities.

PART IX—THE IHR ROSTER OF EXPERTS, THE EMERGENCY COMMITTEE AND THE REVIEW COMMITTEE
(*Articles 47–53: Not relevant for the NQS' relationship with the revised IHR*)

PART X—FINAL PROVISIONS (only the relevant articles)
Article 54 Reporting and review

1. States Parties and the Director-General shall report to the Health Assembly on the implementation of these Regulations as decided by the Health Assembly.

2. The Health Assembly shall periodically review the functioning of these Regulations. To that end it may request the advice of the Review Committee, through the Director-General. The first such review shall take place no later than five years after the entry into force of these Regulations.

3. WHO shall periodically conduct studies to review and evaluate the functioning of Annex 2. The first such review shall commence no later than one year after the entry into force of these Regulations. The results of such reviews shall be submitted to the Health Assembly for its consideration, as appropriate.

Article 57 Relationship with other international agreements

1. States Parties recognize that the IHR and other relevant international agreements should be interpreted so as to be compatible. The provisions of the IHR shall not affect the rights and obligations of any State Party deriving from other international agreements.

2. Subject to paragraph 1 of this Article, nothing in these Regulations shall prevent States Parties having certain interests in common owing to their health, geographical, social or economic conditions, from concluding special treaties or arrangements in order to facilitate the application of these Regulations, and in particular with regard to:

The expanded NQS would be called upon to provide information to fulfill the United States' duty under this article to report on its implementation of the IHR.

Article 57.1 is potentially important should the expanded NQS find itself confronted with a choice between compliance with the revised IHR and compliance with another international legal regime. The likelihood of direct conflicts between the revised IHR and other international legal regimes is not significant for many reasons, including the flexibility built into the revised IHR that allows for health measures to be applied pursuant to other international agreements.

Article 57.2 allows the United States to develop agreements or arrangements with other states parties to facilitate the application of

(continued)

TABLE F.3 Continued

Revised IHR	Implications for Plans to Expand the National Quarantine System (NQS)
(a) the direct and rapid exchange of public health information between neighbouring territories of different States; (b) the health measures to be applied to international coastal traffic and to international traffic in waters within their jurisdiction; (c) the health measures to be applied in contiguous territories of different States at their common frontier; (d) arrangements for carrying affected persons or affected human remains by means of transport specially adapted for the purpose; and (e) deratting, disinsection, disinfection, decontamination or other treatment designed to render goods free of disease-causing agents. 3. Without prejudice to their obligations under these Regulations, States Parties that are members of a regional economic integration organization shall apply in their mutual relations the common rules in force in that regional economic integration organization. *Article 62 Reservations* 1. States may make reservations to these Regulations in accordance with this Article. Such reservations shall not be incompatible with the object and purpose of these Regulations. 2. Reservations to these Regulations shall be notified to the Director-General in accordance with paragraph 1 of Article 59 and Article 60, paragraph 1 of Article 63 or paragraph 1 of Article 64, as the case may be. A State not a Member of WHO shall notify the Director-General of any reservation with its notification of acceptance of these Regulations. States	the IHR. This provision would accommodate the United States concluding agreements to post federal quarantine resources in other countries as part of the plan to expand the NQS. This provision would only affect the expanded NQS in the event that the United States made reservations to the revised IHR. At present, the United States has only indicated that it would make one reservation addressing implementation of the revised IHR under the U.S. federal system of government.

(continued)

formulating reservations should provide the Director-General with reasons for the reservations.

3. A rejection in part of these Regulations shall be considered as a reservation.

4. The Director-General shall, in accordance with paragraph 2 of Article 65, issue notification of each reservation received pursuant to paragraph 2 of this Article. The Director-General shall:

(a) if the reservation was made before the entry into force of these Regulations, request those Member States that have not rejected these Regulations to notify him or her within six months of any objection to the reservation, or

(b) if the reservation was made after the entry into force of these Regulations, request States Parties to notify him or her within six months of any objection to the reservation. States objecting to a reservation should provide the Director-General with reasons for the objection.

5. After this period, the Director-General shall notify all States Parties of the objections he or she has received with regard to reservations. Unless by the end of six months from the date of the notification referred to in paragraph 4 of this Article a reservation has been objected to by one-third of the States referred to in paragraph 4 of this Article, it shall be deemed to be accepted and these Regulations shall enter into force for the reserving State, subject to the reservation.

6. If at least one-third of the States referred to in paragraph 4 of this Article object to the reservation by the end of six months from the date of the notification referred to in paragraph 4 of this Article, the Director-General shall notify the reserving State with a view to its considering withdrawing the reservation within three months from the date of the notification by the Director-General.

TABLE F.3 Continued

Revised IHR	Implications for Plans to Expand the National Quarantine System (NQS)
7. The reserving State shall continue to fullfill any obligations corresponding to the subject matter of the reservation, which the State has accepted under any of the international sanitary agreements or regulations listed in Article 58.	
8. If the reserving State does not withdraw the reservation within three months from the date of the notification by the Director-General referred to in paragraph 6 of this Article, the Director-General shall seek the view of the Review Committee if the reserving State so requests. The Review Committee shall advise the Director-General as soon as possible and in accordance with Article 50 on the practical impact of the reservation on the operation of these Regulations.	
9. The Director-General shall submit the reservation, and the views of the Review Committee if applicable, to the Health Assembly for its consideration. If the Health Assembly, by a majority vote, objects to the reservation on the ground that it is incompatible with the object and purpose of these Regulations, the reservation shall not be accepted and these Regulations shall enter into force for the reserving State only after it withdraws its reservation pursuant to Article 63. If the Health Assembly accepts the reservation, these Regulations shall enter into force for the reserving State, subject to its reservation.	

ANNEX 3

TABLE F.4 Analysis of the WTO's Agreement on the Application of Sanitary and Phytosanitary Measures (SPS Agreement): Implications for Plans to Expand the National Quarantine System

Article of the SPS Agreement	Implications for the Plans to Expand the National Quarantine System (NQS)
Article 1 *General Provisions* 1. This Agreement applies to all sanitary and phytosanitary measures which may, directly or indirectly, affect international trade. Such measures shall be developed and applied in accordance with the provisions of this Agreement. 2. For the purposes of this Agreement, the definitions provided in Annex A shall apply. 3. The annexes are an integral part of this Agreement. 4. Nothing in this Agreement shall affect the rights of Members under the Agreement on Technical Barriers to Trade with respect to measures not within the scope of this Agreement.	As contemplated, the federal government would task the expanded NQS to address threats to U.S. public health posed by goods imported into the United States. Thus, the expanded NQS would apply sanitary and phytosanitary (SPS) measures as defined by the SPS Agreement. Annex A.1 of the SPS Agreement defines a SPS measure to include any measure applied to protect human life or health from risks arising from additives, contaminants, toxins or disease-causing organisms in foods, beverages, or feedstuffs or from risks arising from diseases carried by animals, plants, or products thereof, or from risks arising from the entry and the establishment of pests. All these risks would be part of the mandate of an expanded NQS, thus making the SPS Agreement relevant to the responsibilities the expanded NQS will undertake.
Article 2 *Basic Rights and Obligations* 1. Members have the right to take sanitary and phytosanitary measures necessary for the protection of human, animal or plant life or health, provided that such measures are not inconsistent with the provisions of this Agreement. 2. Members shall ensure that any sanitary or phytosanitary	<u>Article 2.1</u>: This provision states that all WTO members have the right to take SPS measures to protect human health. The expansion of the NQS by the federal government would be an exercise of this sovereign right. Article 2.1 conditions the exercise of this right, however, on WTO members applying SPS measures consistently

(continued)

TABLE F.4 Continued

Article of the SPS Agreement	Implications for the Plans to Expand the National Quarantine System (NQS)
measure is applied only to the extent necessary to protect human, animal or plant life or health, is based on scientific principles and is not maintained without sufficient scientific evidence, except as provided for in paragraph 7 of Article 5. 3. Members shall ensure that their sanitary and phytosanitary measures do not arbitrarily or unjustifiably discriminate between Members where identical or similar conditions prevail, including between their own territory and that of other Members. Sanitary and phytosanitary measures shall not be applied in a manner which would constitute a disguised restriction on international trade. 4. Sanitary or phytosanitary measures which conform to the relevant provisions of this Agreement shall be presumed to be in accordance with the obligations of the Members under the provisions of GATT 1994 which relate to the use of sanitary or phytosanitary measures, in particular the provisions of Article XX(b).	with the other provisions in the SPS Agreement. Article 2.2: This provision sets out the basic science-based disciplines with which SPS measures have to comply—the measures have to be necessary to protect human health, be based on scientific principles, and not maintained without sufficient scientific evidence. SPS measures applied by the expanded NQS will, thus, need to be scientifically grounded and justified for the measure to survive scrutiny under the SPS Agreement. Article 2.3: This provision contains the basic trade-related disciplines that the SPS Agreement applies to the SPS measures of WTO members. The expanded NQS' application of SPS measures will have to comply with not only the science-based disciplines but also the trade-related disciplines in the SPS Agreement. Article 2.4: This provision provides that, if a WTO member's SPS measure complies with the SPS Agreement, that measure is deemed to comply with the provisions of GATT. Thus, the application of SPS measures by the expanded NQS that comply with the SPS Agreement will not be vulnerable to claims that the measures violate GATT.
Article 3 *Harmonization* 1. To harmonize sanitary and phytosanitary measures on as wide a basis as possible, Members shall base their sanitary or phytosanitary measures on international standards, guidelines or recommendations, where they exist, except as otherwise provided for in this Agreement, and in particular in paragraph 3.	Article 3 contains the harmonization disciplines of the SPS Agreement. These provisions involve obligations and incentives for WTO member states to use international standards, guidelines, and recommendations as the basis for their SPS measures. Thus, the expanded NQS is under an obligation to base the SPS measures it

applies on existing international standards, if they exist. Conforming national measures to international standards means that the measures comply with the SPS Agreement.

The expanded NQS can apply a SPS measure that is more protective of health (and restrictive of trade) than an existing international standard if it complies with the other rules of the SPS Agreement (the science-based and trade-related disciplines). Particularly, the more protective measure must have a scientific basis.

2. Sanitary or phytosanitary measures which conform to international standards, guidelines or recommendations shall be deemed to be necessary to protect human, animal or plant life or health, and presumed to be consistent with the relevant provisions of this Agreement and of GATT 1994.

3. Members may introduce or maintain sanitary or phytosanitary measures which result in a higher level of sanitary or phytosanitary protection than would be achieved by measures based on the relevant international standards, guidelines or recommendations, if there is a scientific justification, or as a consequence of the level of sanitary or phytosanitary protection a Member determines to be appropriate in accordance with the relevant provisions of paragraphs 1 through 8 of Article 5.^{a} Notwithstanding the above, all measures which result in a level of sanitary or phytosanitary protection different from that which would be achieved by measures based on international standards, guidelines or recommendations shall not be inconsistent with any other provision of this Agreement.

4. Members shall play a full part, within the limits of their resources, in the relevant international organizations and their subsidiary bodies, in particular the Codex Alimentarius Commission, the International Office of Epizootics, and the international and regional organizations operating within the framework of the International Plant Protection Convention, to promote within these organizations the development and periodic review of standards, guidelines and recommendations with respect to all aspects of sanitary and phytosanitary measures.

5. The Committee on Sanitary and Phytosanitary Measures provided for in paragraphs 1 and 4 of Article 12 (referred to in this Agreement as the "Committee") shall develop a procedure to monitor the process of international harmonization and

(continued)

TABLE F.4 Continued

Article of the SPS Agreement	Implications for the Plans to Expand the National Quarantine System (NQS)
coordinate efforts in this regard with the relevant international organizations.	
Article 4 *Equivalence* 1. Members shall accept the sanitary or phytosanitary measures of other Members as equivalent, even if these measures differ from their own or from those used by other Members trading in the same product, if the exporting Member objectively demonstrates to the importing Member that its measures achieve the importing Member's appropriate level of sanitary or phytosanitary protection. For this purpose, reasonable access shall be given, upon request, to the importing Member for inspection, testing and other relevant procedures. 2. Members shall, upon request, enter into consultations with the aim of achieving bilateral and multilateral agreements on recognition of the equivalence of specified sanitary or phytosanitary measures.	This article of the SPS Agreement would require the expanded NQS to recognize the SPS measures of exporting countries as equivalent if the exporting countries demonstrate objectively to the United States that its measures achieve the level of protection selected as appropriate by the United States. Whether this obligation to recognize the SPS measure of two other WTO members as equivalent restricts the sovereignty of the United States significantly is doubtful because the importing WTO member (here, the United States) remains in control of the process of granting equivalence status to the SPS measures of WTO members exporting products to the United States. The United States has, however, entered into mutual recognition agreements and arrangements with other WTO members, such as the EU; so these equivalence pacts could affect the way in which the NQS deals with products from such countries.
Article 5 *Assessment of Risk and Determination of the Appropriate Level of Sanitary or Phytosanitary Protection* 1. Members shall ensure that their sanitary or phytosanitary measures are based on an assessment, as appropriate to the circumstances, of the risks to human, animal or plant life or health, taking into account risk assessment techniques developed by the relevant international organizations.	This article contains a number of important provisions from the perspective of the operation of the expanded NQS: Risk assessment: SPS measures have to be based on a risk assessment (Article 5.1) that has to take into account a number of factors (Articles 5.2 and 5.3). The expanded NQS cannot, thus,

2. In the assessment of risks, Members shall take into account available scientific evidence; relevant processes and production methods; relevant inspection, sampling and testing methods; prevalence of specific diseases or pests; existence of pest- or disease-free areas; relevant ecological and environmental conditions; and quarantine or other treatment.

3. In assessing the risk to animal or plant life or health and determining the measure to be applied for achieving the appropriate level of sanitary or phytosanitary protection from such risk, Members shall take into account as relevant economic factors: the potential damage in terms of loss of production or sales in the event of the entry, establishment or spread of a pest or disease; the costs of control or eradication in the territory of the importing Member; and the relative cost-effectiveness of alternative approaches to limiting risks.

4. Members should, when determining the appropriate level of sanitary or phytosanitary protection, take into account the objective of minimizing negative trade effects.

5. With the objective of achieving consistency in the application of the concept of appropriate level of sanitary or phytosanitary protection against risks to human life or health, or to animal and plant life or health, each Member shall avoid arbitrary or unjustifiable distinctions in the levels it considers to be appropriate in different situations, if such distinctions result in discrimination or a disguised restriction on international trade. Members shall cooperate in the Committee, in accordance with paragraphs 1, 2 and 3 of Article 12, to develop guidelines to further the practical implementation of this provision. In developing the guidelines, the Committee shall take into account all relevant factors, including the exceptional character of

apply a SPS measure without having based that measure on a risk assessment (but not necessarily a risk assessment carried out by the NQS but by any federal government agency, other WTO member, or nonstate actor).

Trade-related disciplines: Articles 5.4, 5.5, and 5.6 contain trade-related disciplines to ensure that SPS measures applied are the least trade-restrictive measures possible and do not constitute arbitrary or unjustified discrimination or a disguised restriction on international trade.

Precautionary principle: Article 5.7 allows WTO members to apply provisionally a SPS measure when the scientific evidence is insufficient or inconclusive, as long as the WTO member applying such a provisional measure continues to try to obtain more information and reviews the provisional measure periodically.

Transparency: Article 5.8 imposes a duty of transparency on a WTO member with respect to SPS measures that it applies because it requires such WTO member to provide information to other WTO members that request information about SPS measures applied to their exports.

(continued)

TABLE F.4 Continued

Article of the SPS Agreement	Implications for the Plans to Expand the National Quarantine System (NQS)
human health risks to which people voluntarily expose themselves.	
6. Without prejudice to paragraph 2 of Article 3, when establishing or maintaining sanitary or phytosanitary measures to achieve the appropriate level of sanitary or phytosanitary protection, Members shall ensure that such measures are not more trade-restrictive than required to achieve their appropriate level of sanitary or phytosanitary protection, taking into account technical and economic feasibility.[b]	
7. In cases where relevant scientific evidence is insufficient, a Member may provisionally adopt sanitary or phytosanitary measures on the basis of available pertinent information, including that from the relevant international organizations as well as from sanitary or phytosanitary measures applied by other Members. In such circumstances, Members shall seek to obtain the additional information necessary for a more objective assessment of risk and review the sanitary or phytosanitary measure accordingly within a reasonable period of time.	
8. When a Member has reason to believe that a specific sanitary or phytosanitary measure introduced or maintained by another Member is constraining, or has the potential to constrain, its exports and the measure is not based on the relevant international standards, guidelines or recommendations, or such standards, guidelines or recommendations do not exist, an explanation of the reasons for such sanitary or phytosanitary measure may be requested and shall be provided by the Member maintaining the measure.	

(continued)

Article 6
Adaptation to Regional Conditions, Including Pest- or Disease-Free Areas and Areas of Low Pest or Disease Prevalence

1. Members shall ensure that their sanitary or phytosanitary measures are adapted to the sanitary or phytosanitary characteristics of the area—whether all of a country, part of a country, or all or parts of several countries—from which the product originated and to which the product is destined. In assessing the sanitary or phytosanitary characteristics of a region, Members shall take into account, inter alia, the level of prevalence of specific diseases or pests, the existence of eradication or control programmes, and appropriate criteria or guidelines which may be developed by the relevant international organizations.

2. Members shall, in particular, recognize the concepts of pest- or disease-free areas and areas of low pest or disease prevalence. Determination of such areas shall be based on factors such as geography, ecosystems, epidemiological surveillance, and the effectiveness of sanitary or phytosanitary controls.

3. Exporting Members claiming that areas within their territories are pest- or disease-free areas or areas of low pest or disease prevalence shall provide the necessary evidence thereof in order to objectively demonstrate to the importing Member that such areas are, and are likely to remain, pest- or disease-free areas or areas of low pest or disease prevalence, respectively. For this purpose, reasonable access shall be given, upon request, to the importing Member for inspection, testing and other relevant procedures.

From the perspective of the expanded NQS, Article 6 would require that SPS measures applied by the expanded NQS are adapted to the SPS characteristics of the areas from which products come. This obligation exists to prevent WTO members from applying SPS measures to products from regions where the disease or pest in question does not exist (i.e., no public health justification supports the imposition of a SPS measure to prevent the importation of a disease from a country or region where that disease does not exist). Exporting WTO members have transparency obligations to support the compliance of importing WTO members with this requirement of the SPS Agreement.

TABLE F.4 Continued

Article of the SPS Agreement	Implications for the Plans to Expand the National Quarantine System (NQS)
Article 7 *Transparency* Members shall notify of changes in their sanitary or phytosanitary measures and shall provide information on their sanitary or phytosanitary measures in accordance with the provisions of Annex B.	Transparency is an important general principle of the SPS Agreement (and all WTO agreements), so the expanded NQS will have to operate in conformity with its requirements. Annex B of the SPS Agreement contains the detailed set of rules concerning transparency with which the expanded NQS should be concerned.
Article 8 *Control, Inspection and Approval Procedures* Members shall observe the provisions of Annex C in the operation of control, inspection and approval procedures, including national systems for approving the use of additives or for establishing tolerances for contaminants in foods, beverages or feedstuffs, and otherwise ensure that their procedures are not inconsistent with the provisions of this Agreement.	Article 8 combined with Annex C imposes on WTO members obligations in how they operate their procedures for control, inspection, and approval of goods pursuant to the application of SPS measures. These obligations would affect how the expanded NQS would operate its control, inspection, and approval procedures concerning SPS measures it applied.
Article 9 *Technical Assistance* 1. Members agree to facilitate the provision of technical assistance to other Members, especially developing country Members, either bilaterally or through the appropriate international organizations. Such assistance may be, inter alia, in the areas of processing technologies, research and infrastructure, including in the establishment of national regulatory bodies, and may take the form of advice, credits, donations and grants, including for the purpose of seeking technical expertise, training and	This provision is not directly relevant to the federal government's to expand the NQS because those plans do not, to Consultant's knowledge, involve providing technical assistance to developing-country WTO members concerning their application of SPS measures. The federal government could, however, involve the expanded NQS in providing technical assistance to developing-country WTO members.

equipment to allow such countries to adjust to, and comply with, sanitary or phytosanitary measures necessary to achieve the appropriate level of sanitary or phytosanitary protection in their export markets.

2. Where substantial investments are required in order for an exporting developing country Member to fulfill the sanitary or phytosanitary requirements of an importing Member, the latter shall consider providing such technical assistance as will permit the developing country Member to maintain and expand its market access opportunities for the product involved.

Article 10
Special and Differential Treatment

1. In the preparation and application of sanitary or phytosanitary measures, Members shall take account of the special needs of developing country Members, and in particular of the least-developed country Members.

2. Where the appropriate level of sanitary or phytosanitary protection allows scope for the phased introduction of new sanitary or phytosanitary measures, longer time-frames for compliance should be accorded on products of interest to developing country Members so as to maintain opportunities for their exports.

3. With a view to ensuring that developing country Members are able to comply with the provisions of this Agreement, the Committee is enabled to grant to such countries, upon request, specified, time-limited exceptions in whole or in part from obligations under this Agreement, taking into account their financial, trade and development needs.

4. Members should encourage and facilitate the active participation of developing country Members in the relevant international organizations.

This provision requires WTO members to "take account of" the special needs of developing-country and particularly least-developed-country WTO members in the application of SPS measures. This obligation would apply to the expanded NQS, but the obligation does not significantly affect U.S. sovereignty in terms of the SPS measures it applies.

(continued)

TABLE F.4 Continued

Article of the SPS Agreement	Implications for the Plans to Expand the National Quarantine System (NQS)
Article 11 *Consultations and Dispute Settlement* 1. The provisions of Articles XXII and XXIII of GATT 1994 as elaborated and applied by the Dispute Settlement Understanding shall apply to consultations and the settlement of disputes under this Agreement, except as otherwise specifically provided herein. 2. In a dispute under this Agreement involving scientific or technical issues, a panel should seek advice from experts chosen by the panel in consultation with the parties to the dispute. To this end, the panel may, when it deems it appropriate, establish an advisory technical experts group, or consult the relevant international organizations, at the request of either party to the dispute or on its own initiative. 3. Nothing in this Agreement shall impair the rights of Members under other international agreements, including the right to resort to the good offices or dispute settlement mechanisms of other international organizations or established under any international agreement.	This provision gives jurisdiction over disputes under the SPS Agreement to the WTO Dispute Settlement Understanding (DSU). The importance of this provision for the expanded NQS is that the obligations of the SPS Agreement can be enforced by other countries through the DSU, which heightens the importance for the United States of the expanded NQS complying with the requirements of the SPS Agreement.
Article 12 *Administration* 1. A Committee on Sanitary and Phytosanitary Measures is hereby established to provide a regular forum for consultations. It shall carry out the functions necessary to implement the provisions of this Agreement and the furtherance of its objectives, in particular with respect to harmonization. The Committee shall reach its decisions by consensus.	This provision addresses the establishment and responsibilities of the SPS Committee and is not directly relevant to the expanded NQS' anticipated responsibilities.

(continued)

2. The Committee shall encourage and facilitate ad hoc consultations or negotiations among Members on specific sanitary or phytosanitary issues. The Committee shall encourage the use of international standards, guidelines or recommendations by all Members and, in this regard, shall sponsor technical consultation and study with the objective of increasing coordination and integration between international and national systems and approaches for approving the use of food additives or for establishing tolerances for contaminants in foods, beverages or feedstuffs.

3. The Committee shall maintain close contact with the relevant international organizations in the field of sanitary and phytosanitary protection, especially with the Codex Alimentarius Commission, the International Office of Epizootics, and the Secretariat of the International Plant Protection Convention, with the objective of securing the best available scientific and technical advice for the administration of this Agreement and in order to ensure that unnecessary duplication of effort is avoided.

4. The Committee shall develop a procedure to monitor the process of international harmonization and the use of international standards, guidelines or recommendations. For this purpose, the Committee should, in conjunction with the relevant international organizations, establish a list of international standards, guidelines or recommendations relating to sanitary or phytosanitary measures which the Committee determines to have a major trade impact. The list should include an indication by Members of those international standards, guidelines or recommendations which they apply as conditions for import or on the basis of which imported products conforming to these standards can enjoy access to their markets. For those cases in which a Member does not apply an international standard,

TABLE F.4 Continued

Article of the SPS Agreement	Implications for the Plans to Expand the National Quarantine System (NQS)
guideline or recommendation as a condition for import, the Member should provide an indication of the reason therefor, and, in particular, whether it considers that the standard is not stringent enough to provide the appropriate level of sanitary or phytosanitary protection. If a Member revises its position, following its indication of the use of a standard, guideline or recommendation as a condition for import, it should provide an explanation for its change and so inform the Secretariat as well as the relevant international organizations, unless such notification and explanation is given according to the procedures of Annex B.	
5. In order to avoid unnecessary duplication, the Committee may decide, as appropriate, to use the information generated by the procedures, particularly for notification, which are in operation in the relevant international organizations.	
6. The Committee may, on the basis of an initiative from one of the Members, through appropriate channels invite the relevant international organizations or their subsidiary bodies to examine specific matters with respect to a particular standard, guideline or recommendation, including the basis of explanations for non-use given according to paragraph 4.	
7. The Committee shall review the operation and implementation of this Agreement three years after the date of entry into force of the WTO Agreement, and thereafter as the need arises. Where appropriate, the Committee may submit to the Council for Trade in Goods proposals to amend the text of this Agreement having regard, inter alia, to the experience gained in its implementation.	

Article 13
Implementation

Members are fully responsible under this Agreement for the observance of all obligations set forth herein. Members shall formulate and implement positive measures and mechanisms in support of the observance of the provisions of this Agreement by other than central government bodies. Members shall take such reasonable measures as may be available to them to ensure that non-governmental entities within their territories, as well as regional bodies in which relevant entities within their territories are members, comply with the relevant provisions of this Agreement. In addition, Members shall not take measures which have the effect of, directly or indirectly, requiring or encouraging such regional or non-governmental entities, or local governmental bodies, to act in a manner inconsistent with the provisions of this Agreement. Members shall ensure that they rely on the services of non-governmental entities for implementing sanitary or phytosanitary measures only if these entities comply with the provisions of this Agreement.

This provision is important for the expanded NQS because it reiterates that the SPS Agreement's provisions are obligations that must be observed. The expanded NQS will become an important component of how the United States complies with its duties under the SPS Agreement.

Article 14
Final Provisions

The least-developed country Members may delay application of the provisions of this Agreement for a period of five years following the date of entry into force of the WTO Agreement with respect to their sanitary or phytosanitary measures affecting importation or imported products. Other developing country Members may delay application of the provisions of this Agreement, other than paragraph 8 of Article 5 and Article 7, for two years following the date of entry into force of the WTO Agreement with respect to their existing sanitary or phytosanitary measures affecting importation or imported products, where such application is prevented by a lack of technical expertise, technical infrastructure or resources.

This provision does not apply to the United States.

(continued)

TABLE F.4 Continued

Article of the SPS Agreement	Implications for the Plans to Expand the National Quarantine System (NQS)
ANNEX A: DEFINITIONS*c* *1. Sanitary or phytosanitary measure—any measure applied:* (a) to protect animal or plant life or health within the territory of the Member from risks arising from the entry, establishment or spread of pests, diseases, disease-carrying organisms or disease-causing organisms; (b) to protect human or animal life or health within the territory of the Member from risks arising from additives, contaminants, toxins or disease-causing organisms in foods, beverages or feedstuffs; (c) to protect human life or health within the territory of the Member from risks arising from diseases carried by animals, plants or products thereof, or from the entry, establishment or spread of pests; or (d) to prevent or limit other damage within the territory of the Member from the entry, establishment or spread of pests. Sanitary or phytosanitary measures include all relevant laws, decrees, regulations, requirements and procedures including, inter alia, end product criteria; processes and production methods; testing, inspection, certification and approval procedures; quarantine treatments including relevant requirements associated with the transport of animals or plants, or with the materials necessary for their survival during transport; provisions on relevant statistical methods, sampling procedures and methods of risk assessment; and packaging and labelling requirements directly related to food safety.	This annex defines many of the important terms and concepts that are at the heart of obligations in the SPS Agreement, including definitions of what constitutes a SPS measure; what counts as an international standard, guideline, or recommendation; and what "risk assessment" means. These definitions will be important to the expanded NQS' compliance with the SPS Agreement.

2. *Harmonization*—The establishment, recognition and application of common sanitary and phytosanitary measures by different Members.

3. *International standards, guidelines and recommendations*
   (a) for food safety, the standards, guidelines and recommendations established by the Codex Alimentarius Commission relating to food additives, veterinary drug and pesticide residues, contaminants, methods of analysis and sampling, and codes and guidelines of hygienic practice;
   (b) for animal health and zoonoses, the standards, guidelines and recommendations developed under the auspices of the International Office of Epizootics;
   (c) for plant health, the international standards, guidelines and recommendations developed under the auspices of the Secretariat of the International Plant Protection Convention in cooperation with regional organizations operating within the framework of the International Plant Protection Convention; and
   (d) for matters not covered by the above organizations, appropriate standards, guidelines and recommendations promulgated by other relevant international organizations open for membership to all Members, as identified by the Committee.

4. *Risk assessment*—The evaluation of the likelihood of entry, establishment or spread of a pest or disease within the territory of an importing Member according to the sanitary or phytosanitary measures which might be applied, and of the associated potential biological and economic consequences; or the evaluation of the potential for adverse effects on human or animal health arising from the presence of additives, contaminants, toxins or disease-causing organisms in food, beverages or feedstuffs.

(continued)

TABLE F.4 Continued

Article of the SPS Agreement	Implications for the Plans to Expand the National Quarantine System (NQS)
5. *Appropriate level of sanitary or phytosanitary protection*—The level of protection deemed appropriate by the Member establishing a sanitary or phytosanitary measure to protect human, animal or plant life or health within its territory. NOTE: Many Members otherwise refer to this concept as the "acceptable level of risk."	
6. *Pest- or disease-free area*—An area, whether all of a country, part of a country, or all or parts of several countries, as identified by the competent authorities, in which a specific pest or disease does not occur. NOTE: A pest- or disease-free area may surround, be surrounded by, or be adjacent to an area—whether within part of a country or in a geographic region which includes parts of or all of several countries—in which a specific pest or disease is known to occur but is subject to regional control measures such as the establishment of protection, surveillance and buffer zones which will confine or eradicate the pest or disease in question.	
7. *Area of low pest or disease prevalence*—An area, whether all of a country, part of a country, or all or parts of several countries, as identified by the competent authorities, in which a specific pest or disease occurs at low levels and which is subject to effective surveillance, control or eradication measures.	

This annex provides the detailed obligations for making sure the application of SPS measures by WTO members is transparent. These rules would apply to the operation of the expanded NQS in each of the areas identified: publication of regulations, inquiry points, and notification procedures.

ANNEX B: TRANSPARENCY OF SANITARY AND PHYTOSANITARY REGULATIONS

Publication of regulations

1. Members shall ensure that all sanitary and phytosanitary regulations[d] which have been adopted are published promptly in such a manner as to enable interested Members to become acquainted with them.

2. Except in urgent circumstances, Members shall allow a reasonable interval between the publication of a sanitary or phytosanitary regulation and its entry into force in order to allow time for producers in exporting Members, and particularly in developing country Members, to adapt their products and methods of production to the requirements of the importing Member.

Enquiry points

3. Each Member shall ensure that one enquiry point exists which is responsible for the provision of answers to all reasonable questions from interested Members as well as for the provision of relevant documents regarding:

(a) any sanitary or phytosanitary regulations adopted or proposed within its territory;

(b) any control and inspection procedures, production and quarantine treatment, pesticide tolerance and food additive approval procedures, which are operated within its territory;

(c) risk assessment procedures, factors taken into consideration, as well as the determination of the appropriate level of sanitary or phytosanitary protection;

(d) the membership and participation of the Member, or of relevant bodies within its territory, in international and

(continued)

TABLE F.4 Continued

Article of the SPS Agreement	Implications for the Plans to Expand the National Quarantine System (NQS)
regional sanitary and phytosanitary organizations and systems, as well as in bilateral and multilateral agreements and arrangements within the scope of this Agreement, and the texts of such agreements and arrangements.	
4. Members shall ensure that where copies of documents are requested by interested Members, they are supplied at the same price (if any), apart from the cost of delivery, as to the nationals[e] of the Member concerned.	
Notification procedures	
5. Whenever an international standard, guideline or recommendation does not exist or the content of a proposed sanitary or phytosanitary regulation is not substantially the same as the content of an international standard, guideline or recommendation, and if the regulation may have a significant effect on trade of other Members, Members shall:	
(a) publish a notice at an early stage in such a manner as to enable interested Members to become acquainted with the proposal to introduce a particular regulation;	
(b) notify other Members, through the Secretariat, of the products to be covered by the regulation together with a brief indication of the objective and rationale of the proposed regulation. Such notifications shall take place at an early stage, when amendments can still be introduced and comments taken into account;	
(c) provide upon request to other Members copies of the proposed regulation and, whenever possible, identify the parts which in substance deviate from international standards, guidelines or recommendations;	

(continued)

(d) without discrimination, allow reasonable time for other Members to make comments in writing, discuss these comments upon request, and take the comments and the results of the discussions into account.

6. However, where urgent problems of health protection arise or threaten to arise for a Member, that Member may omit such of the steps enumerated in paragraph 5 of this Annex as it finds necessary, provided that the Member:

(a) immediately notifies other Members, through the Secretariat, of the particular regulation and the products covered, with a brief indication of the objective and the rationale of the regulation, including the nature of the urgent problem(s);

(b) provides, upon request, copies of the regulation to other Members;

(c) allows other Members to make comments in writing, discusses these comments upon request, and takes the comments and the results of the discussions into account.

7. Notifications to the Secretariat shall be in English, French or Spanish.

8. Developed country Members shall, if requested by other Members, provide copies of the documents or, in case of voluminous documents, summaries of the documents covered by a specific notification in English, French or Spanish.

9. The Secretariat shall promptly circulate copies of the notification to all Members and interested international organizations and draw the attention of developing country Members to any notifications relating to products of particular interest to them.

10. Members shall designate a single central government authority as responsible for the implementation, on the national level, of the provisions concerning notification procedures according to paragraphs 5, 6, 7 and 8 of this Annex.

TABLE F.4 Continued

Article of the SPS Agreement	Implications for the Plans to Expand the National Quarantine System (NQS)
General reservations 11. Nothing in this Agreement shall be construed as requiring: (a) the provision of particulars or copies of drafts or the publication of texts other than in the language of the Member except as stated in paragraph 8 of this Annex; or (b) Members to disclose confidential information which would impede enforcement of sanitary or phytosanitary legislation or which would prejudice the legitimate commercial interests of particular enterprises. ANNEX C CONTROL, INSPECTION AND APPROVAL PROCEDURES*f* 1. Members shall ensure, with respect to any procedure to check and ensure the fulfilment of sanitary or phytosanitary measures, that: (a) such procedures are undertaken and completed without undue delay and in no less favourable manner for imported products than for like domestic products; (b) the standard processing period of each procedure is published or that the anticipated processing period is communicated to the applicant upon request; when receiving an application, the competent body promptly examines the completeness of the documentation and informs the applicant in a precise and complete manner of all deficiencies; the competent body transmits as soon as possible the results of the procedure in a precise and complete manner to the applicant so that corrective action may be taken if necessary; even when the	This annex applies obligations concerning how WTO members implement control, inspection, and approval procedures with respect to products subject to SPS measures. These duties would affect the way in which the expanded NQS operates because the expanded NQS will be involved with control, inspection, and approval actions concerning products that might pose health threats.

(continued)

application has deficiencies, the competent body proceeds as far as practicable with the procedure if the applicant so requests; and that upon request, the applicant is informed of the stage of the procedure, with any delay being explained;

(c) information requirements are limited to what is necessary for appropriate control, inspection and approval procedures, including for approval of the use of additives or for the establishment of tolerances for contaminants in food, beverages or feedstuffs;

(d) the confidentiality of information about imported products arising from or supplied in connection with control, inspection and approval is respected in a way no less favourable than for domestic products and in such a manner that legitimate commercial interests are protected;

(e) any requirements for control, inspection and approval of individual specimens of a product are limited to what is reasonable and necessary;

(f) any fees imposed for the procedures on imported products are equitable in relation to any fees charged on like domestic products or products originating in any other Member and should be no higher than the actual cost of the service;

(g) the same criteria should be used in the siting of facilities used in the procedures and the selection of samples of imported products as for domestic products so as to minimize the inconvenience to applicants, importers, exporters or their agents;

(h) whenever specifications of a product are changed subsequent to its control and inspection in light of the applicable regulations, the procedure for the modified product is limited to what is necessary to determine whether adequate confidence exists that the product still meets the regulations concerned; and

TABLE F.4 Continued

Article of the SPS Agreement	Implications for the Plans to Expand the National Quarantine System (NQS)
(i) a procedure exists to review complaints concerning the operation of such procedures and to take corrective action when a complaint is justified. Where an importing Member operates a system for the approval of the use of food additives or for the establishment of tolerances for contaminants in food, beverages or feedstuffs which prohibits or restricts access to its domestic markets for products based on the absence of an approval, the importing Member shall consider the use of a relevant international standard as the basis for access until a final determination is made. 2. Where a sanitary or phytosanitary measure specifies control at the level of production, the Member in whose territory the production takes place shall provide the necessary assistance to facilitate such control and the work of the controlling authorities. 3. Nothing in this Agreement shall prevent Members from carrying out reasonable inspection within their own territories.	

a For the purposes of paragraph 3 of Article 3, there is a scientific justification if, on the basis of an examination and evaluation of available scientific information in conformity with the relevant provisions of this Agreement, a Member determines that the relevant international standards, guidelines or recommendations are not sufficient to achieve its appropriate level of sanitary or phytosanitary protection.

b For purposes of paragraph 6 of Article 5, a measure is not more trade-restrictive than required unless there is another measure, reasonably available taking into account technical and economic feasibility, that achieves the appropriate level of sanitary or phytosanitary protection and is significantly less restrictive to trade.

c For the purpose of these definitions, "animal" includes fish and wild fauna; "plant" includes forests and wild flora; "pests" include weeds; and "contaminants" include pesticide and veterinary drug residues and extraneous matter.

d Sanitary and phytosanitary measures such as laws, decrees or ordinances which are applicable generally.

e When "nationals" are referred to in this Agreement, the term shall be deemed, in the case of a separate customs territory Member of the WTO, to mean persons, natural or legal, who are domiciled or who have a real and effective industrial or commercial establishment in that customs territory.

f Control, inspection and approval procedures include, inter alia, procedures for sampling, testing, and certification.

G

Excerpts from a Standard Memorandum of Agreement Between CDC and Local Hospitals

and treatment for persons affected by other diseases of urgent public health significance for which federal quarantine is not yet authorized.

DESCRIPTION OF SERVICES

The hospital agrees to provide the following services:

1. Provide the referred individual such clinical evaluation, examination, diagnostic, and treatment services as indicated, based on consultation with CDC, for
   the disease(s) or abnormality(ies) for which the individual was referred.
2. Admit the referred individual for care and subject to the availability of beds.
3. Provide care for the individual using isolation and other standard infection control precautions. . . .
4. Upon request, provide to CDC appropriate medical information and clinical
   specimens obtained from the referred individual.
5. Consult with CDC on all decisions related to the care of the referred individual
   which may have a public health impact, including the discontinuation of isolation precautions and discharge from the hospital.
6. Communicate information related to the referred individual to local or state public health authorities, as required by applicable state and local laws related to
   the reporting of persons with communicable diseases.
7. Provide to CDC, within sixty days of execution of this agreement, a written statement outlining the fulfillment of the minimal criteria for hospitalization and care of
   persons with specified communicable diseases as outlined in Appendix 1.

CDC agrees to provide the following services:

[The first two items in this section are perfunctory and therefore were omitted from
this abbreviated MOA.]

3. Provide appropriate input and consultation related to the epidemiology, clinical
   and laboratory diagnosis, management, and prevention of transmission of
   disease(s) for which the referral was made.
4. Collaborate with state and local public health authorities to assist with the design and implementation of appropriate infection control practices at the Hospital and in the community.
5. Provide guidance to the Hospital on personal protective equipment and other
   measures to be used by healthcare workers in the care of referred individuals.

SCOPE OF AUTHORITY

The Hospital and CDC acknowledge that the Hospital retains primary responsibility for the clinical care of the referred individual, and that CDC will serve in a
consultative capacity. The Hospital and CDC further acknowledge that CDC retains full authority for determining when to institute and/or discontinue isolation of
individuals referred under this agreement. The Hospital and CDC finally acknowledge that CDC represents interests of public health, and that the Hospital may be
asked to assist in the implementation of communicable disease control and prevention measures.

EFFECT ON PROCEDURES AND LAWS

. . . This agreement does not supersede any requirements or obligations of the Hospital that otherwise exist in federal, state, or local law. . . .

REIMBURSEMENT OF COST

Pursuant to section 322 of the Public Health Service Act, persons whose care and treatment is authorized in accordance with quarantine laws may receive such care and treatment at the expense of CDC subject to the following:

1. Payment of such expenses shall be made in CDC's sole discretion and subject to the availability of appropriated funds.
2. Any payment of expenses shall be secondary to the obligation of the United States or any third party (including any State or local governmental entity, private insurance carrier, or employer), under any other law or contractual agreement, to pay for such care and treatment, and shall only be paid by CDC after all other available coverage from all third-party payers have made payment.
3. Payment shall be limited to those amounts Hospital would customarily bill the Medicare system using the International Classification of Diseases, Clinical Modification (ICD-CM), and relevant federal regulations promulgated by the Centers for Medicare and Medicaid Services in existence at the time of billing.
4. For diseases specified in an Executive Order of the President for which quarantine/isolation is authorized pursuant to section 361 of the Public Health Service Act, payment shall be limited to costs for services and items reasonable and necessary for the care and treatment of the person for the time period commencing when CDC refers the person to Hospital and ending when, as determined by CDC, the period of isolation or quarantine expires.
5. For diseases other than those described in paragraph (4) above, such payment shall be limited to costs for services and items reasonable and necessary for care and treatment of the person for the time period commencing when CDC refers the person to Hospital and ending when the person's condition is diagnosed, as determined by CDC, with a nonquarantinable disease.

CONFIDENTIALITY

Hospital agrees that it will not disclose the nature of this effort or the terms of this agreement to any person or entity, except as may be necessary to fulfill its obligations hereunder or pursuant to written agreement from CDC. To the extent permitted by federal law, CDC will not disclose the nature of this effort or the terms of this agreement to any person or entity, except as may be necessary to fulfill its mission and statutory and regulatory responsibilities.

RELEASE OF HEALTH INFORMATION

Pursuant to 45 CFR § 164.512(b) of the Health Insurance Portability and Accountability Act (HIPAA) Standards for Privacy of Individually Identifiable Health Information; Final Rule (Privacy Rule) (45 CFR § 164.501), the Hospital may disclose without individual authorization protected health information to public health authorities. CDC is authorized by law to collect or receive such information for the purpose of preventing or controlling disease, injury, or disability

[Sections of MOA omitted here: Settlement of Disputes; No Private Right Created; Amendment, Termination, and Duration; Effective Date; Approving Authorities (signatories)]

POINTS OF CONTACT

The following Hospital and CDC representatives will serve as the points of contact to implement this agreement:

[Name and address of Hospital representative]
[Name and address of CDC Quarantine Station]

APPENDIX I

Preparedness Criteria for Healthcare Facilities

The healthcare facility should be equipped and prepared to care for a limited number of patients with a communicable disease as specified in the Memorandum of Agreement as part of routine operations. The purpose of this document is to establish the preparedness criteria that healthcare facilities must meet in order to comply with the terms of the agreement.

[Twenty specific criteria are outlined in a total of six areas: preparedness planning; clinical evaluation; infection control, isolation, and environmental controls; exposure reporting and evaluation of risk; communication and reporting; and administrative issues.]

APPENDIX II

Certification of Satisfaction of Preparedness Standards

Number of private rooms _____

Number of airborne infection isolation (AII) rooms _____

Number of isolation beds _____

Number of infectious disease physicians _____

Number of infection control practitioners _____

Hospital 24-hour phone number _____

Number of ICU nurses _____

Number of ICU beds _____

Number of critical care physicians _____

Number of critical care nurses _____

EMS Services

Does hospital have a relationship with EMS that will require a separate MOA?

Yes _ No _

If yes,

EMS Contact Name _____

EMS Telephone _____

EMS Email _____

On behalf of the hospital/healthcare facility named below, I certify that we are in full compliance with the Preparedness Standards as outlined in Appendix I.
[signature]

_____

SOURCE: Centers for Disease Control and Prevention, 2004.

H

Committee Biographies

Georges C. Benjamin, M.D., FACP, *Chair,* has been Executive Director of the American Public Health Association (APHA) since December 2002. Prior to joining APHA, Dr. Benjamin was Secretary of the Maryland Department of Health and Mental Hygiene, where he played a key role in developing the state's bioterrorism plan. From 1995 to 1999, he served as Deputy Secretary for Public Health Services. Dr. Benjamin has also worked extensively in the field of emergency medicine. He was Chief of the Acute Illness Clinic at Madigan Army Medical Center in Tacoma, WA; Chief of Emergency Medicine at Walter Reed Army Medical Center; and Chairman of the Community Health and Ambulatory Care Department at the District of Columbia General Hospital. From 1990 to 1991, he served as the District of Columbia's Commissioner of Public Health. He has taught emergency medicine at Georgetown University in Washington, DC and the Uniformed Services University of the Health Sciences in Bethesda, MD. He is a fellow of the American College of Physicians and a former fellow of the American College of Emergency Physicians. Dr. Benjamin has held a variety of positions with the American College of Emergency Physicians, including President and Vice President of the DC chapter, Chairman of the Injury Control Committee, member of the Governmental Affairs Committee, and member of the Health Policy Committee. He also served as President of the Association of State and Territorial Health Officials (2001-2002) and has sat on the editorial board of the *Journal of the National Medical Association.*

Barbara A. Blakeney, M.S., R.N., is President of the American Nurses Association (ANA). She is currently on leave from her role as Director of Health Services for the Homeless at the Boston Public Health Commission. Previously, she had served as the principal health nurse for homeless services and addiction services at the Division of Public Health, Department of Health and Hospitals in Boston, MA. She has held numerous ANA positions, including two terms as ANA Second Vice President and ANA First Vice President. In addition, she has been an adjunct professor in the Department of Family and Community Nursing, University of Massachusetts at Boston. She is the recipient of numerous awards, including ANA's Pearl McIver Public Health Nurse Award for significant contributions to the field of public health on the national level.

Lawrence O. Gostin, J.D., is Associate Dean for Research and Academic Programs and Professor of Law at Georgetown University, as well as Professor of Public Health at the Johns Hopkins School of Hygiene and Public Health. He also directs the Center for Law and the Public's Health at Johns Hopkins and Georgetown Universities. In the wake of September 11, 2001, he led the drafting of the Emergency Health Powers Act to combat bioterrorism and other emerging health threats. Prior to joining the faculties at Georgetown and Johns Hopkins, he served as Executive Director of the American Society of Law, Medicine, and Ethics and as an adjunct professor at the Harvard Law School and the Harvard School of Public Health. From 1974 to 1985, Professor Gostin was the head of the National Council of Civil Liberties (United Kingdom), legal director of the National Association of Mental Health (U.K.), and a faculty member at Oxford University. He is the Health Law and Ethics Editor of the *Journal of the American Medical Association (JAMA)* and author of *Public Health Law: Power, Duty, Restraint* (University of California Press and the Milbank Memorial Fund, 2001) and *Public Health Law and Ethics: A Reader* (University of California Press and the Milbank Memorial Fund, 2002), as well as of articles on international infectious disease law, ethical challenges in combating bioterrorism, and the legal ramifications of the SARS outbreak. He is a member of the Institute of Medicine.

Margaret A. Hamburg, M.D., recently became a Senior Scientist at the Nuclear Threat Initiative (NTI), Washington, DC, after serving for four years as NTI's Vice President for Biological Programs. Prior to joining NTI, Dr. Hamburg was the Assistant Secretary for Planning and Evaluation, U.S. Department of Health and Human Services, serving as principal policy advisor to the Secretary of Health and Human Services. From 1991 to 1997, she held the position of Commissioner of Health for the City of New York. As commissioner, Dr. Hamburg's accomplishments included the creation of the first public health bioterrorism preparedness program in the nation. Dr. Hamburg has also served in the U.S. Office of Disease Prevention and Health Promotion and at the National Institute of Allergy and Infectious Diseases. She is a member of the New York Academy of Medicine and the Council on Foreign Relations and is a fellow of the American Association of the Advancement of Science and the American College of Physicians. She was elected to the Institute of Medicine in 1994.

Farzad Mostashari, M.D., M.S.P.H., is Assistant Commissioner for the Bureau of Epidemiology Services, New York City Department of Health and Mental Hygiene, overseeing research and development of a citywide health information network of outpatient facilities, emergency rooms, 911 dispatches, and pharmacies. An innovator in nontraditional disease surveillance and outbreak detection, Dr. Mostashari was a lead investigator in the outbreaks of West Nile virus and anthrax in New York. He received his graduate training from the Harvard School of Public Health and the Yale Medical School and completed the CDC's Epidemic Intelligence Service. He is a Clinical Assistant Professor of Public Health at Cornell Weill Medical College, a Visiting Research Scientist at the New York Academy of Medicine, and a Clinical Assistant Professor at Tufts University School of Medicine. Dr. Mostashari served as Chair of the 2002 National Syndromic Surveillance Conference and as Co-Chairperson of the 2003 and 2004 conferences. He is a member of the Advisory Committee of the National Bioterrorism Demonstration Project and of the Steering Committee of the Models of Disease Agent Study (MIDAS), NIH.

William A. Petri, Jr., M.D., Ph.D., is Wade Hampton Frost Professor of Epidemiology and Chief, Division of Infectious Disease and International Health, University of Virginia (UVA), Charlottesville. He is also Professor of Medicine, Pathology, and Microbiology. Dr. Petri joined the university's faculty in 1988 after earning both his M.D. and Ph.D. there; his doctorate is in microbiology. To pursue his interest in the molecular mechanisms of pathogenesis of parasitic infection, his laboratory studies *Entamoeba histolytica*, a parasite that destroys host immune cells and causes approximately 50 million illnesses and 100,000 deaths annually around the world. Through complementary field studies in Bangladesh, he is investigating the human immune response to *E. histolytica* and identifying strain-associated differences in virulence. A past president of the American Society of Tropical Medicine and Hygiene, Dr. Petri was selected by the National Institute of Allergy and Infectious Disease (NIAID) to serve on the Blue Ribbon Panel on Bioterrorism and its Implications for Biomedical Research in 2002. He has been a member since 2001 of the Microbiology and Infectious Diseases Research Committee at NIAID. In addition, he sat on the Infec-